JB JOSSEY-BASS

HEALTH COMMUNICATION

From Theory to Practice

Renata Schiavo

John Wiley & Sons, Inc.

Published by Jossey-Bass
A Wiley Imprint
989 Market Street, San Francisco, CA 94103-1741   www.josseybass.com

Jossey-Bass books and products are available through most bookstores. To contact Jossey-Bass directly
call our Customer Care Department within the U.S. at 800-956-7739, outside the U.S. at 317-572-3986,
or fax 317-572-4002.

Jossey-Bass also publishes its books in a variety of electronic formats. Some content that appears in
print may not be available in electronic books.

Library of Congress Cataloging-in-Publication Data

Schiavo, Renata.
  Health communication : from theory to practice / Renata Schiavo. — 1st ed.
      p.; cm.
  Includes bibliographical references and index.
  ISBN 978-0-7879-8205-8 (pbk.)
1. Communication in medicine—United States. 2. Health promotion—United States. 3. Health
planning—United States. I. Title.
  [DNLM: 1. Delivery of Health Care. 2. Communication. 3. Health Planning. 4. Program
Development. W 84.1 S329h 2007]
  R118.S33 2007
  610.1'4—dc22
                                                                                    2006101792

Printed in the United States of America
FIRST EDITION
PB Printing   10 9 8 7 6 5 4 3 2 1

CONTENTS

TABLES, FIGURES, EXHIBITS, AND NUMBERED BOXES

TABLES

FIGURES

EXHIBITS

NUMBERED BOXES

*For my daughters, Oriana and Talia, and,
of course, my husband, Roger Ullman*

PREFACE

When my child will grow up, he will walk on his own, he will walk on his own two feet, and that is the greatest gift of all.
<small>A MOTHER WHOSE CHILD RECEIVED THE POLIO VACCINE AS PART OF THE ONGOING POLIO ERADICATION CAMPAIGN IN INDIA (WORLD HEALTH ORGANIZATION AND GLOBAL POLIO ERADICATION INITIATIVE, 2004A)</small>

"I first became familiar with the importance and impact of health communication while working on the polio eradication campaign in India," relates one of my students, Prarthana Shukla, who holds a medical degree from Ahmedabad, India, and moved to the United States to complete a master's in public health at New York University (interview with the author, 2006). As a member of one of the medical teams that administered the oral polio vaccine to infants and unimmunized children in India, she attributes the long lines of people waiting to be immunized to a widespread and well-designed communication campaign that used multiple channels to convey the importance and safety of immunization. Despite her lack of experience in health communication, several analyses and postintervention evaluations (Waisbord, 2004; Favin, 2004) agree with her observation and contribute to the bulk of evidence in many disease areas that has recently propelled health communication to the forefront of the public health arena.

Health communication has been defined as "the main currency of healthcare in the 21st century" (Clancy, quoted in Krisberg, 2004). Ready access to relevant, reliable, and culturally appropriate information enables the general public, patients, health care providers, public health professionals, and others to address personal and public health concerns far more effectively than in the past (U.S. Department of Health and Human Services, 2001). In the wake of the anthrax crisis in 2001, communication was defined by the U.S. Centers for Disease Control (CDC) and other federal authorities as the most important health-care-related science of the twenty-first century (White House, 2004; Prue, Lackey, Swenarski, and Gantt, 2003). For the first time, health communication is part of the Healthy People 2010 objectives, the official public health agenda of the U.S. federal government.

Health communication courses as well as specific health communication programs have been flourishing in the United States and around the rest of the world. This has created the need for comprehensive and up-to-date tools to train students and staff on health communication theory and practice.

The need for this book became clear while I was looking for a textbook for my health communication course. I wanted a book that combined a theoretical and practice-based overview of current issues and topics in health communication with a step-by-step practical section that would help readers acquire technical skills in program planning, implementation, and evaluation. Conversations with other health communication practitioners and colleagues confirmed the need for this kind of book.

For the past eighteen years, I have been focusing on international health care. I have had the opportunity to work on staff or as a consultant for nonprofit organizations, pharmaceutical companies, communication agencies, governments, universities, and research laboratories in the United States and several countries in Europe, Latin America, and Africa. I know that health communication is a powerful tool that can help improve health outcomes, contribute to eliminating health disparities, and promote behavioral and social change. I wanted this book to reflect my practice-based perspective and convey to readers my enthusiasm and trust in the enormous potential of well-designed and well-implemented health communication programs to improve individual and public health outcomes.

The recent health communication "renaissance," as it has been called by a few authors (including Bernhardt, 2004, p. 2051), has also been accompanied by a passionate attempt to redefine health communication and its role in public health, as well as to encourage health professionals around the world to take advantage of this tool whenever possible. In doing so, most authors and practitioners seem to agree that health communication is an approach drawing on multiple disciplines, including mass communication, social marketing, health education, anthropology, and sociology (Bernhardt, 2004; Institute of Medicine, 2003; World Health Organization, 2003). I wanted this book to contribute to this debate by capturing and summarizing recent trends and opinions, as well as my own practical and teaching experience. Ultimately the goal is to help create new generations of health communication experts and contribute to expanding the pool of health professionals who will use this approach.

ACKNOWLEDGMENTS

A great number of colleagues, friends, and family members have contributed to the creation of this book. My first heartfelt thanks go to my editors, Andy Pasternack and Seth Schwartz of Jossey-Bass, for their invaluable help and guidance with the many questions related to this project. Special thanks also to Sally Guttmacher of New York University for her encouragement when the idea of this book was in its infancy.

Thanks to my anonymous reviewers for their invaluable suggestions that have considerably contributed to the significance of this book. My appreciation also goes to all professional friends and colleagues who provided suggestions on early drafts or helped secure relevant case studies and interviews. Among them are Doug Arbesfeld, Joe Casey, Lenore Cooney, Amanda Crowe, Gustavo Cruz, Chris Elias, Everold Hosein, Sherry Michelstein, Elil Renganathan, and Lisa Weiss. I am very grateful to Prarthana Shukla, one of my students who worked as a research assistant for this project, for her dedication and hard work. Thanks to other students who have contributed feedback, most notably Lawrence Fung and Ellen Sowala.

There are many people to whom I owe my practical experience in health communication. These include my colleagues, clients, and partners with whom I have had the privilege to work over the years. I spent endless nights with many of them brainstorming about new or old projects and learned a great deal from all of them.

Finally, many thanks to my husband, Roger Ullman, for his endless support and lifetime partnership, and to our daughters, Oriana and Talia, for inspiring my work ethics and life. And to my mother, Amalia Ronchi, many thanks for understanding that I had no time to chat during the many months dedicated to this project.

ABOUT THE AUTHOR

Renata Schiavo, Ph.D., M.A., is a senior health communications consultant. She is also an adjunct assistant professor of public health at New York University's Steinhardt School of Education, Department of Nutrition, Food Studies and Public Health, where she teaches health communication.

Schiavo has over eighteen years of international health care experience in the United States and several countries in Europe, Latin America, and Africa. She has worked on staff or as a consultant for nonprofit organizations, universities, pharmaceutical companies, communications agencies, research laboratories, and governments. Her communication work has focused on oncology, HIV/AIDS, malaria, leishmaniasis, central nervous system disorders, cardiovascular diseases, women's health, respiratory diseases, obesity, biotechnology, infectious diseases, childhood immunization, Lyme disease, and primary nocturnal enuresis.

Schiavo's fields of expertise include strategic planning, behavior communications, marketing communications, communication training, patient and professional medical communications, constituency relations, public relations, media relations, audience and market research, corporate communications, Internet-based communications, and strategic partnerships.

Schiavo served as an executive vice president at the Cooney/Waters Group (CWG), one of the largest independent health care communications agencies in the United States. Prior to joining CWG, she formed and headed the corporate and marketing communications department of Rhodia Farma, the Brazilian affiliate of Rhone-Poulenc Rorer (now Sanofi-Aventis). Previously she worked in the health care divisions of the New York–based communications agencies Manning Selvage & Lee and Noonan/Russo

Communications. She also worked as a senior consultant to UNICEF-Angola and the local ministry of health on malaria prevention strategies as well as evaluating local communications programs.

Formerly, Schiavo was a postdoctoral research scientist at Columbia University and New York University, where she worked on numerous molecular and cell biology projects.

Schiavo is a member of the American Public Health Association as well as the Steering Committee of its Health Communication Working Group. She serves on the advisory board of *Cases in Public Health Communication and Marketing,* an online peer-reviewed journal. Schiavo has also contributed with articles and opinions to the Communication Initiative and is a member of the Communication for Behavioral Impact Global Technical Network, which is maintained by the World Health Organization.

INTRODUCTION

Convincing people to adopt healthy behaviors or policymakers and professionals to introduce and change practices in support of better health has never been an easy task. Childhood immunization, for example, is one of the greatest medical and scientific successes of recent times. Because of immunization, many diseases that were once a threat to the life and well-being of children have become rare or have been eradicated in many countries in the world. Yet as for most other health-related issues and interventions, changing public and professional minds and convincing parents to immunize their healthy children against diseases that may occur has taken a worldwide multidisciplinary effort. Health communication has played a fundamental role in this effort since the introduction of the first childhood vaccine. Consider the case of Bonnie, the mother of a newborn child, who is offered a vaccine for her baby at birth or a few days after.

Bonnie, an American, is the twenty-five-year-old mother of a beautiful baby girl. She is thrilled about her child but quite fearful because parenting is new to her. She has read about the benefits of immunization but is too young to remember any of the diseases against which she should immunize her child. She does not know anyone who had polio or whooping cough or Hib (*Haemophilus influenzae* type B) disease. She has also heard conflicting information about the potential adverse events or risks that may be associated with immunization and is unsure about which of the available information is correct. She is confused and does not know whether she wants to immunize her child.

Bonnie's case is a typical example of issues or informational needs that health communication interventions can successfully address. These include:

- Providing Bonnie with research-based and reliable information that will reassure her about the importance of immunization and its low risk
- Improving communication with her pediatrician or health care provider by teaching her what questions to ask and raising awareness among health care providers of patients' needs and most frequent concerns
- Developing tools such as brochures, posters, Web pages, and other informational vehicles from reputable sources that will reinforce the information Bonnie will hear from her health care provider
- Encouraging peer-to-peer support by establishing venues and events where new mothers can discuss immunization
- Raising disease awareness by targeting consumer media, parenting publications, and other vehicles so that Bonnie and other parents can become familiar with the severity of vaccine-preventable diseases and the benefits of immunization

Health communication approaches will work only if they rely on an in-depth understanding of Bonnie's and other new mothers' lifestyles, concerns, beliefs, attitudes, barriers to change, and sources of information about newborns and immunization. It would also be important to research and understand the cultural, social, and ethnic environment in which Bonnie lives. What kind of support does she get from family, friends, and her working environment? Who most influences her decisions on her child's well-being and upbringing? What does she fear about immunization? Is there any existing program in her community that focuses on childhood immunization? What are the lessons learned? These are just some of the many questions that need to be answered before developing a health communication program intended for Bonnie and her peers.

ABOUT THIS BOOK

The example about Bonnie should make clear that health communication is "a part of everyday life" (du Pré, 2000, p. 3). Therefore, health communication programs should be based on information and facts that draw on the everyday lives of their audiences, as well as the environment where they live and work. One of the fundamental premises of this book is the importance of a research- and practice-based approach to developing theories, models, and methods that should guide and inform health communication planning and management.

The goal of this book is to provide a comprehensive introduction to health communication by combining the theory and practice of this field with a hands-on guide to program development and implementation. This book is a much-needed introductory text on health communication that addresses the needs of students and professionals who are pursuing a career in health care. It also incorporates many advanced topics that can help health communication practitioners and researchers, as well as experts in related areas, reflect on current issues and trends and advance their behavioral, practice, or policy change goals in a more efficient manner.

One of the primary themes of this book is the evolving nature of health communication and the importance of recognizing that there is no single magical health communication intervention. On the contrary, health communication is a multidisciplinary approach that relies on different action areas, such as interpersonal communications, public relations, public advocacy, community mobilization, professional communications, and constituency relations, among others (see Chapter One or the Glossary for a definition of all these terms). It is the blend of these areas that allows practitioners to involve communities, individuals, professional audiences, policymakers, and the general public with communication interventions that will prompt them to consider, analyze, and eventually adopt the behavior, policy, or practice suggested by a given health communication program or approach.

Over the years I have developed a practice-based definition of *health communication* that has inspired my work for this book. I believe that health communication is a multifaceted and multidisciplinary approach to reach different audiences and share health-related information with the goal of influencing, engaging, and supporting individuals, communities, health professionals, special groups, policymakers, and the public to champion, introduce, adopt, or sustain a behavior, practice, or policy that will ultimately improve health outcomes.

WHO SHOULD READ THIS BOOK

This book is primarily aimed at two audiences. The first of these audiences includes all professionals and individuals who are new to this field, such as graduate and undergraduate students in health communication, public health, public health education, public health nursing, community health and preventive medicine, communication, marketing, or nursing, as well as young and middle-career practitioners and researchers in this field. It also includes health and medical professionals, public health experts, funders, nonprofit board members and staff, physicians, nurses, and other health care providers with experience in related disciplines and a professional interest in health communication.

In the second audience are practicing managers, researchers, and instructors who can benefit from the strategic and step-by-step approach this book offers to implement health communication programs and train students and staff on this topic in a more efficient, effectual, and time-saving manner.

OVERVIEW OF THE CONTENTS

Two of the fundamental premises of this book are the multidisciplinary and multifaceted nature of health communication, as well as the interdependence of the individual, social, political, and disease-related factors that influence health communication interventions, and health care in general. With these premises in mind, the division of topics in parts and chapters is only instrumental to the text's readability and clarity. Readers should always consider the connection among the different theoretical and practical aspects of health communication as well as all external factors (political, social, cultural, economic, market, and other influences that shape or contribute to a specific situation or health problem as well as influence key program audiences) that influence this field. This introduction is an essential part of the book and is instrumental to maximize use and understanding of the text.

This book is divided in three parts. Part One focuses on defining health communication—its theoretical basis as well as its contexts and key action areas. Part One also establishes the importance of considering cultural, geographical, socioeconomic, ethnic, age, and gender influences on people's concepts of health and illness, as well as their approach to health problems and their solutions. Finally, this part addresses the role of health communication in public health as well as in the marketing or private sector contexts.

Part Two focuses on the different areas of health communication defined in Part One: interpersonal communications, public relations and public advocacy, community mobilization, professional medical communications, and constituency relations.

In all chapters in Part Two, key health communication issues are raised in the form of a question or brought to life in a case study. This is followed by a discussion of a specific communication approach or area. All chapters discuss specific communication areas in the context of the multidisciplinary nature of health communication and the need for an integrated approach. Special emphasis is placed on the importance of selecting and adapting health communication tools to a fast-changing social, political, market, and public health environment. Case studies and testimonials from experts and practitioners in the field are included in many of the chapters in Part Two.

Part Three provides a step-by-step guide to the development and implementation of a health communication plan. Each chapter covers specific steps of the health communication planning process or implementation and evaluation phases. Case studies, practical tips, and specific examples aim to facilitate readers' understanding of the planning process, as well as to build technical skills in health communication planning. Recent methodologies and trends in measuring and evaluating results of health communication programs are explored here.

Appendix A contains resources and worksheets on health communication planning. Online resources listed in Appendix B point to job listings, conferences, journals, organizations, centers, and programs in the health communication field.

The Glossary of key health communication planning terms at the end of the text should be used as a reference while reading this book, as well as a way to recap key definitions in health communication planning. Some of the key terms from the glossary are highlighted in bold type and briefly defined the first time they are mentioned in the text, so that readers can become familiar with them before approaching the chapters in Part Three that more specifically cover these topics. Other topic-specific definitions are included in relevant chapters.

Many chapters start with a practical example or case study. This is often used to establish the need for communication approaches that should be based on an in-depth understanding of intended audiences' perceptions, beliefs, attitudes, behavior, and barriers to change, as well as the cultural, social, and ethnic context in which they live. While referring to current theories and models, the book also reinforces the importance of the experience of health communication practitioners in developing theories, models, and approaches that should guide and inform health communication planning and management.

Each chapter ends with discussion questions for readers to reflect on, practice, and implement key concepts. Finally, all chapters are interconnected but are also designed to stand alone and provide a comprehensive overview on the topic they cover.

AUTHOR'S NOTE

As a health communication practitioner and instructor, I fully understand the complexity of communicating about health and illness. Changing human and social behavior to attain better health outcomes is often a lifetime endeavor.

My heartfelt appreciation and admiration go to all professionals, students, patients, policymakers, and ordinary people who every day dedicate their time to make a difference on their own health outcomes or those of their families, communities, special groups, or populations. These include all professionals and researchers in the health care and public health fields, the students or young practitioners who have committed themselves to a rewarding but demanding career, the patients who strive to keep themselves informed and make the right health decisions, the health care providers who dedicate their lives to alleviate and manage human sufferance, the mass media, government officers, associations, advocacy groups, and everyone else who may have an impact on health care.

I believe that being aware of current health communication theories and experiences may ease the process of communicating about health and illness and make it more approachable for all of these groups and individuals. I hope this book will help.

HEALTH COMMUNICATION

From Theory to Practice

PART ONE

INTRODUCTION TO HEALTH COMMUNICATION

CHAPTER ONE

WHAT IS HEALTH COMMUNICATION?

IN THIS CHAPTER

- Defining Health Communication
- Health Communication in the Twenty-First Century: Key Characteristics and Defining Features
- The Role of Health Communication in the Marketing Mix
- Health Communication in Public Health
- Overview of Key Communication Areas
- What Health Communication Can and Cannot Do
- Key Concepts
- For Discussion and Practice

Health communication is an evolving and increasingly prominent field in both public health and the nonprofit and commercial sectors. Therefore, many authors and organizations have been attempting to define or redefine it over time. Because of the multidisciplinary nature of health communication, many of the definitions may appear somewhat different from each other. Nevertheless, when they are analyzed, most point to the role that health communication can play in influencing and supporting individuals, communities, health care professionals, policymakers, or special groups to adopt and sustain a behavioral practice or a social or policy change that will ultimately improve health outcomes.

Understanding the true meaning of health communication and establishing the right context for its implementation may help communication managers and other health care professionals identify early on the training needs of staff and others who are involved in the communication process. It will also help create the right organizational mind-set and capability that should lead to a successful use of communication approaches to reach audience-specific goals.

This chapter sets the stage to discuss current health communication contexts. It also positions the importance of health communication in public health as well as in the private sector. Finally, it describes key elements, action areas, and limitations of the health communication approach.

DEFINING HEALTH COMMUNICATION

There are several definitions of health communication. For the most part, all of them point to a similar role of this approach in the process of advocating for and improving individual or public health outcomes. This section analyzes and aims to consolidate different definitions for health communication. This analysis starts from the literal and historical meaning of the word *communication*.

WHAT IS COMMUNICATION?

An understanding of health communication theory and practice requires reflection on the literal meaning of the word *communication*. *Communication* is defined in this way: "1. *Exchange of information,* between individuals, for example, by means of speaking, writing, or using a common system of signs and behaviors; 2. *Message*—a spoken or written message; 3. *Act of communicating*; 4. *Rapport*—a sense of mutual understanding and sympathy; 5. *Access*—a means of access or communication, for example, a connecting door" (Encarta Dictionary: English, North America).

In fact, all of these meanings can help define the modalities of well-designed health communication programs. As with other forms of communication, health communication should be based on a two-way exchange of information that uses a "common system of signs and behaviors." It should be accessible and create "mutual feelings of understanding and sympathy" among members of the communication team and **intended audiences** (all audiences the health communication program is seeking to influence and engage in the communication process; also referred to as *target audiences*). Finally, **communication channels** (the means or path used to reach intended audiences with health communication messages and materials, such as the mass media) and messages are the "connecting doors" that allow health communication interventions to reach intended audiences.

Communication has its roots in people's need to share and transmit meanings and ideas. A review of the origin and interpretation of early forms of communication, such as writing, shows that many of the reasons for which people may have started developing graphic notations and other early forms of writing are similar to those we can list for health communication.

One of the most important questions about the origins of writing is, "Why did writing begin and for what specific reasons?" (Houston, 2004, p. 234). Although the answer is still being debated, many established theories suggest that writing developed because of state and ceremonial needs (Houston, 2004). More specifically, in ancient Mesoamerica, early forms of writing may have been introduced to help local rulers "control the underlings and impress rivals by means of propaganda" (Houston, 2004, p. 234; Marcus, 1992) or "capture the dominant and dominating message within self-interested declarations" (Houston, 2004, p. 234) with the intention of "advertising" (p. 235) such views. In other words, it is possible to speculate that the desire and need to influence and connect with others are among the most important reasons for the emergence of early forms of writing. This need is also evident in many other forms of communication that seek to create feelings of approval, recognition, or friendliness, among others.

HEALTH COMMUNICATION DEFINED

One of the key objectives of health communication is to influence individuals and communities. The goal is admirable since health communication aims to improve health outcomes by sharing health-related information. In fact, the Centers for Disease Control and Prevention (CDC) define *health communication* as "the study and use of communication strategies to inform and influence individual and community decisions that enhance health" (2001;

U.S. Department of Health and Human Services, 2005). The word *influence* is also included in the *Healthy People 2010* definition of health communication as "the art and technique of informing, influencing, and motivating individual, institutional, and public audiences about important health issues" (U.S. Department of Health and Human Services, 2005, p. 11-2).

Another important role of communication is to create a receptive and favorable environment in which information can be shared, understood, absorbed, and discussed by the program's intended audiences. This requires an in-depth understanding of the needs, beliefs, taboos, attitudes, lifestyle, and social norms of all key communication audiences. It also demands that communication is based on messages that are easily understood. This is well characterized in the definition of *communication* by Pearson and Nelson (1991), who view it as "the process of understanding and sharing meanings" (p. 6).

A practical example that illustrates this definition is the difference between making an innocent joke about a friend's personality trait and doing the same about a colleague or recent acquaintance. The friend would likely laugh at the joke, while the colleague or recent acquaintance might be offended. In communication, understanding the context of the communication effort is interdependent with becoming familiar with target audiences. This increases the likelihood that all meanings are shared and understood in the way communicators intended them. Therefore, communication, especially about life-and-death matters such as in health care, is a long-term strategic process. It requires a true understanding of target audiences as well as the communicator's willingness and ability to adapt and redefine the goals, strategies, and activities of communication on the basis of audience feedback.

Health communication interventions have been successfully used for many years by nonprofit organizations, the commercial sector, and others to advance public, corporate, or product-related goals in relation to health. As many authors have noted, health communication draws from numerous disciplines, including health education, mass and speech communication, marketing, social marketing, psychology, anthropology, and sociology (Bernhardt, 2004; Institute of Medicine, 2003; World Health Organization, 2003). It relies on different communication activities or action areas, including interpersonal communications, public relations, public advocacy, community mobilization, and professional communications (World Health Organization, 2003; Bernhardt, 2004).

Table 1.1 provides some of the most recent definitions of health communication and is organized by key words most commonly used to characterize health communication and its role. It is evident that "sharing meanings or information," "influencing individuals or communities," "informing," "motivating target audiences," "exchanging information," and "changing behaviors," are among the most common attributes of health communication.

Another important attribute of health communication should be "to support and sustain change." In fact, key elements of successful health communication programs or campaigns always include long-term program sustainability, as well as the development of communication tools and steps that make it easy for individuals, communities, and other audiences to adopt or sustain a recommended behavior, practice, or policy change. If we integrate this practice-based perspective with many of the definitions in Table 1.1, the following new definition emerges:

Health communication is a multifaceted and multidisciplinary approach to reach different audiences and share health-related information with the goal of influencing, engaging, and supporting individuals, communities, health professionals, special groups, policymakers and the public to champion, introduce, adopt, or sustain a behavior, practice, or policy that will ultimately improve health outcomes.

HEALTH COMMUNICATION IN THE TWENTY-FIRST CENTURY: KEY CHARACTERISTICS AND DEFINING FEATURES

Health communication is about improving health outcomes by encouraging behavior modification and social change. It is increasingly considered an integral part of most public health interventions (U.S. Department of Health and Human Services, 2005; Bernhardt, 2004). It is a comprehensive approach that relies on the full understanding and involvement of its target audiences.

TABLE 1.1. HEALTH COMMUNICATION DEFINITIONS

Key Words	Definitions
To inform and influence (individual and community) decisions	"Health communication is a key strategy to *inform* the public about health concerns and to maintain important health issues on the public agenda" (New South Wales Department of Health, Australia, 2006).
	"The study or use of communication strategies to *inform and influence* individual and community decisions that enhance health" (CDC, 2001; U.S. Department of Health and Human Services, 2005).
	Health communication is a "means to disease prevention through behavior modification" (Freimuth, Linnan, and Potter, 2000, p. 337). It has been defined as the study and use of methods to *inform and influence* [italics added throughout table] individual and community decisions that enhance health" (Freimuth, Linnan, and Potter, 2000, p. 338; Freimuth, Cole, and Kirby, 2000, p. 475).
	"Health communication is a process for the development and diffusion of messages to specific audiences in order to *influence* their knowledge, attitudes and beliefs in favor of healthy behavioral choices" (Exchange, 2006; Smith and Hornik, 1999).
	"Health communication is the use of communication techniques and technologies to (positively) *influence* individuals, populations, and organizations for the purpose of promoting conditions conducive to human and environmental health" (Maibach and Holtgrave, 1995, pp. 219–220; Health Communication Unit, 2006). "It may include diverse activities such as clinician-patient interactions, classes, self-help groups, mailings, hot lines, mass media campaigns, and events" (Health Communication Unit, 2006).
Motivating individuals	"The art and technique of informing, influencing and *motivating* individual,

TABLE 1.1. HEALTH COMMUNICATION DEFINITIONS, CONT'D.

Key Words	Definitions
	institutional, and public audiences about important health issues. Its scope includes disease prevention, health promotion, health care policy, and business, as well as enhancement of the quality of life and health of individuals within the community" (Ratzan and others, 1994, p. 361).

"Effective health communication is the art and technique of *informing, influencing, and motivating* individuals, institutions, and large public audiences about important health issues based on sound scientific and ethical considerations" (Tufts University Student Services, 2006). |
| Change behaviors | "Health communication, like health education, is an approach which attempts to *change a set of behaviors* in a large-scale target audience regarding a specific problem in a predefined period of time" (Clift and Freimuth, 1995, p. 68). |
| Increase knowledge and understanding of health-related issues | "The goal of health communication is to *increase knowledge and understanding* of health-related issues and to improve the health status of the intended audience" (Muturi, 2005, p. 78).

"Communication means a process of *creating understanding* as the basis for development. It places emphasis on people interaction" (Agunga, 1997, p. 225). |
| Empowers people | "Communication *empowers* people by providing them with knowledge and understanding about specific health problems and interventions" (Muturi, 2005, p. 81). |
| Exchange, interchange of information, two-way dialogue | "A process for partnership and participation that is based on *two-way dialogue,* where there is an interactive *interchange of information,* ideas, techniques and knowledge between senders and receivers of information on an equal |

TABLE 1.1. HEALTH COMMUNICATION DEFINITIONS, CONT'D.

Key Words	Definitions
	footing, leading to improved understanding, shared knowledge, greater consensus, and identification of possible effective action" (Exchange, 2005).
	"Health communication is the scientific development, strategic dissemination, and critical evaluation of relevant, accurate, accessible, and understandable health *information communicated to and from intended audiences* to advance the health of the public" (Bernhardt, 2004, p. 2051).

Health communication theory draws on a number of additional disciplines and models. Health communication and its theoretical basis have evolved and changed in the past fifty years (Piotrow, Kincaid, Rimon, and Rinehart, 2003; Bernhardt, 2004). With increasing frequency, it is considered "the avant-garde in suggesting and integrating new theoretical approaches and practices" (Drum Beat, 2005).

Most important, communicators are no longer viewed as those who write press releases and other media-related communications, but as fundamental members of the public health or health industry teams. Communication is no longer considered a skill (Bernhardt, 2004) but a science-based discipline that requires training and passion and relies on the use of different **vehicles** (materials, activities, events, and other tools used to deliver a message through communication channels; Health Communication Unit, 2003b) and channels. According to Saba (2006):

> In the past and this is probably the most prevalent trend even today, health communication practitioners were trained "on-the-job." People from different fields (sociology, demography, public health, psychology, communication with all its different specialties, such as filmmaking, journalism and advertising) entered or were brought into health communication programs to meet the need

for professional human resources in this field. By performing their job and working in teams, they learned how to adapt their skills to the new field and were taught by other practitioners about the common practices and basic "lingo" of health communication.

In the mid 90s, and in response to the increasing demand for health communication professionals, several schools in the United States started their own curricular programs and/or "concentrations" in Health Communication. This helped bring more attention from the academic world to this emerging field. The number of peer-reviewed articles and several other types of health communication publications increased. The field moved from in-service training to pre-service education.

As a result, there is an increasing understanding that "the level of technical competence of communication practitioners can affect outcomes. A structured approach to health communications planning, a spotless program execution and a rigorous evaluation process are the result of adequate training. In health communication, the learning process is a lifetime endeavor and should be facilitated by the continuous development of new training initiatives and tools" (Schiavo, 2006). Training may start in the academic setting but should always be influenced and complemented by practical experience and observations, as well as other learning and training opportunities, including in-service training and continuing professional education.

Health communication can reach its highest potential when it is discussed and applied within a team-oriented context that includes many other health care and public health professionals. Teamwork and mutual agreement on the intervention's ultimate objectives and expected results are key to the successful design, implementation, and impact of any program.

Finally, it is important to remember that there is no magic bullet that can address health issues. Health communication is an evolving discipline and should always seek to incorporate lessons learned as well to use a multidisciplinary approach to all interventions. This is in line with one of the fundamental premises of this book that recognizes the experience of practitioners as a key factor in developing theories, models, and approaches that should guide and inform health communication planning and management.

Table 1.2 lists the key elements of health communication, which are further analyzed below.

AUDIENCE CENTERED

Health communication is a long-term process that begins and ends with the audience's desires and needs. In health communication, the audience is not merely a target (even if this terminology is very well established and used by practitioners around the world) but an active participant in the process of analyzing the health issue and finding culturally appropriate and cost-effective solutions. It is a common practice in health communication not only to research intended audiences and other key constituencies but also to strive to engage them in defining and implementing key strategies and activities. This is often accomplished by working together with organizations and leaders who represent them. For example, if a health communication program aims to reach breast cancer survivors, all strategies and key program elements should be designed, discussed, tested, and implemented together with membership organizations, patient groups, leaders, and audience samples representing this target audience. Most important, these audiences need to feel invested and well represented. They should be the key protagonists of the action-oriented process that will lead to behavioral or social change.

TABLE 1.2. KEY CHARACTERISTICS OF HEALTH COMMUNICATION

Audience-centered

Research-based

Multidisciplinary

Strategic

Process oriented

Cost-effective

Creative in support of strategy

Audience and media specific

Relationship building

Aimed at behavioral or social change

RESEARCH BASED

Health communication is grounded in research. Successful health communication programs are based on a true understanding not only of the intended audience but also of the situational environment. This includes existing programs and lessons learned, policies, social norms, key issues, and obstacles in addressing the specific health problem.

The overall premise of health communication is that behavioral change is conditioned by the environment in which people live, as well as by those who influence them. Creating a receptive environment in which the target audience can discuss a health issue and be supported in its intention to change by key influentials (for example, family members, health care providers) is often one of the aims of health communication programs. This requires a comprehensive research approach that relies primarily on traditional research techniques for the formal development of a **situation analysis** (a planning term that describes the analysis of individual, social, political, and behavior-related factors that can affect attitudes, behaviors, social norms, and policies about a health issue) and **audience profile** (a comprehensive, research-based, and strategic description of all key audiences' characteristics, demographics, needs, values, attitudes, and behavior). Situation analysis and audience profile are fundamental and interrelated steps of health communication planning (the audience profile is described in this book as a component of the situation analysis) and are described in detail in Chapter Ten.

MULTIDISCIPLINARY

Health communication is "transdisciplinary in nature" (Bernhardt, 2004, p. 2051; Institute of Medicine, 2003) and draws on multiple disciplines (Bernhardt, 2004; World Health Organization, 2003). Health communication recognizes the complexity of attaining behavioral and social change and uses a multifaceted approach that is grounded in the application of several theoretical frameworks and disciplines, including health education, social marketing, and behavioral and social change theories (see Chapter Two for a comprehensive discussion of key theories and models). It draws on principles successfully used in the private and commercial sectors and also on the audience-centered approach of other disciplines, such as psychology, sociology, and anthropology (World Health Organization, 2003). It is not anchored to a single specific theory or model. With the audience always at the core of each intervention, it uses a case-by-case approach in selecting those models, theories, and strategies that are best suited to reach people's hearts; secure their involvement in the health issue, and, most important, its solutions; and support and facilitate their journey on a path to better health.

Piotrow, Rimon, Payne Merritt, and Saffitz (2003) identify four different "eras" of health communication:

> (1) The clinic era, based on a medical care model and the notion that if people knew where services were located they would find their way to the clinics; (2) the field era, a more proactive approach emphasizing outreach workers, community-based distribution, and a variety of information, education, and communication (IEC) products; (3) the social marketing era, developed from the commercial concepts that consumers will buy the products they want at subsidized prices; and, (4) today, the era of strategic behavior communications, founded on behavioral science models that emphasize the need to influence social norms and policy environments to facilitate and empower the iterative and dynamic process of both individual and social change [pp. 1–2].

However, even in the context of strategic behavior communications, many of the theoretical approaches of the different eras of health communication still find a use in program planning or execution. For example, the situation analysis of a health communication program uses primarily commercial and social marketing tools and models (see Chapters Two and Ten for a detailed description) to analyze the environment in which change should occur. Instead, in the early stages of approaching key opinion leaders and other key **stakeholders** (individuals and groups who have an interest or share responsibilities in a given health issue), keeping in mind McGuire's communication for persuasion steps (1984; see Chapter Two) may help communicators gain stakeholder support for the importance or the urgency of adequately addressing a health issue. This theoretical flexibility should keep communicators focused on their audiences and always on the lookout for the best approach and planning framework to influence people's core beliefs and behaviors and engage them in the communication process. In concert with the other features previously discussed, it also enables the overall communication process to be truly fluid and suited to respond to audiences' needs.

The importance of a somewhat flexible theoretical basis, which should be selected on a case-by-case basis (National Cancer Institute, 2005a), is already supported by reputable organizations and authors. For example, a publication by the U.S. Department of Health and Human Services, National Institutes of Health, National Cancer Institute (2002), points to the importance of selecting planning frameworks that "can help [communicators] identify the social sciences theories most appropriate for understanding the problem and the situation" (p. 218). These theories, models, and constructs include several theoretical concepts and frameworks (see Chapter Two) that are also used in motivating change at an individual level, interpersonal level, or organizational, community, and societal level (National Cancer Institute, 2002) by related or complementary disciplines.

The goal here is not to advocate for a lack of theoretical structure in communication planning and execution. On the contrary, planning frameworks, models, and theories should be consistent at least until preliminary steps of the evaluation phase of a program are completed. This allows communicators to take advantage of lessons learned and redefine theoretical constructs and **communication objectives** (the intermediate steps that need to be achieved in order to meet program goals and outcome objectives; National Cancer Institute, 2002) by comparing **program outcomes**, which measure changes in knowledge, attitudes, skills, behavior, and other parameters, with those that were anticipated in the planning phase. However, the ability to draw on multiple disciplines and theoretical constructs is a definitive advantage of the health communication approach and one of the keys to the success of well-planned and well-executed communication programs.

STRATEGIC

Health communication programs need to display a sound strategy and plan of action. All activities need to be well planned and respond to a specific audience-related need. Consider again the example of Bonnie, the twenty-five-year-old mother who is not sure about whether to immunize her newborn child. Activities in support of a strategy that focuses on facilitating communication between Bonnie and her health care provider make sense only if research shows all or any of the following points: (1) Bonnie is likely to be influenced primarily, or at least significantly, by her health care provider and not by family or other new mothers; (2) there are several gaps in the understanding of patients' needs that prevent health care providers from communicating effectively; and (3) providers lack adequate tools to talk about this topic with patients in a time-effective and efficient manner.

Communication strategies (the overall approach that is used to accomplish the communication objectives) need to be research based, and all activities should serve such strategies. Therefore, program planners should not rely on any workshop, press release, brochure, video, or anything else to provide effective communication without making sure that their content and format reflect the selected approach (the strategy) and is a priority in reaching the audience's heart. For this purpose, health communication strategies need to respond to an actual need that has been identified by preliminary research and confirmed by the intended audience.

PROCESS ORIENTED

Communication is a long-term process. Influencing people and their behaviors requires an ongoing commitment to the health issue and its solutions. This is rooted in a deep understanding of target audiences and their environments and aims at building consensus among audience members about the potential plan of action.

Most, if not all, health communication programs change or evolve from what communication experts had originally devised due to the input and participation of key opinion leaders, patient groups, professional associations, policymakers, audience members, and other key stakeholders.

In health communication, educating target audiences about health issues and ways to address them is only the first step of a long-term, audience-centered process. This process often requires theoretical flexibility to accommodate the needs of interested groups and audiences.

While in the midst of many process-oriented projects, many practitioners may have noticed that health communication is often misunderstood. Health communication uses multiple channels and approaches, which, despite what some people may think, include but are not limited to the use of the mass media. Moreover, health communication aims at improving health outcomes and in the process help advance public health goals or create market share (depending on whether health communication strategies are used for nonprofit or for-profit goals). Finally, health communication cannot focus only on channels, messages, and tools. It also should be process oriented and attempt to persuade, involve, and create consensus and feelings of ownership among intended audiences.

Exchange, a networking and learning program on health communication for development that is based in the United Kingdom and has multiple partners, views health communication as "a process for partnership and participation that is based on two-way dialogue, where there is an interactive interchange of information, ideas, techniques, and knowledge between senders and receivers of information on an equal footing, leading to improved understanding, shared knowledge, greater consensus, and identification of possible effective action" (2005). This definition makes sense in all settings and situations, but it assumes a greater relevance for health communication programs that aim to improve health outcomes in developing countries. Communication for development often needs to rely on creative solutions that compensate for the lack of local capabilities and infrastructures. These solutions usually emerge after months of discussion with local community leaders and organizations, government officials, and members of target audiences. Word of mouth and the ability of the community leaders to engage members of their communities is often all that communicators have at hand.

Consider the case of Maria, a mother of four children who lives in a small village in sub-Saharan Africa together with her seventy-five-year-old father. Her village is almost completely isolated from major metropolitan areas, and very few people in town have a radio or know how to read. Maria is unaware that malaria, which is endemic in that region, poses a higher risk to children than to the elderly. Since elderly people benefit from a high hierarchical status in that region, if Maria is able to find money to purchase mosquito nets to protect someone in her family from mosquito bites and the consequent threat of malaria, she would probably choose that her father sleep under them, leaving her children unprotected. This is in spite of the high mortality rate from malaria among children in her village. If her village's community leaders told her to do otherwise, she would likely change her practice and protect her children.

Involving Maria's community leaders in the communication process that would lead to a change in her habits requires a long-term commitment. Such effort demands the involvement of local organizations and authorities who are respected and trusted by community leaders, as well as an open mind in listening to suggestions and seeking solutions with the help of all key stakeholders. Because of the lack of local capabilities and widespread access to adequate communication channels, this process is likely to take longer than any similar initiative in the developed world. Therefore, communicators should view this as an ongoing process and applaud every small step forward.

COST-EFFECTIVE

Cost-effectiveness is a concept that health communication borrows from commercial and social marketing. It is particularly important in the competitive working environment of nonprofit organizations, where the lack of sufficient funds or adequate economic planning can often undermine important initiatives. It implies the need to seek solutions that allow communicators to advance their goals with minimal use of human and economic resources. Nevertheless, concerns related to cost-effectiveness should never prompt a significant reduction of the program's objectives unless resources are not adequate to support all of them. Communicators should use their funds as long as they are well spent and advance their research-based strategy. They should also seek creative solutions that minimize the use of internal funds and human resources by seeking partnerships, using existing materials or programs as a starting point, and maximizing synergies with the work of other departments in their organization or external groups and stakeholders in the same field.

CREATIVE IN SUPPORT OF STRATEGY

Creativity is a significant attribute of communicators since it allows them to consider multiple options, formats, and channels to reach target audiences. It also helps them devise solutions that preserve the sustainability and cost-effectiveness of specific health communication interventions. However, even the greatest ideas or the best-designed and best-executed communication tools may fail to achieve behavioral or social change goals if they do not respond to a strategic need identified by marketing and audience-specific research and endorsed by key stakeholders from target groups. Too often communication programs and resources fail to make an impact because of this common mistake.

For example, providing a brochure to a target audience on how to use insecticide-treated nets (ITNs) makes sense only if the audience is already aware of the cycle of malaria transmission, as well as the need for protection from mosquito bites. If this is not the case and members of target communities still believe that malaria is contracted by bathing in the river or is a complication of some other fevers (Pinto,1998; Schiavo, 1998, 2000), the first strategic imperative is disease awareness, with a specific focus on the cycle of transmission and subsequent protective measures. All communication materials and activities need to address this basic information before talking about the use of ITNs and potential reasons to use them instead of other protection measures. The communicator's creativity should come into play by devising the most suitable and culturally friendly tools to engage intended groups in the process of changing their behaviors, beliefs, and attitudes toward the disease and its prevention. However, creativity should never be used to develop and implement great, sensational, or innovative ideas that do not respond to actual needs and strategic priorities.

AUDIENCE AND MEDIA SPECIFIC

The importance of audience-specific messages and channels became one of the most important lessons learned after the anthrax-by-mail bioterrorist attacks that rocked the United States in October 2001.

At the time, several letters containing the lethal agent *Bacillus anthracis* were mailed to senators and representatives of the media (Jernigan and others, 2002; Blanchard and others, 2005). The attack also exposed government staff workers, including U.S. postal workers in the U.S. Postal Service facility in Washington, D.C., and other parts of the country, to anthrax. Two workers in the Washington facility died as a result of inhalation anthrax (Blanchard and others, 2005).

Communication during this emergency was perceived by several members of the medical, patient, and worker communities as well as public figures and the media to be often inconsistent and disorganized (Blanchard and others, 2005; Vanderford, 2003). Equally important, postal workers and U.S. Senate staff have reported erosion of their trust in public health agencies (Blanchard and others, 2005). Several analyses point to the possibility that the one message–one behavior approach to communication (UCLA, 2002)—in other words, using the same message and strategic approach for all audiences—led to feelings of being left out among postal workers, who in the Brentwood facility in Washington, D.C., were primarily African Americans or individuals with a severe hearing impairment (Blanchard and others, 2005). They also point to the need for public health officials to develop the relationships that are needed to communicate with groups of different racial and socioeconomic backgrounds, as well as "those with physical limitations that could hinder communication, such as those with hearing impairments" (Blanchard and others, 2005, p. 494; McEwen and Anton-Culver, 1988).

The lessons learned from the anthrax scare support some of the fundamental principles of good health communication practices. Messages need to be audience specific and tailored to channels allowing the most effective reach to target audiences. Since it is very likely that communication efforts always aim at producing multiple audience-appropriate behaviors, the one message–one behavior approach should be avoided (UCLA, 2002) even when time and resources are lacking. As highlighted by the anthrax case study, in developing audience-specific messages and activities, the contribution of local advocates and community representatives is fundamental to increase the likelihood that messages will be heard, understood, and trusted by target audiences.

RELATIONSHIP BUILDING

Communication is a relationship business. Establishing and preserving good relationships is critical to the success of health communication interventions, and, among other things, can help build long-term and successful partnerships and coalitions, secure credible stakeholder endorsement of the health issue, and expand the pool of ambassadors on behalf of the health cause.

Most important, good relationships help create the environment of "shared meanings and understanding" (Pearson and Nelson, 1991, p. 6) that is central to seeking social or behavioral change at the individual and community levels. Good relationships should be established with key stakeholders and representatives of target audiences, health organizations, governments, and many other critical members of the extended health communication team. (A detailed discussion of the dos and don'ts of successful partnerships and relationship building efforts is included in Chapters Eight and Twelve.)

AIMED AT BEHAVIORAL AND SOCIAL CHANGE

Today we are in the "era of strategic behavior communications" (Piotrow and others, 2003, p. 2). Although the ultimate goal of health communication has always been influencing behaviors and social norms, there is a renewed emphasis on the importance of establishing behavioral and social objectives early in the design of health communication interventions.

"What do you want people to do?" is the first question that should be asked in communication planning meetings. Do you want them to immunize their children before age two? Become aware of their risk for heart disease and behave accordingly to prevent it? Ask their dentists about oral cancer screening? Want local legislators to support a stricter law on the use of infant car seats? Create an environment of peer-to-peer support designed to discourage adolescents from initiating smoking? Answering these kinds of questions is the first step in identifying suitable and research-based objectives of a communication program.

Although different theories (see Chapter Two) support the importance of behavioral or social change as key indicators for success, these two parameters are actually interconnected. In fact, social change typically takes place as the result of a series of behavioral changes at the individual, group, or community level.

THE ROLE OF HEALTH COMMUNICATION IN THE MARKETING MIX

Health communication strategies are extensively used in the commercial and nonprofit sectors to support and motivate behavioral change, product adoption, or the endorsement of a health issue or cause. In the private sector, health communication strategies are primarily used in a marketing context. Still, many of the other behavioral and social constructs of health communication—and definitely all of these models and tools that position the audience at the center of any intervention—are considered and used at least at an empirical level. As in other settings (for example, public health), health communication functions tend to be similar to those described in the "What Health Communication Can and Cannot Do" section of this chapter.

Many in the private sector regard health communication as a critical component of the marketing mix, which is traditionally defined by the key four Ps of social marketing (see Chapter Two for a more detailed description): product, price, place, and promotion—in other words, "developing, delivering, and promoting a superior offer" (Maibach, 2003).

When looking at the health communication environment where change should occur and be sustained (Figure 1.1), it becomes clear that effective communication can be a powerful tool in seeking to influence all of the factors that are highlighted in the figure. It is also clear that regardless of whether these factors are related to the audience, health behavior, product, service, social, or political environment, all of them are interconnected and can mutually affect each other. At the same time, health communication interventions can tip the existing balance among these factors and change the weight they may have in defining a specific health issue and its solutions.

Figure 1.1 also reflects some of the key principles of marketing models as well as the socioecological model (Morris, 1975) and

FIGURE 1.1. HEALTH COMMUNICATION ENVIRONMENT

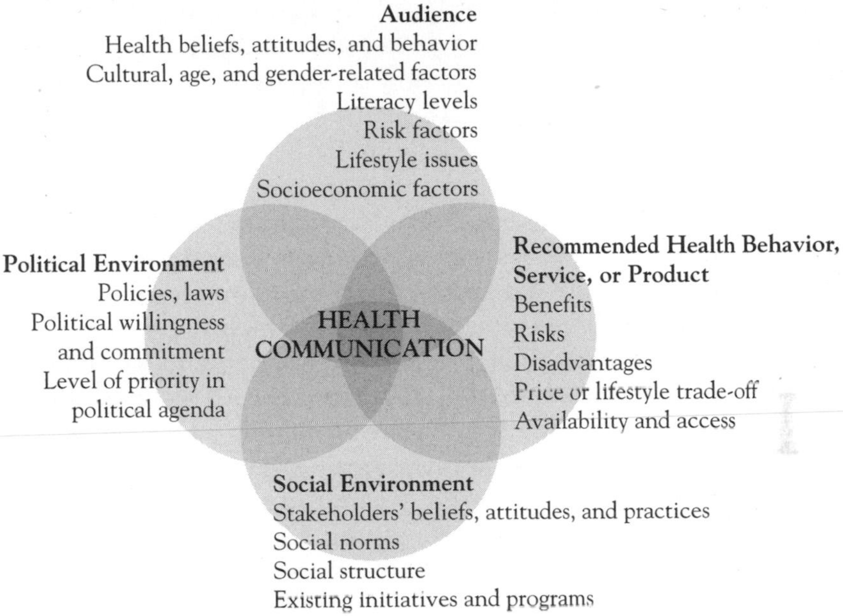

Audience
Health beliefs, attitudes, and behavior
Cultural, age, and gender-related factors
Literacy levels
Risk factors
Lifestyle issues
Socioeconomic factors

Political Environment
Policies, laws
Political willingness
and commitment
Level of priority in
political agenda

HEALTH
COMMUNICATION

**Recommended Health Behavior,
Service, or Product**
Benefits
Risks
Disadvantages
Price or lifestyle trade-off
Availability and access

Social Environment
Stakeholders' beliefs, attitudes, and practices
Social norms
Social structure
Existing initiatives and programs

other theoretical models (VanLeeuwen, Waltner-Toews, Abernathy, and Smit, 1999) that are used in public health to show the connection and influence of different factors (individual, interpersonal, community, organizational, and public policy) on individual, group, and community behavior as well as to understand the process that may lead to behavioral and social change.

HEALTH COMMUNICATION IN PUBLIC HEALTH

Prior to the recent call to action by many federal and multilateral organizations, which encouraged a strategic and more frequent use of communication, health communication has been used only marginally in public health. It has been perceived more as a skill than a discipline and confined to the mere dissemination of scientific and medical findings by public health professionals (Bernhardt, 2004).

Fortunately, most public health organizations and leaders (Freimuth, Cole, and Kirby, 2000; U.S. Department of Health and Human Services, 2005; Institute of Medicine, 2003; Bernhardt, 2004; National Cancer Institute and National Institutes of Health, 2002; Piotrow and others, 1997) now recognize the role that health communication can play in advancing health outcomes and the general health status of interested populations and special groups. Most important, there is a new awareness of the reach of health communication, as well as its many strategic action areas (for example, interpersonal communications, professional medical communications, and public relations).

As defined by *Healthy People 2010* (U.S. Department of Health and Human Services, 2005), the U.S. public health agenda, the scope of health communication in public health "includes disease prevention, health promotion, health care policy, and the business of health care as well as enhancement of the quality of life and health of individuals within the community" (p. 11–20; Ratzan, 1994). Health communication "links the domains of communication and health" (p. 11–3) and is increasingly regarded as a science (Freimuth and others, 2000), of great importance in public health, especially in the era of emerging infectious diseases, global threats, bioterrorism, and a new emphasis on a preventive and patient-centered approach to health.

OVERVIEW OF KEY COMMUNICATION AREAS

Global health communication is a term increasingly used to include different communication approaches and action areas, such as interpersonal communications, social and community mobilization, and advocacy (Haider, 2005; Waisbord and Larson, 2005). Well-planned health communication programs rely on an integrated blend of different action areas that should be selected in consideration of expected behavioral and social outcomes (World Health Organization, 2003; O'Sullivan, Yonkler, Morgan, and Merritt, 2003; Health Communication Partnership, 2005e). Long-term results can be achieved only through a participatory process that involves all interested audiences and uses all culturally appropriate action areas and communication channels. Remember that there is no magic bullet in health communication.

Message repetitiveness and frequency are also important factors in health communication. Often the resonance effect, which can be defined as the ability to create a snowball effect for message delivery by using multiple vehicles, sources, and messengers, can help motivate people to change by reminding them of the desired behavior (for example, complying with childhood immunization requirements, using mosquito nets for protection against malaria, attempting to quit smoking) and its benefits. To this end, several action areas are normally used in health communication and are described in detail in the topic-specific chapters in Part Two:

• *Interpersonal communications,* which uses interpersonal channels (for example, one-on-one or group meetings) and is based on active listening, social and behavioral theories, and the ability to relate to and identify with the audience's needs and cultural preferences and efficiently addressing them. This includes "personal selling and counseling" (World Health Organization, 2003, p. 2), which takes place during one-on-one encounters with members of interested audiences and other key stakeholders, as well as during group events and in locations where materials and services are available. It also includes provider-patient communications, which has been identified as one of the most important areas of health communication (U.S. Department of Health and Human Services, 2005) and should aim at improving health outcomes by optimizing the relationships between providers and their patients.

• *Public relations, public advocacy, and government relations,* which relies on the skillful use of culturally competent and audience-appropriate mass media, as well as other communication channels to place a health issue on the public agenda, advocate for its solutions, or highlight the importance that the government and other key stakeholders take action.

• *Community mobilization,* a bottom-up and participatory process. By using multiple communication channels, community mobilization seeks to involve community leaders and the community at large in addressing a health issue, becoming part of the key steps to behavioral or social change, or practicing a desired behavior.

• *Professional medical communications,* a peer-to-peer approach targeting health care professionals that, among others, aims to (1) promote the adoption of best medical and health practices; (2)

establish new concepts and standards of care; (3) publicize recent medical discoveries, beliefs, parameters, and policies; (4) change or establish new medical priorities; and (5) advance health policy changes.

• *Constituency relations,* a critical component of all other areas of health communication as well as a communication area of its own. Constituency relations refer to the process of (1) creating consensus among key stakeholders about health issues and their potential solutions, (2) expanding program reach by involving key constituencies, (3) developing alliances, (4) managing and anticipating criticisms and opponents, and (5) maintaining key relationships with other health organizations or stakeholders.

WHAT HEALTH COMMUNICATION CAN AND CANNOT DO

Health communication cannot work in a vacuum and is normally a critical component of larger public health interventions or corporate efforts. Because of the complexity of health issues, it may "not be equally effective in addressing all issues or relaying all messages" (National Cancer Institute and National Institutes of Health, 2002, p. 3), at least in a given time frame.

Health communication cannot replace the lack of local infrastructure (such as the absence of appropriate health services or hospitals) or capability (such as an inadequate number of health care providers in relation to the size of the population being attended). It cannot compensate for inadequate medical solutions to treat, diagnose, or prevent any disease. But it can help advocate for change and create a receptive environment to support the development of new health services or the allocation of additional funds for medical and scientific discovery, access to existing treatments or services, or the recruitment of health care professionals in new medical fields or underserved geographical areas. In doing so, it helps secure political commitment, stakeholder endorsement, and community involvement to encourage change and improve health outcomes.

Because of the evolving role of health communication, other authors and organizations have been defining the potential contribution of health communication to the health care and public health fields. For example, the U.S. National Cancer Institute

(2002) has a homonymous section, which partly inspired the need for this section, in one of its publications on the topic.

Understanding the role and the potential impact of health communication on different aspects of public health, and health care in general, is important to take full advantage of the contribution of this emerging field to health outcomes as well as to set realistic expectations on what can be accomplished among team members, program partners, intended audiences, and other key stakeholders. Table 1.3 lists what health communication can and cannot do.

TABLE 1.3. WHAT HEALTH COMMUNICATION CAN AND CANNOT DO

Health Communication Can Help. . .	*Health Communication Cannot. . .*
Raise awareness of health issues to drive policy or practice changes.	Work in a vacuum, independent from other larger public health or marketing interventions.
Secure stakeholder endorsement of health issues.	Replace the lack of local infrastructure or capability.
"Influence perceptions, beliefs and attitudes that may change social norms" (NCI, 2002, p. 3).	Compensate for the absence of adequate treatment or diagnostic or preventative options.
Promote data and emerging issues to establish new standards of care.	"Be equally effective in addressing all issues or relaying all messages", at least in the same time frame (NCI, 2002, p. 3).
"Increase demand for health services" (NCI, 2002, p. 3) and products.	
Show benefits of behavior change.	
"Demonstrate healthy skills" (NCI, 2002, p. 3).	
Provoke public discussion to drive disease diagnosis, treatment, or prevention.	
Suggest and "prompt action" (NCI, 2002, p. 3).	
Build constituencies to support health practice changes.	
Support the need for additional funds for medical and scientific discovery.	
Advocate for equal access to existing health products and services.	
Create a climate of receptivity for new health services or products.	
Strengthen third-party relationships.	
Improve provider-patient relationships, and ultimately, patient compliance and outcomes.	

KEY CONCEPTS

- Health communication is a multifaceted and multidisciplinary approach to reach different audiences and share health-related information with the goal of influencing, engaging, and supporting individuals, communities, health professionals, special groups, policymakers, and the public to champion, introduce, adopt, or sustain a behavior, practice, or policy that will ultimately improve health outcomes.
- Health communication is an increasingly prominent field in public health, as well as in the private sector (both nonprofit and commercial).
- One of the key characteristics of health communication is its multidisciplinary nature, which allows the theoretical flexibility that is needed to consider each situation and audience for their unique characteristics and needs and select the best approach and planning framework to reach out to people and involve them in the health issue and its solutions.
- Health communication is an evolving discipline that should always incorporate lessons learned and practical experiences. Practitioners should have a key role in defining theories and models to inform health communication planning and management.
- It is important to be aware of key features and limitations of health communication (and more specifically what communication can and cannot do).
- Health communication relies on several action areas.
- Well-designed programs are the result of an integrated blend of different areas that should be selected in the light of expected behavioral and social outcomes.

FOR DISCUSSION AND PRACTICE

1. Did you have any preliminary idea about the definition and role of health communication prior to reading this chapter? If yes, how does it compare to what you have learned in this chapter?
2. In your opinion, what are the two most important defining features of health communication, and why? How do they relate to the other key characteristics of health communication that are discussed in this chapter?

3. Can you recall a personal experience in which a health communication program, message, or health-related encounter (for example, a physician visit) has influenced your decisions or perceptions about a specific health issue? Describe the experience, and emphasize key factors that affected your decision and health behavior.
4. Did you ever participate in the development or implementation of a health communication campaign? If yes, what were some of the key learnings, and how do they relate to the attributes of health communication as described in this chapter?

CHAPTER TWO

CURRENT HEALTH COMMUNICATION THEORIES AND ISSUES

IN THIS CHAPTER

- Key Theoretical Influences in Health Communication
- Select Models for Strategic Behavior and Social Change Communication
- Other Theoretical Influences and Planning Frameworks
- Current Issues and Topics in Health Care: Implications for Health Communication
- Key Concepts
- For Discussion and Practice

In the past fifty years, the field of health communication has experienced a dramatic growth and evolution, which is still continuing. The multidisciplinary nature of health communication has been recognized by several organizations and leaders (Institute of Medicine, 2003; Bernhardt, 2004; World Health Organization, 2003) and is also one of the most important characteristics of health communication.

While several authors and organizations have been trying to define the theoretical basis of health communication, the intersection among many different disciplines (for example, behavioral and social sciences, social marketing and health education) as well as between social sciences and the humanities is still a growing field of research and practical application (Health Communication Partnership, 2005a). Some authors have been referring to a "family tree" (Waisbord, 2001, p. 1) of communication theories and models; others do not emphasize the chronological sequence and interdependence of communication theories but focus primarily on the impact such theories may have on potential program design and outcomes (Institute of Medicine of the National Academies, 2002).

Theories and planning models are particularly important for students and young practitioners in this field. Theories help clarify how to approach a health issue and try to address it through a health communication intervention. They also have a significant weight at all levels in communication research, donor-sponsored programs, retrospective analyses, outcome and impact evaluation, and all other circumstances that demand a rigorous program design. Theories can also provide a powerful tool to organize one's thoughts and design interventions that clearly have in mind specific behavioral or social outcomes. Communication theories and frameworks are used in a less rigorous way in the commercial, nonprofit, and private sectors in the interest of time. The downside to this approach is that it may become more difficult to link any specific behavioral or social outcome to the actual health communication program, which is already a notably complex task in health communication (see Chapter Twelve).

This chapter provides a brief overview of major theories and planning frameworks and their implications in health communication. Models and theoretical constructs are often used in these ways:

- Provide a basis for communication planning and evaluation.
- Inspire specific communication approaches.
- Help implement a specific phase of a health communication program.
- Support a true understanding of target audiences and groups as well as the health communication environment among health communication practitioners and other members of the communication team.

While reviewing these theories and models, junior health communication practitioners and students should remember that these are just selected references, which ideally should prompt further inquiries and readings on the theory of health communication.

They should also keep in mind that theories, models, and planning frameworks should (1) be considered part of a tool kit and selected on a case-by-case basis; (2) respond to an audience's needs; (3) address the specific health situation and all factors that play a role in determining it; (4) inform and guide message development as well as the identification of appropriate communication channels; and (5) be revisited in the light of emerging factors and needs. This selection process should take into account expected program outcomes and the desired behavioral or social impact of the program. For all other readers (including current health communication practitioners, researchers, and other health professionals), the following overview should provide an updated summary of selected theories and models that currently inspire this field as well as health-related issues and topics that influence its practice.

KEY THEORETICAL INFLUENCES IN HEALTH COMMUNICATION

Health communication is influenced by different disciplines and theoretical approaches. Some of the most important theories can be divided into the following categories: behavioral and social science theories, mass communications theories, marketing and social marketing, and other theoretical influences, including medical models, sociology, and anthropology. In addition, several planning frameworks and models have been developed to reflect or incorporate key principles from some or all of these categories. The overview that follows focuses on select theories and models as well as their potential or actual impact on health communication practice.

SELECTED BEHAVIORAL AND SOCIAL SCIENCES THEORIES

Behavioral and social sciences theories seek to analyze and explain how change occurs at the individual, community, or social levels. Some of these theories focus on only the key steps that may lead to behavioral or social change. Most of them also emphasize the interconnection and mutual dependence of individual and external factors. As previously mentioned, this connection is of great importance in health communication.

Diffusion of Innovation Theory

Initially developed by Everett Rogers (1962, 1983, 1995), the diffusion of innovation theory addresses how new ideas, concepts, or practices can spread within a community or "society or from one society to another" (National Cancer Institute and National Institutes of Health, 2002, p. 226). The theory identifies and defines five subgroups on the basis of the audience's characteristics and propensity to accept and adopt innovation (Beal and Rogers, 1960):

- Innovators
- Early adopters
- Early majority
- Late majority
- Laggards

The overall premise of this theory is that change occurs over time and is dependent on the following stages (Rogers, 1962, 1983, 1995; Waisbord, 2001; Health Communication Partnership, 2005b):

- Awareness
- Knowledge and interest
- Decision
- Trial or implementation
- Confirmation or rejection of the behavior

It also observes that innovators usually decide much faster than any other subgroup on whether to adopt new ideas, concepts, or practices (Beal and Rogers, 1960; see Figure 2.1). Therefore, innovators can act as role models and persuade other subgroups (including laggards) to accept and adopt new behaviors and social practices.

Like many other theories in any field, diffusion of innovation has been misused and misinterpreted at times (Health Communication Partnership, 2005b). Some critics have observed that the trickle-down approach, from the innovators to the laggards, may not work in all situations (Waisbord, 2001). Rogers himself modified the theory to change the focus from "a persuasion approach

FIGURE 2.1. ATTRIBUTES OF THE AUDIENCE

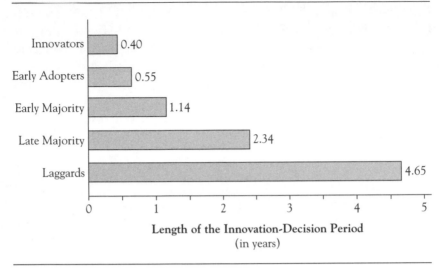

Length of the Innovation-Decision Period
(in years)

Beal, G. M., and Rogers, E. M. *The adoption of two farm practices in a central Iowa community.* Special report no. 26, p. 14. Ames, Iowa: Agricultural and Home Economics Experiment Station, Iowa State University, 1960. Used by permission.

(transmission of information between individuals and groups)" to "a process by which participants create and share information with one another in order to reach a mutual understanding" (Waisbord, 2001, p. 5; Rogers, 1976).

Nevertheless, diffusion of innovation still plays a role in health communication and is widely used by a variety of communication practitioners and organizations for program research and planning. The major contribution of the theory is its early audience segmentation model, which supports the importance of looking at intended audiences as a complex puzzle of different subgroups, stages, and needs that should be considered in developing communication messages and activities.

Finally, the individuals' stage model provides a perspective on the time and the external conditions that are needed to achieve behavioral or social change. It is a useful tool in thinking about the levels of awareness, knowledge, and interest among target groups (Health Communication Partnership, 2005b). It is also a valid reminder that continuing to engage innovators and early adopters or their representatives in program planning and evaluation is essential to program sustainability as well as to the involvement of larger segments of the intended population in accepting and adopting innovative behaviors or social practices. For a practical example about the application of this theory, see Box 2.1.

Box 2.1

Diffusion of Innovation Theory: A Practical Example

Luciana, a nineteen-year-old college student, lives in a coastal town in southern Italy and loves going to the beach. During her summer vacation and many of the late spring weekends, she spends four to six hours each day basking in the sun while talking with her friends or playing beach volleyball or swimming. She uses sunscreen lotion with a low sunscreen protection factor (SPF) and only at the beginning of the season to avoid sunburn. Once she is tanned, she may not use it at all. Most of her friends rarely use any sunscreen protection and, if they do, use the same kind with a low SPF. During the winter, Luciana keeps her tan by using artificial ultraviolet sunlamps.

In the summer, getting a nice *tintarella*, the Italian word for suntan, is one of Italians' favorite pastimes and is considered very attractive. People compliment each other on their *tintarella*. While Luciana and some of her friends may be somewhat aware that prolonged and continuous sun exposure is a risk factor for skin cancer, the aesthetic appeal and social approval of a tanned skin allay her doubts about sun exposure. She also feels she is too young to worry about skin cancer, does not know enough about it, and therefore does not feel the need to use much stronger sunscreen protection.

A review of the literature on the subject (for example, Monfrecola, Fabbrocini, Posteraro, and Pini, 2000) shows that Luciana's fictional profile is somewhat representative of frequent beliefs and behavior among a percentage of Italian young people who live on the Mediterranean coast.

According to the diffusion of innovations theory, Luciana could be considered an innovator or early adopter in her peer group if she starts using higher sunscreen protection and limiting her use of sunlamps. Ideally, she could talk with her peers and circle of friends about following her example. In fact, most of them do not use any sunscreen and may be slower to change than Luciana.

There are a few facts that are good indicators that she could become an innovator or early adopter: her education level (she is a college student), socioeconomic background (both of her parents hold advanced degrees and professional jobs and have raised Luciana to question existing behaviors in the light of new information), personality (she is rational, resourceful, and charming and often perceived as a leader in her peer group), exposure to media (she is well read and relies on a variety of media for information and entertainment), attitude toward change (she is willing to experiment with new things and behaviors if she understands them and perceives their benefits), and social involvement (she is an active member of several student organizations and other social and political groups).

If we look at the different stages of the diffusion of innovation theory (awareness, knowledge and interest, decision, trial or implementation, confirmation or rejection of the behavior), the first step is to make Luciana aware of skin cancer's severity, recent increase, and strong link to sun exposure and sunlamp use. Recent facts and incidence data should be used to reinforce her awareness and point to the need for sunscreen use.

If research shows that Luciana is already aware of the disease severity and related risk factors, communication messages and interactions should focus on making skin cancer relevant to her and her peers (the second stage of the diffusion theory). Knowledge that skin cancer can also occur among young people and the sun's damaging effects begin at an early age (National Cancer Institute, 2005b) may help increase Luciana's concern about sun exposure. Still, her perception that a tanned body is more attractive than an untanned one may prevent her from taking action and should be addressed early as part of the overall intervention. Focusing on the damaging effects of sun exposure on the skin's appearance and overall aging process may appeal to Luciana's aesthetic values.

Social support as well as the ability to sustain the recommended behavior should be encouraged by using adequate communication tools and activities while Luciana goes through the three remaining stages of the diffusion of innovation theory as she decides, tries, and, ideally, continues to use sunscreen and limit her use of sunlamps. In these stages, Luciana will need to perceive the advantages of behavioral change, find it acceptable for her lifestyle, and find it easy to implement and sustain. Sunscreen samples and detailed instructions on when to apply the sunscreen (not only to prevent skin burning) can facilitate use.

The program should also address her other concerns: the appeal of an untanned or lightly tanned body (Monfrecola, Fabbrocini, Posteraro, and Pini, 2000), which could be reinforced by celebrities, institutions, older family members, or others who could act as role models; and the reduced risk for a potentially life-threatening disease. Change would occur only if all tools and activities are designed by taking into account Luciana's needs and make her feel she is a key actor in the overall change process. If these needs are adequately met, Luciana may become an ambassador (innovator) for the importance of sunscreen use among her circle of friends, peers, and social groups. (An example on the topic of skin cancer is given in Weinreich, 1999.)

In approaching the rest of this chapter, readers may find it helpful to apply Luciana's fictional example or other examples to all theories and models that are discussed in this chapter. At a minimum, this would prompt awareness of different ways of organizing one's thoughts when dealing with the same health issue using different theoretical frameworks. It will also provide a tool to organize audience-related research.

Health Belief Model

The health belief model (HBM; Becker, Haefner, and Maiman, 1977; Janz and Becker, 1984; Strecher and Rosenstock, 1997) was originally intended to explain why people did not participate in programs that could help them diagnose or prevent diseases (National Cancer Institute and National Institutes of Health, 2002). The major assumption of this model is that in order to engage in healthy behaviors, intended audiences need to be aware of their risk for severe or life-threatening diseases and perceive that the benefits of behavior change outweigh potential barriers or other negative aspects of recommended actions. HBM is one of the first theories developed to explain the process of change in relation to health behavior. It has also inspired—among many other influences and models—the field of health education. Health education is defined as "any planned combination of learning experiences designed to predispose, enable, and reinforce voluntary behavior conducive to health in individuals, groups, or communities" (*Healthy People 2010,* p. 11-20; Green and Kreuter, 1999).

HBM has the following key components:

- *Perceived susceptibility:* The individual's perception on whether he or she is at risk for contracting a specific illness or health problem
- *Perceived severity:* The subjective feeling on whether the specific illness or health problem can be severe (for example, permanently impair physical or mental functions) or life threatening and therefore worthy of one's attention
- *Perceived benefits:* The individual's perceptions of the advantages of adopting recommended actions that would eventually reduce the risk for disease severity, morbidity, and mortality
- *Perceived barriers:* The individual's perceptions of the costs of and obstacles to adopting recommended actions (includes economic costs as well other kinds of lifestyle sacrifices)
- *Cues to action:* Public or social events that can signal the importance of taking action (for example, a neighbor who is diagnosed with the same disease or a mass media campaign)
- *Self-efficacy:* The individual's confidence in his or her ability to perform and sustain the recommended behavior with little or no help from others

In describing the HBM, Pechmann (2001) referred to it as a "risk learning model because the goal is to teach new information about health risks and the behaviors that minimize those risks" (p. 189). The overall premise of the HBM is that knowledge will bring change. Knowledge is brought to target audiences through an educational approach that primarily focuses on messages, channels, and spokespeople (Andreasen, 1995).

"Some authors caution that the HBM does not pre-suppose or imply a strategy for change" (Rosenstock and Kirscht, 1974, p. 472; Andreasen, 1995, p. 10). Nevertheless, the major contribution of the HBM to the health communication field is its emphasis on the importance of knowledge, a necessary but *not* sufficient step to change. HBM can also be used for audience-related research since it provides a useful framework to organize one's thoughts in developing an audience profile.

Social Cognitive Theory

Also known as social learning theory, social cognitive theory (SCT; Bandura, 1977, 1986, 1997) explains behavior as the result of three reciprocal factors: behavior, personal factors, and outside events. Any change in any of these three factors is expected to determine changes in the remaining ones (National Cancer Institute and National Institutes of Health, 2002). Behavior is viewed as influenced by a combination of personal and outside factors and events.

One of SCT's key premises is its emphasis on the outside environment, which becomes a source of observational learning. According to SCT, the environment is a place where individuals can observe an action, understand its consequences, and, as a result of personal and interpersonal influences, become motivated to repeat and adopt it. SCT has these key components (Bandura, 1977, 1986, 1997; National Cancer Institute and National Institutes of Health, 2002; Health Communication Partnership, 2005c):

- *Attention*—people's awareness of the action being modeled and observed.
- *Retention*—people's ability to remember the action being modeled and observed.
- *Reproduction (Trial)*—people's ability to reproduce the action being modeled and observed.
- *Motivation*—people's internal impulse and intention to perform the action. Motivation depends on a number of social, affective, and physiological influences (for example, the support of peers and family members to perform the action, the knowledge that the action will improve physical performance) as well as the perception of self-efficacy.
- *Performance*—the individual's ability to perform the action on a regular basis.
- *Self-efficacy*—the individual's confidence in his or her ability to perform and sustain the action with little or no help from others, which plays a major role in actual performance.

SCT can provide a framework to approach several different questions in program research and planning, but its major contribution to health communications is to understand the mechanisms and factors that can influence retention, reproduction, and motivation (Health Communication Partnership, 2005c) on a given behavior.

Theory of Reasoned Action

The theory of reasoned action (TRA; Ajzen and Fishbein, 1980) suggests that behavioral performance is primarily determined by the strength of the person's intention to perform a specific behavior. It identifies two major factors that contribute to such intentions (Ajzen and Fishbein, 1980; Health Communication Partnership, 2005d; Coffman, 2002):

- A person's attitude toward the behavior. In general, attitudes can be defined as positive or negative emotions or feelings toward a behavior, a person, a concept, or an idea (for example: "I . . . eating fruit and vegetables"; "I . . . my friend's boyfriend").
- A person's subjective norms about the behavior. In the TRA, subjective norms are defined as the opinion or judgment, positive or negative, that loved ones, friends, family, colleagues, professional organizations, or other key influentials may have about a potential behavior (for example, "My friends do not approve that I smoke marijuana"; "My doctor recommends that I exercise at least twice per week").

Under the TRA, attitudes toward a specific behavior are a function of the person's beliefs about the consequences of such behavior (for example, "smoking marijuana may have a negative impact on my concentration and work performance"). These are called *behavioral beliefs*.

Subjective norms are influenced by *normative beliefs*, which refer to whether a person may think significant others will approve or not of his or her behavior (for example, "I think that if I start to smoke marijuana, some of my friends may not approve of it"). Another component of normative beliefs is the person's motivation to comply with other people's ideas and potential approval (Coffman, 2002). For example, if the normative belief is the one above ("I think that if I start to smoke marijuana, some of my friends may not approve it"), the person's motivation to comply can be assessed by asking the following question: "Do I care enough about these specific friends to avoid smoking marijuana?"

TRA is currently one of the most influential theories in health communication and is frequently used also in program evaluation (Coffman, 2002). However, it is important to maintain some caution in concluding that the intention of adopting a certain behavior always translates in actual behavioral performance. Communication can play an important role in supporting behavioral intentions and increasing the likelihood that they would become actual behaviors. This requires the development of adequate tools that would facilitate and make it easy for people to try, adopt, and integrate new health behaviors in their lifestyle.

TRA is particularly useful in analyzing and identifying reasons for action and messages that can change people's attitudes. It is also a good tool in profiling **primary audiences** (the people whom the program seeks to influence more directly and would primarily benefit from change) and **secondary audiences** (individuals and groups who can have an influence on the primary audience) (Health Communication Partnership, 2005d).

Ideation

The ideation theory (Kincaid, Figueroa, Storey, and Underwood, 2001; Rimon, 2002; Cleland and Wilson, 1987) refers to "new ways of thinking and diffusion of those ways of thinking by means of social interaction in local, culturally homogenous communities" (O'-Sullivan, Yonkler, Morgan, and Merritt 2003, pp. 1–3; Bongaarts and Watkins, 1996). This theory is used in strategic behavior communications to identify and influence ideational elements (Rimon, 2002; Kincaid, Figueroa, Storey, and Underwood, 2001), such as attitudes, knowledge, self-efficacy, social and peer approval, and other factors that can affect and determine health behavior (see Figure 2.2).

One of the key premises of the ideation theory is "that the more ideational elements that apply to someone, the greater the probability that they will adopt a healthy behavior" (Kincaid and Figueroa, 2004).

Convergence Theory

Like other theories in the social process category (O'Sullivan, Yonkler, Morgan, and Merritt, 2003), the convergence theory (Kincaid, 1979; Rogers and Kincaid, 1981) emphasizes the importance "of information sharing, mutual understanding and mutual agreement" on any collective or group action that would bring social change (Figueroa, Kincaid, Rani, and Lewis, 2002, p. 4). It is based on the perspective that an individual's perceptions and behavior are influenced by the perceptions and behaviors of members of the same group, such as members of professional associations,

FIGURE 2.2. IDEATION THEORY

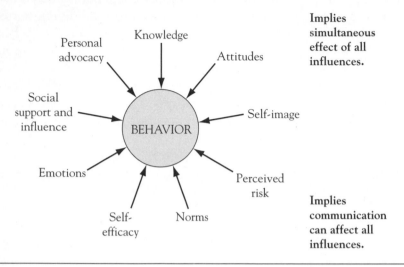

Sources: Kincaid, D. L., and Figueroa, M. E. *Ideation and Communication for Social Change.* Health Communication Partnership Seminar, April 23, 2004. Used by permission. Rimon, J. G. *Behaviour Change Communication in Public Health. Beyond Dialogue: Moving Toward Convergence.* The Communication Initiative, 2002. http://www.comminit.com/strategicthinking/stnicroundtable/sld-1744.html. Retrieved Nov. 2005. Used by permission.

work colleagues, and family members, and by people "in one's personal networks," such as peers, friends, or personal or professional acquaintances (O'Sullivan, Yonkler, Morgan, and Merritt, 2003, pp. 1–4).

This theory is characterized by three distinctive features (Kincaid, 1979; Rogers and Kincaid, 1981; Figueroa, Kincaid, Rani, and Lewis, 2002):

• Information is shared using a participatory process in which there is no sender or receiver but everyone creates and shares information. Participants in this process include individuals or groups and institutions such as professional associations, community organizations, churches, and schools.
• Communication emphasizes individual perceptions and interpretations of the information being shared, encourages an ongoing dialogue, and fosters mutual understanding and agreement on common meanings.

- Communication is horizontal and involves two or more participants. In a horizontal model of communication, all participants
are equal and aim to reach mutual agreement that may stimulate a group action.

This theory has contributed to redefining communication as a
process in which all participants need to respect and take into account other people's feelings, emotions, and beliefs. It has also
highlighted the importance of social networks and key influentials
in defining the path to social change.

Stages of Behavior Change Model
The stages of behavior change model, also known as transtheoretical model (Prochaska and DiClemente, 1983; Grimley, Gabrielle,
Bellis, and Prochaska, 1993; Prochaska and Vellicer, 1997), defines
behavioral change as a process that goes through different stages
or steps. Each stage describes different "levels of motivation or
readiness to change" (National Cancer Institute and National Institutes of Health, 2002, p. 221; Prochaska and Vellicer, 1997). The
model identifies five stages of change (Prochaska and Vellicer,
1997; Weinreich, 1999):

1. Precontemplation, in which individuals have no intention of
adopting a recommended health behavior but are learning
about it
2. Contemplation, in which individuals are considering adopting
the recommended behavior
3. Decision, in which people decide to adopt the recommended
health behavior
4. Action, in which people try to adopt the recommend behavior
for a short period of time
5. Maintenance, in which people continue to perform the recommended health behavior for a long period of time (at least
above six months) and, ideally, incorporate it in their routine
and lifestyle

In health communication, these stages of change can be used
in the segmentation phase of intended audiences (see Chapter
Ten) to identify groups that, among other related characteristics,
will also have similar levels of motivation and readiness for behavioral change (Weinrich, 1999). Therefore, this theory can be

instrumental in designing communication objectives, messages, and strategies for each of these groups (National Cancer Institute and National Institutes of Health, 2002).

Communication for Persuasion Theory

This theory was developed by social psychologist William McGuire and focuses on how people process information. McGuire (1984) highlighted twelve interdependable steps in the process of persuasive communications (McGuire, 1984; National Cancer Institute and National Institutes of Health, 2002; Alcalay and Bell, 2000). He suggested that in order to assimilate and perform a new behavior, a person should (McGuire, 1984; National Cancer Institute and National Institutes of Health, 2002):

1. Be exposed to the message.
2. Pay attention to it.
3. Find it interesting or personally relevant.
4. Understand it.
5. Figure out how the new behavior could fit in his or her life.
6. Accept the change that is being proposed.
7. Remember and validate the message.
8. Be able to think of the message in relevant contexts or situations.
9. Make decisions on the basis of the retrieved information or message.
10. Behave in line with that decision.
11. Receive positive reinforcement for that behavior.
12. Integrate the new behavior into his or her life.

This model also suggests that these twelve steps are interdependent. Achieving any of them is strictly contingent on success at all prior steps. Message design, messenger credibility, communication channels, and the characteristics of both the intended audiences and the recommended behavior, which should be intended to fit easily in people's lives, all influence behavioral outcomes.

While the current focus of health communication is more on engaging intended audiences than persuading them, keeping in mind McGuire's steps for persuasion can provide a valid framework for approaching key audiences and stakeholders to secure their initial involvement and input in the health issue. In doing so, it is also important to remember that an audience's characteristics and needs may change over time. This should prompt communicators to incorporate these changes in message design and delivery as well as redefine recommended behaviors in function of people's lifestyles and needs.

MASS COMMUNICATION THEORIES

No one can dispute the ability of the mass media to reach significant percentages of interested groups and audiences. If adequately used and selected in response to audience's needs and preferences, radio, television, printed media, and the Internet are powerful connectors between communicators and their audiences.

Mass communication theories include research and studies that focus on the impact of the mass media on target populations. However, many of their key principles and observations can apply in general to the overall field of global health communication. The following definitions are important when looking at this family of theories and can help improve understanding of the overall topic:

- *Media effects* are simply the consequences [on target audiences] of what the mass media do, whether intended or not.
- *Media power,* on the other hand, refers to a general potential on the part of the media to have effects, especially of a planned kind.
- *Media effectiveness* is a statement about the efficiency of media in achieving a given aim and always implies intention or some planned communication goal [McQuail, 1994, p. 333].

While several authors divide mass communication theories into different eras and subgroups (McQuail, 1994; Health Communication Partnership, 2005a), a comprehensive discussion of all of them is beyond the scope of this book. Therefore, the theory presented next represents only an example of models and studies in this category.

Cultivation Theory of Mass Media

Developed by George Gerbner, the cultivation theory "specifies that repeated, intense exposure to deviant definitions of 'reality' in the mass media leads to perceptions of the 'reality' as normal"

(Communication Initiative, 2003a; Gerbner, 1969; Gerbner, Gross, Morgan, and Signorielle, 1980). "The result is a social legitimization of the reality depicted in the mass media, which can influence behavior" (Communication Initiative, 2003a; Gerbner, Gross, Morgan, and Signorielle, 1980). In other words, the media have the power to portray a behavior and make it socially acceptable by shaping public perceptions and feelings toward that behavior. *Cultivation* refers to the ability of the mass media to produce long-term effects on target audiences by nurturing their feelings through continuous message exposure. This process also relies on the ability of the mass media to "transcend traditional barriers of time, space and social grouping" (Communication Initiative, 2003a; Gerbner, 1969).

Cultivation is a concept that transcends the mass media and applies to the overall field of health communication. In fact, nurturing the feelings of key stakeholders and interested audiences through continuous message exposure, using all kinds of communication channels including the mass media, is a practice that frequently helps secure their involvement in the health issue and its solutions.

MARKETING-BASED MODELS

In the private (commercial and nonprofit) sector, the field of marketing refers to strategic activities that encourage the use of products or services by consumers or special groups. Over time, marketing-based models have also inspired public health interventions that aim at the endorsement of new health products, services, or behaviors. The two models that are presented next have many similar features and contribute to the theoretical basis of health communication.

Social Marketing

Social marketing has been defined as "the application of commercial marketing technologies to the analysis, planning, execution, and evaluation of programs designed to influence the voluntary behavior of target audiences in order to improve their personal welfare and that of their society" (Andreasen, 1995, p. 7). Similar to commercial marketing, behavior change is the ultimate goal of social marketing. However, in commercial marketing, behavior change is sought primarily to benefit the sponsoring organizations (Andreasen, 1995), even if, in some cases, marketing activities also encourage the adoption of healthy behaviors, such as immunization or compliance to medication, that can improve the health conditions of target populations.

Social marketing practices are consumer centered (Andreasen, 1995; Kotler and Roberto, 1989) and stress the importance of four elements, referred to as the four Ps of social marketing:

- *Product*—the behavior, service, product, or policy that the organization or program seeks to see adopted by target audiences. In social marketing, products can be tangible (for example, condoms or mosquito nets being sold and distributed as part of a social marketing campaign) or intangible (for example, the behavior being recommended and adopted by target audiences).
- *Price*—the price of the product that is being promoted or the emotional, physical, community, or social cost of adopting the new behavior, policy, or practice.
- *Place*—the product distribution channels (for example, point-of-service locations, wholesale distributors) or the place where it is most appropriate to expose target audiences to communication messages and tools to facilitate the adoption of the new behavior.
- *Promotion*—how a message is conveyed. It thus refers to how to motivate intended audiences so they try and perform the recommended behavior or adopt a new policy or practice.

Social marketing is also considered a planning framework to be used with other theories and models in health communication planning (National Cancer Institute and National Institutes of Health, 2002). Additional theoretical constructs should closely fit the specific health issue and its potential solutions and, most important, sustain community participation and involvement (Waisbord, 2001).

Critics of social marketing view this approach as a top-down model that does not allow the level of community participation required for effective change, especially in the case of developing countries: "For them, social marketing is a non-participatory strategy because it treats most people as consumers rather than protagonists" (Waisbord, 2001, p. 9).

Social marketing major's contribution to the health communication field is a systematic audience-centered and market-driven approach to program research. Social marketing techniques and tools are particularly helpful in developing audience profiles, situation and marketing analysis, and defining the health problem and potential solutions. Even when these analyses occur in a participatory context, which involves members of intended audiences and should be always encouraged, many research tools and techniques are imported from social marketing and marketing practices (see Chapter Ten).

Another contribution is related to the importance of cost-effectiveness and competitive analyses. The social marketing approach to competition encourages the analysis and understanding of all alternatives, such as alternative behaviors or programs or products, that people may have (Andreasen, 1995). This helps develop a desirable "product" that is likely to be adopted and to fit people's lifestyle, beliefs, and needs. However, in health communication, "products" are always intangible and should coincide with behavioral or social outcomes (for example, changes in immunization or AIDS prevention practices or policies).

Finally, social marketing strategies have been shown to be helpful in raising disease and risk awareness (see the example in Box 2.2). In public health, other models and techniques should complement the social marketing framework in order to encourage program sustainability as well as a long-lasting community involvement and the building of local capacity (Waisbord, 2001).

Box 2.2

Raising Awareness of Infant Mortality Disparities in San Francisco

In San Francisco, African American infants suffer a mortality rate 2 to 3 times higher than white infants. In an attempt to address this disparity, the San Francisco Public Health Department (SFDPH) partnered with community based organizations and the Family Health Outcomes Project at the University of California, San Francisco, and, with funding from the Centers for Disease Control REACH 2010 initiative, created the Seven Principles Project. The project included a social marketing campaign aimed at (1) raising awareness of the gap in infant mortality rates among African Americans who live in San Francisco; (2) increasing knowledge of specific practices and risk factors that have been associated with higher incidence of sudden infant death syndrome (SIDS); and (3) encouraging families to take action.

Methods

Working together with African American residents and using focus groups to secure program feedback, the Seven Principles Project developed three multi-media campaigns. The three campaigns all used the same media to disseminate information. These included advertorials on buses and at bus stops in the neighborhoods where the majority of African Americans reside, posters, cards, brochures, handouts, church fans, and radio public service announcements on radio stations that are popular with the African American community. Main messages included: (1) Black babies die at twice the rate of all babies in San Francisco; (2) To reduce the chance of SIDS, babies sleep best on their backs: and (3) STOP Black Babies from dying—take action. The campaign also provided a telephone number that people could call to get involved with the project.

The campaign's main concepts and activities were based on research findings on knowledge, attitudes and beliefs about infant mortality and SIDS among African Americans. Prior to the design of the Seven Principles Project, the SFDPH conducted several focus groups to assess existing awareness levels and to help develop effective intervention strategies. Focus groups included 250 African American community members. Focus group findings revealed that prior to the campaign, over half of the participants did not know about any disparity in infant mortality in San Francisco. In addition, a baseline telephone survey of 804 African Americans ages 18–64 showed that only 39.6% knew about the disparity. Moreover, 28.5% of survey respondents were not aware that placing an infant on its back to sleep may reduce the risk of SIDS. Since the disparity in infant mortality rates has persisted for years, clearly this message had not been effectively communicated to the African American community. Project Seven Principles aimed at addressing this information gap.

Results

A follow-up telephone survey conducted with 654 African Americans indicated substantial community exposure to the awareness campaign. . . . It also revealed a statistically significant increase in awareness about the existing disparity in infant mortality when compared to the data collected prior to the campaign (62.7% of respondents who participated in the post-survey were aware of the disparity versus only 39.6% of respondents in the pre-campaign survey). While there was no overall significant increase (70.4% vs. 71.7%) in knowledge about proper sleep positions to prevent SIDS, respondents who reported any exposure to this campaign were more likely to know about proper sleep positions (79.7% vs. 64.3%).

Source: Rienks, J., Smyly, V., Oliva, G., Mack Burch, L., and Belfiori, J. "Evidence That Social Marketing Campaigns Can Effectively Increase Awareness of Infant Mortality Disparities." Paper presented at the Annual Meeting of the American Public Health Association, Philadelphia, Dec. 13, 2005. Used by permission.

Integrated Marketing Communications

Integrated marketing communications (IMC) is a strategic approach used in the private sector to develop, implement, and evaluate brand communication programs. It takes into account and addresses the consumer's perspective, needs, beliefs, and perceptions and relies on the strategic integration of measurable objectives and approaches (Schultz and Schultz, 2003; Nowak and others, 1998). It is considered an avant-garde marketing approach, has been incorporated in several academic programs, and forms part of the curricula of many departments (New York University, 2006; University of Utah, 2006; Emerson College, 2006). IMC principles are also reflected in some models for strategic behavior communications.

IMC recognizes that the flow and volume of information is constantly increasing for most audiences around the world (Schultz, Tannerbaum, and Lauterborn, 1994; Renganathan and others, 2005). Therefore, message clarity and consistency, as well as "an integrated and coordinated approach with credibility is vital" (Renganathan and others, 2005, p. 310). The most important contribution of IMC to health communication is its emphasis on the significance of a multifaceted and strategic approach based on the intended audiences' point of view and addressing their key needs.

Select Models for Strategic Behavior and Social Change Communication

Several models incorporate or combine behavioral, social, or marketing theories described in this chapter. Select examples of these models and planning frameworks are described next.

Communication for Behavioral Impact

Communication for behavioral impact (COMBI) is an integrated communication approach developed and implemented by the World Health Organization (2003) in collaboration with many partners around the world. Although COMBI has been applied primarily in the health care field, its key principles and methodologies may be relevant to other areas. For example, COMBI has been used as part of UNICEF's programs on child protection and juvenile justice in Moldovia (E. Hosein, personal communications with the author, 2005, 2006).

With its emphasis on behavioral impact, COMBI is a model for strategic behavior communications. It is a research-based, participatory approach that seeks to identify and address behavioral issues that may have an impact on health outcomes (Renganathan and others, 2005; E. Hosein, personal communications with the author, 2005, 2006).

COMBI is based on two fundamental principles. "First: Do nothing—produce no T-shirt, no posters, no leaflets, no videos, until you have set out clear, precise, specific behavioral objectives. Second: Do nothing—produce no T-shirts, no posters, no leaflets, no videos, until you have successfully undertaken a situational 'market' analysis in relation to preliminary behavioral objectives" (Renganathan and others, 2005). The situational market analysis calls for taking the recommended behavior back into the community and listening to its members to identify the "communication keys" to help secure their involvement (E. Hosein, personal communication with the author, 2005, 2006). According to COMBI principles, an example of behavioral objectives is: "Prompt X number of people to swallow 4–6 tablets a day at home in the presence of Filaria Prevention Assistant (or go to the distribution point) on Filaria Day" (Renganathan and others, 2005). Evaluation of

COMBI programs is specific to the achievement of the behavioral objectives specified early in program planning.

COMBI focuses on addressing specific diseases and related health behaviors, but it also may have an impact on social change. For example, the initial focus of COMBI has been primarily on communicable diseases that have been jeopardizing the socioeconomic development of entire communities and countries, especially in the developing world (World Health Organization, 2003; Renganathan and others, 2005). With this in mind, COMBI's contribution to development and social change is its potential to "remove a significant obstacle that keeps people in poverty" (Renganathan and others, 2005, p. 318), as well as to reduce the mortality rates of diseases that affect entire families and communities. It also contributes to strengthen people's health literacy and disease-related self-reliance.

As with most other kinds of interventions and models, COMBI alone is not sufficient to address development issues (Renganathan and others, 2005) and public health deficiencies. Yet it can help make a difference. Addressing broader social issues such as health disparities, poverty, and injustice, all factors contributing to poor health, requires many different kinds of public health strategies and interventions, which should all rely on long-term commitment, a step-by-step approach, people's participation, and a series of behavioral changes at the policymaker, stakeholder, funding agency, population, community, and individual levels. COMBI operates within this larger context as an approach to minimize the burden of disease and strengthen health services. In doing so, it supports one of the fundamental goals of public health.

COMBI integrates principles and methodologies from multiple disciplines, including marketing, mass communications, information-education-communication, social mobilization, anthropology, and sociology. It models its integrated approach on recent developments and lessons learned from IMC, which is widely used in the private and commercial sectors. As in IMC, COMBI uses a strategic blend of activities, channels, and audience-specific messages to address people's perceptions, attitudes, and behaviors (World Health Organization, 2003; Renganathan and others, 2005).

COMBI takes into account key IMC learnings, including the influence of people's perceptions—in other words, what people "believe to be important or true" (Renganathan and others, 2005, p. 309)—have on attitudes and behaviors. It also stresses the importance of clear, credible, and consistent communication messages in reference to the healthy behaviors, products, or services that people are asked to endorse and use (World Health Organization, 2003; Renganathan and others, 2005).

PRECEDE-PROCEED MODEL

Designed by Lawrence Green and Marshall Kreuter (Green and Kreuter, 1991, 1999; Green and Ottoson, 1999), the precede-proceed model "is an approach to planning that analyzes the factors contributing to behavior change" (National Cancer Institute and National Institutes of Health, 2002, p. 219). The model is based on the principle that long-lasting change always occurs voluntarily (Communication Initiative, 2003b; National Cancer Institute, 2005a) and is determined by the individual motivation to become directly involved with the process of change. Individuals need to feel empowered to change their quality of life (National Cancer Institute, 2005a) and in doing so are influenced by their community and social structure.

The key factors influencing behavior change are divided in three categories:

- *Predisposing factors*—the individual's knowledge, attitudes, behavior, beliefs, and values before intervention that affect willingness to change
- *Enabling factors*—factors in the environment or community of an individual that facilitate or present obstacles to change
- *Reinforcing factors*—the positive or negative effects of adopting the behavior (including social support) that influence continuing the behavior [National Cancer Institute and National Institutes of Health, 2002, p. 219].

This model fits well with current thinking and reinforces the importance of considering the individual as part of the social environment. It also supports the notion of individual empowerment and capacity building at both the individual and community levels, one of the most important components of sustainable behavior and social change.

COMMUNICATION FOR SOCIAL CHANGE

Communication for social change (CFSC) is a participatory model for communication planning, implementation, and evaluation. It was developed with the original input and sponsorship of the Rockefeller Foundation, which in 1997 convened a conference to explore the connection between communication and social change. The actual model was developed on the basis of the recommendations from all participants at this initial conference as well as follow-up meetings (Figueroa, Kincaid, Rani, and Lewis, 2002).

CFSC is defined as "a process of public and private dialogue through which people define who they are, what they want and how they can get it" (Gray-Felder and Dean, 1999, p. 15). It is an integrated model that describes an "iterative process" to community dialogue that "starts with a catalyst/stimulus that can be external or internal to the community," and "when effective, leads to collective action and the resolution of a common problem" (Figueroa, Kincaid, Rani, and Lewis, 2002, p. iii).

In this model, outcome indicators of social change include "leadership, degree and equity of participation, information equity, collective self-efficacy, sense of ownership, and social cohesion" (Figueroa, Kincaid, Rani, and Lewis, 2002 p. iv). Although the model is evolving, it is important to recognize that social change (for example, less poverty, less HIV/AIDS) can take a long time and demands intermediate evaluation parameters to assess progress (Rockefeller Foundation Communication and Social Change Network, 2001).

Social change is always the result of a series of gradual behavioral changes at the individual, group, and community level. Therefore, behavioral outcomes should remain an important evaluation parameter in health communication even in the context of social change models.

OTHER THEORETICAL INFLUENCES AND PLANNING FRAMEWORKS

Several other models and planning frameworks influence the theory and practice of health communication. A few examples, including medical models and logic models, are discussed next.

MEDICAL MODELS

Communication is also influenced by general beliefs about the intrinsic causes of health and illness. Over time, two medical models have been influencing communication in the provider-patient setting and in relation to how health organizations and professionals perceive what kinds of topics and factors should be addressed as part of a public health intervention.

The first of the two models, the biomedical model, has been around for many centuries and is based on the assumption that poor health is a physical phenomenon that "can be explained, identified, and treated with physical means" (du Pré, 2000, p. 8; Twaddle and Hessler, 1987). Therefore, the biomedical model does not take into account the person's psychological conditions, individual and social beliefs, attitudes and norms, or other factors that can affect health and illness. As a result, communication efforts that are based on this model tend to be informative, strictly scientific, doctrinarian, authoritarian, "efficient" and "focused" (du Pré, 2000, p. 9). Communication relies on a top-down approach in which medical providers or health organizations limit their efforts to transferring their knowledge on the medical and scientific causes of an illness and to prescribing a solution.

This approach lacks empathy with the patient or target audience's feelings and social experiences (Friedman and DiMatteo, 1979; Laine and Davidoff, 1996; du Pré, 2000). Moreover, it does not take into account current knowledge that most diseases and their prognoses are heavily influenced by social and cultural habits, as well as the individual's psychological status. For example, health conditions such as obesity, diabetes, and depression are clearly influenced by external factors, which can include lifestyle issues, emotional stress, and cultural beliefs and preferences. Finally, disease prevention is not considered under this model since its practice is closely related to the ability of health professionals and organizations to engage interested individuals and communities in the act of prioritizing a recommended behavior by reaching out to their core beliefs, feelings, and needs.

The second model, the biopsychosocial model, is based on the premise that poor health is not only a physical phenomenon but "is also influenced by people's feelings, their ideas about health, and the events of their lives" (du Pré, 2000, p. 9; Engel, 1977).

Given the recent emphasis on a patient-centered approach to health, the biopsychosocial model has been gradually substituted for the biomedical model. Many professional societies and institutions, including the American Medical Association, American Academy of Family Physicians, and several hospitals and universities, have guidelines and courses on provider-patient communications that highlight the importance of relating to patients' feelings, literacy levels, needs, and other key factors that can improve patient compliance and outcomes. More broadly, the model also fits well with many of the current practices and theories in health communication, including most of the theoretical constructs discussed in this chapter. Under this model, communication tends to be empathetic, sensible to the audience's needs and feelings, aimed at generating understanding of scientific and medical issues, motivational, and truly interdependent.

LOGIC MODELING

Logic modeling is a flexible framework (Morzinski and Montagnini, 2002) that has been used for program planning and evaluation in the fields of education (Harvard Family Research Project, 2005), public-private partnerships (Watson, 2000), health education (University of Wisconsin, Extension Program Development, 2005), and many other programmatic areas. In general, it is a one-page summary of the program's key components, the rationale used in defining program strategies, objectives and key activities, and expected program outcomes and measurement parameters that will be used in evaluating them (Harvard Family Research Project, 2005). In sum, logic models are used to explain the relationship about all program components and related outcomes.

More recently, logic models have been considered a helpful tool in the planning and evaluation of public communication campaigns (Coffman, 2002) and other communication interventions. They are tools for organizing one's thoughts in considering all programmatic options as well as to provide key stakeholders, partners, and team members with a quick snapshot of a specific program and its rationale. Logic models can be constructed using different theories and assumptions (Harvard Family Research Project, 2005), so they fit the health issues and the needs of the audiences under consideration.

The first step in logic modeling is analyzing the situation and the environment in which the program would occur (Morzinski and Montagnini, 2002). This planning and evaluation framework encompasses the following categories (University of Wisconsin, Extension Program Development, 2005):

- An overview of all human and economic resources used for the program
- A list of all audience-centered activities, services, events, or products
- An outcome analysis, including all results and changes at the individual, community, and organizational levels
- Overall program assumptions, that is, the beliefs that guide and inform program planning
- All external factors that may influence the health issue and its potential solutions

Appendix A provides online resources on the development of logic models for health communication planning.

CURRENT ISSUES AND TOPICS IN HEALTH CARE: IMPLICATIONS FOR HEALTH COMMUNICATION

In addition to theories and models, a number of issues influence the practice of health communication. Many of them are specific to a certain country, environment, political situation, health issue, or population, among others. Because of the large variety and number of such issues, a comprehensive discussion of all of them is beyond the reach of this book. Therefore, the topics explored next are just examples of some of the issues that are currently influencing health communication practice.

HEALTH DISPARITIES

The concept of health equity has rightly emerged worldwide as a primary guiding principle for the work of most organizations that operate in the health care field. Health equity addresses the importance of eliminating health disparities by minimizing or removing differences in the well-being and health status of diverse populations and groups. As Dr. Martin Luther King Jr. is often quoted to have said, "Of all forms of inequality, injustice in health is the most shocking and the most inhuman" (Randall, 2006).

"The United States National Institutes of Health (NIH) defines health disparities as the 'differences in the incidence, prevalence, mortality, and burden of diseases and other adverse health conditions that exist among specific population groups in the United States'" (Center for Health Equity Research and Promotion, 2005). In practice, most health disparities refer to differences in quality of health care received as well as overall access to health services and products among different populations or subgroups of the same population. These differences may result in unfavorable patient outcomes or reduced life expectancy in underserved or minority populations.

Income, education, socioeconomic conditions, literacy levels, ethnicity, geographical location, race, health care provider understanding (or the lack of) of cultural differences, and language barriers are some of the underlying factors that can influence health equity or create health disparities. Some health disparities are also related to "genetic and biological differences among ethnic groups or between men and women" (Center for Health Equity Research and Promotion, 2005).

Health communication can contribute to reducing or eliminating health disparities by addressing the above factors through audience-specific campaigns and programs. *Cultural competence,* which can be defined as the ability to relate to the unique characteristics of each population or ethnic group and to address them in an efficient way, is an important prerequirement for strategic programming. If used as part of larger public health interventions, culturally competent health communication strategies can affect change at the individual, community, organizational, and policy levels (Freimuth and Quinn, 2004).

PATIENT EMPOWERMENT

Patient empowerment is an important concept in modern medicine and one of the central pillars of health communication strategies. However, definitions and the expectations this term may generate vary by health settings, contexts, and environments. For example, the term can refer to patient awareness about a disease and its treatment, which allows patients to engage in informed discussions with their health care providers and therefore participate in treatment and prevention decisions. It can imply the patient's ability to feel competent to adhere to recommended treatment or prevention measures or to engage in behaviors that may improve health outcomes. And it can include the patient's involvement in the public debate about policies, health care regulations, medical practices, research funding, and social change.

Partnering for Patient Empowerment Through Community Awareness (2005) and the Standing Committee of European Doctors (2004) are two of the organizations that are focusing on expanding consumer awareness about diseases and health resources or improving patient-provider communications. Others have effectively mobilized and engaged patient groups in the process of policy and social change. AIDS and other life-threatening conditions have taught patients around the world important lessons. Over time, AIDS activists have had a tremendous impact on drug approval regulations, research funding, policies, and access to AIDS drugs, as well as public perception of AIDS, just to name a few topics.

Because of the variety and levels of patient involvement, it is important to refrain from using the term *patient empowerment* in a general way. When a planned health communication intervention is targeted to patients or the general public, consideration should be given to what patients should ideally be able to do and what kind of empowerment is expected from them.

LIMITS OF PREVENTIVE MEDICINE AND HABITS

Despite the medical and scientific advances of the past few centuries, preventive medicine cannot eliminate disease. However, preventive medicine and habits have contributed to extending life expectancy and improving the overall quality of life of many populations and groups.

Still, preventive medicine does not work all the time. This concept may be troublesome for some people and therefore should be considered in designing health communication interventions. Consider the example of Eduardo, a fifty-year-old low- to middle-class

Puerto Rican man who smokes and is being pressured by his family to quit because of the risk of oral cancer. They also want him to have regular checkups with his doctor and break his habit of seeking medical help only when he is seriously ill. The family has been alarmed by the recent death of a close cousin who was a heavy smoker and developed oral cancer. However, Eduardo has a very good friend who never smoked in his life and still developed oral cancer. He makes several arguments against his family's request to change his health-seeking habits:

- Quitting smoking will not guarantee that he will not get cancer.
- He enjoys smoking and drinking alcohol.
- Why is his family worried about oral cancer? What happened to their cousin is a rare event.
- He is too busy for regular checkups with his doctor.

Eduardo is right about the limits of preventive medicine and habits. However, there are a few facts that may help him see his family's point of view if discussed as part of a comprehensive and culturally competent health communication intervention:

- Oral cancer incidence is two times higher among men in Puerto Rico than among mainland U.S. Hispanics (Hayes and others, 1999) and higher than that observed in white males living on the mainland United States (Parkin and others, 1997).
- Together with alcohol consumption, tobacco use is a primary risk factor for oral cancer (Blot and others, 1988). Actually, their joint effect appears to be more than additive, if not multiplicative. The risk for oral and pharyngeal cancers is between six and fifteen times greater for smokers who are also heavy drinkers compared to individuals who neither smoke nor drink (Mashberg and Samit, 1995).
- Smoking cessation is a standard preventive measure against the risk for oral cancer (Matiella, 1991; U.S. Department of Health and Human Services, 1986, 1994).

Of course, many other issues need to be considered and addressed in order to convince Eduardo to quit smoking—for example, his social context, the potential difficulty of succeeding in quitting smoking, and the priority assigned by his health care provider to oral cancer screening. Still, it is important to remember that most people are not aware of disease risk factors and other relevant information.

Incorporating disease statistics and information in health communication interventions legitimizes the quest for behavior and social change. It also helps attract people's attention by positioning the health issue in a larger context than the family and circle of friends in which they live. Finally, it may help them accept the limits of preventive medicine and behavior by showcasing whenever possible the high percentage of cases in which disease can be prevented.

Prevention does not work in all cases, but it still works in most cases.

THE EMERGENCE OF E-HEALTH

The Internet and related technologies have significantly extended "the scope of health care beyond its traditional boundaries" (Eysenbach, 2001, p. e20) and consequently affected the practice of health communication. Increasingly, patients, health care professionals, the general public, and the overall health care community rely on the Internet for a variety of services and communications, which include advice on health issues, virtual pharmacies, distance learning for practitioners, medical or public health information systems (for example, disease surveillance systems), and health records, to name a few applications (Gantenbein, 2001; Eysenbach, 2001).

E-health has emerged as "a field in the intersection of medical informatics, public health and business, referring to health services and information delivered or enhanced through the Internet and related technologies" (Eysenbach, 2001, p. e20). In health communication, the increasing reliance on the Internet by consumers and professionals has opened the way to the use of interactive health communication tools (for example, Web sites, Internet-based games, online press rooms, disease symptoms simulations, opinion polls, seminars), which are often designed as part of larger health communication interventions. It has also prompted several initiatives and research studies that attempt to analyze the impact of the Internet on health beliefs, behaviors, outcomes, and policies, as well as health-related encounters and communications such as patient-provider interactions. Finally, it has raised questions about the accuracy of sources of information on the Internet, as well as the importance of understanding the implications of Internet use in relation to issues of patient privacy and equal access to information by those who may not have the resources or skills to take advantage of new technologies (Eysenbach, 2001; Cline and Haynes, 2001). Some of these topics as well as the use of the Internet and its implications in health communication are briefly discussed throughout relevant chapters of this book in relation to different health communication areas and planning phases.

Interactive health communication has been defined as the "interaction of an individual—consumer, patient, caregiver or professional—with or through an electronic device or communication technology to access or transmit health information or to receive guidance and support on a health-related issue" (Robinson, Patrick, Eng, and Gustafson, 1998, p. 1264). Several other disciplines influence or contribute to interactive health communication (Gantenbein, 2001). These include areas of public health informatics, defined as "the systematic application of information and computer science and technology to public health practice, research and learning" (U.S. Department of Health and Human Services, 2005, p. 23–23); medical informatics, "the field that concerns itself with the cognitive, information processing, and communication tasks of medical practice, education and research" (Greenes and Shortliffe, 1990, p. 1114); and consumer health informatics, "the branch of medical informatics that analyzes consumers' needs for information; studies and implements methods of making information accessible to consumers; and models and integrates consumers' preferences into medical information systems" (Eysenbach, 2000, p. 1713).

In addition to extending the outreach of health communication programs, the rising use of the Internet and other new technologies provides health communication practitioners with an opportunity to contribute to public awareness and policy efforts that can expand access to this new channel for health information as well as limit the potential harm to individual and public health that may derive from inaccurate Internet-based sources.

LOW HEALTH LITERACY

"Low health literacy is the inability to read, understand and act on health information" (Zagaria, 2004, p. 41). It is one of the most important issues in health communication. No matter how accurate, compelling, or graphically appealing information appears to be, the overall purpose of any materials or verbal communication is defeated if people cannot understand it.

Low health literacy affects all different age groups and ethnic backgrounds. "Nearly half of all American adults—90 million people—have difficulty understanding and acting upon health information" (Institute of Medicine, 2004, p. 1). In Canada, a significant percentage of the population lacks basic literacy skills (for example, the ability to work well with words and numbers, or read and understand printed materials) that are needed to process complex information, including health information (Gillis, 2005).

In addition to inadequate reading, writing, or math skills, other factors contribute to low health literacy (Institute of Medicine, 2004; Zorn, Allen, and Horowitz, 2004):

- Poor or insufficient speaking, listening, or comprehension ability
- Language barriers
- Low ability to advocate for oneself or navigate the health care system
- Inadequate background information
- Low socioeconomic status

More recently, the increasing role of the Internet as a key source of health information has been creating a divide between those who can take advantage of this additional resource and those who cannot (U.S. Department of Health and Human Services, 2006a). Therefore, Internet access and computer skills, or the lack thereof, may also affect health literacy levels.

Healthy People 2010 describes health literacy as "the degree to which individuals have the capacity to obtain, process, and understand basic health information and services needed to make appropriate health decisions" (U.S. Department of Health and Human Services, 2005, pp. 11–20; Selden and others, 2000). Health communication can help improve this capacity by taking into account literacy levels in all phases of strategic planning and program implementation. As part of broader public health and literacy interventions, health communication can contribute to breaking down barriers to the understanding of health-related issues using culturally relevant messages, materials, and activities that reflect the language capability and preferences of target audiences.

Health communication interventions can also play a key role in building the skills needed to improve overall health literacy levels. They can help sensitize health care providers, public health officers, industry representatives, and others in the health care field about the need to reach out to patients and the general public in these audiences' own terms. (Resources on selected methods to assess health literacy and to evaluate literacy levels of communication messages, materials, and activities are included in Appendix A.)

IMPACT OF MANAGED CARE AND OTHER COST-CUTTING INTERVENTIONS ON HEALTH

The advent of managed care in the United States has had an overall impact on provider-patient relationships, as well as the way health care may be perceived by the media, the general public, and health care providers. This is not only a U.S.-based phenomenon. Cost-cutting interventions are being implemented in many places around the world. For example, several countries in Asia are increasingly adopting managed care plans (Gross, 2001).

Managed care organizations essentially manage the costs and the delivery of health services to patients. Many aspects of health care (for example, the choice of a primary care physician, the eligibility for medical tests and other procedures) that traditionally were decided only by the health care provider or the patient are now scrutinized and influenced by managed care. Other worldwide cost-cutting interventions are part of the same trend that over the past few decades has been shifting responsibilities for health care from the government to companies (such as managed care organizations) or individuals.

The time that providers can dedicate to an individual patient has been reduced by the need to see an increasing number of patients each workday. From the patient's perspective, the quality of care may seem inferior and lacking the human touch that much longer conversations with physicians and indiscriminate access to tests and other medical procedures may provide.

While the debate on the pros and cons of cost-cutting interventions is beyond the scope of this book, it may be worth considering the implications of the current health care environment for health communication interventions:

- Health communication planning should take into account both the provider's and patient's opinion on cost-saving interventions and their perceived impact on their professional and personal lives.
- Health communication activities can help health care providers improve their communication skills and optimize their time with patients by managing expectations, addressing questions in a brief but efficient manner, and showing empathy with patients' needs and worries.
- Through advocacy, mass media campaigns, professional and government relations, and other strategic activities, health communication can help create a climate in which managed care organizations, legislators, and other key audiences would feel compelled to preserve the right balance between quality of care and cost-saving measures.

These are just a few examples of the kinds of considerations that should be given to the current cost-saving environment and how this could be incorporated in strategic health communication planning.

REEMERGENCE OF COMMUNICABLE DISEASES

The reemergence of many infectious diseases that had started to decline or disappear has influenced health communication in two different but related ways. First, it is one of the reasons for the health communication renaissance. Because of the rising incidence of several reemerging diseases such as cholera and tuberculosis (Centers for Disease Control, 1994a), many authors and organizations have pointed to the need to raise awareness of the ongoing risk for communicable diseases by using the health communication approach (Freimuth, Cole, and Kirby, 2000).

In fact, many infectious diseases may again become a public threat in the absence of effective prevention and communication strategies. For examples, pediatricians in the United States and many other countries have been witnessing increasing parental complacency about the need for childhood vaccines. Vaccines have become victims of their own success since many parents have never seen the devastating effects of diseases (National Foundation for Infectious Diseases, 1997) such as polio or *Haemophilus influenzae* type B, the leading cause of bacterial meningitis and acquired mental retardation in American children before the vaccine was introduced (National Association of Pediatric Nurse Practitioners, 2005).

Still, five cases of polio among children in an Amish dairy farm community in Minnesota in 2005 (Harris, 2005) are a powerful reminder that even vaccine-preventable infectious diseases remain a threat everywhere, including the developed world. In most cases, they are just a train ride or flight away. Communicating about the ongoing risk for infectious diseases has become a strategic imperative.

The second implication of this topic in health communication is related to the attempt by the health care community to redefine health risk communications, which are assuming greater prominence. Risk communications has been identified by *Healthy People 2010* as one of the relevant contexts of health communication. It is defined as "the dissemination of individual and population health risk information" (U.S. Department of Health and Human Services, 2005, p. 11–3).

Health communication has traditionally used strategies that raise awareness of disease severity and risk among interested groups and populations, so that people can relate to this risk and learn how to minimize it. Now, a more systematic approach to risk communications has been dictated by new attitudes toward disease prevention (or the lack of) that have led to the reemergence of many infectious diseases.

THE THREAT OF BIOTERRORISM

The threat of bioterrorism has forced public health officials, governments, and key community leaders and organizations to revisit their communication strategy in the light of the possibility of an emergency situation. A few general principles about the key characteristics of communications efforts aimed at averting a potential public health disaster have emerged from the lessons learned from the 2001 anthrax-by-mail bioterrorist attacks in the United States (see Chapter One). These include:

- Clear, timely, accurate, and audience-specific messages
- Credible spokespeople
- Strategic planning
- Coordinated efforts
- Adequate channels
- Culturally competent attitude to communication

Although all of these elements are standard attributes of well-designed and well-implemented health communication programs, the issue of preparedness assumes a greater importance in emergencies. In health communication, preparedness relates to:

- A standard protocol for crisis communications that organizations and agencies across the country can use in a coordinated effort
- Early selection and training of key spokespeople who can address target audiences in a crisis
- A standard document addressing potential questions from different audiences or from the mass media
- Other audience- and issue-specific tools and materials

CAPACITY AND INFRASTRUCTURE BUILDING IN THE DEVELOPING WORLD

Health communication cannot replace the lack of adequate local capacity, training, or infrastructure. When health services are unavailable or too distant from a significant percentage of interested audiences, health communication interventions should help create the political and social willingness that is needed to build hospitals, recruit and train local health care providers, and make health products available.

This is a major issue in developing countries. Nevertheless, lack of capability or training often affects health care in developed

countries too. For example, underserved populations around the
world may be faced with a shortage of medical supplies in local
hospitals or inadequate numbers of nurses or physicians per number of patients (Physicians for Human Rights, 2004; Colwill and
Cultice, 2003). Among others, health communication can play a
role in the process of expanding local capacity and infrastructure
in these ways:

- Engaging local leaders and government officers in the process
  of assessing local needs and subsequently creating or updating
  health services
- Raising awareness among local health care providers of standard medical practices that they may not use routinely
- Training patients and family caregivers so they can ask the
  right questions in physicians' offices, local meetings, and all
  other venues where health care–related decisions are made
- Increasing the visibility of leaders and organizations that focus
  on a specific health issue, disease, or local need
- Creating local awareness of disease severity and risk so that the
  issue can be prioritized and addressed in the community
  through adequate services and training

Lack of local capacity and training should force communicators to reflect on the limits of communication interventions. It
should make them prioritize those strategies that together with
other public health interventions would help develop critical
masses, political willingness, and innovative processes to address
existing deficiencies.

INTERNATIONAL ACCESS TO ESSENTIAL DRUGS

The HIV/AIDS crisis in Africa and other developing regions,
where the high incidence of AIDS has been threatening not only
lives but also the regions' economic and social development, has
dramatically pointed to the importance of equal access to life-
saving medications (Ruxin and others, 2005). It would certainly be
a failure of modern medicine if treatment could not be delivered
to those most in need of it.

In developing countries, access to medications is primarily influenced by cost, capacity for storage and drug delivery, adequate medical training, local infrastructure for drug distribution, hospitals' and treatment centers' conditions, and political willingness (Ruxin and others, 2005). All of these factors are equally important in ensuring that medications are available to people and can be effectively used to treat them.

While many different efforts and campaigns have been developed and implemented by several organizations in the AIDS and public health field (for example, Doctors Without Borders, Medicus Mundi, World Health Organization), we are still in the process of developing a model that can work in multiple countries and bring together local governments, pharmaceutical companies, local nongovernmental organizations, and other key stakeholders in sharing responsibility for guaranteeing access. This is a complex issue that deserves a book of its own and has been shaping interactions among different key players in the health care field. The overall point is that health communication, together with other kinds of interventions, can help advance this debate by creating consensus and raising awareness about adequate strategies, lessons learned from previous experiences, as well as the importance of a cohesive approach where different stakeholders would assume their share of responsibility. It is a topic that those who enter the health care field cannot ignore.

KEY CONCEPTS

- The theoretical basis of health communication has been influenced by the behavioral and social sciences, health education, social marketing, mass and speech communication, medical models, anthropology, and sociology.
- In this chapter, the most prominent theories and models are divided into the following categories: behavioral and social science theories, mass communication theories, marketing-based models, and other theoretical influences and planning frameworks, including medical models and logic modeling.
- There is a recognition of the multidisciplinary nature of health communication.

- Theories, models, and planning frameworks can influence different aspects and phases of health communication planning, evaluation, and management. They should all be considered as part of a comprehensive tool kit and selected in response to situational and audience-related issues and needs.
- A number of issues and topics influence the practice of health communication and need to be considered in the analysis of the current health care environment.

FOR DISCUSSION AND PRACTICE

1. Select a theory addressed in this chapter, and use a practical example on a health issue of your choice to show how changes in health behaviors may occur according to the steps highlighted by the theory you selected. Box 2.1 provides a practical example on the diffusion of innovation theory. This example can be used as a model for this exercise.
2. In your opinion, what is the main benefit of using theoretical frameworks and planning models in health communication? Do you have experience with any theory-based health communication interventions? If yes, identify key learnings.
3. Of the examples in this chapter of current issues that affect health communication practice, what do you consider the two most important issues, and why? Do you have any experience in addressing these issues or participating in health-related programs that focus on them? What, if anything, have you recently heard in the news about these topics? Is there any other issue that you think may shape the practice of health communication in the near future?

CHAPTER THREE

CULTURAL, GENDER, ETHNIC, RELIGIOUS, AND GEOGRAPHICAL INFLUENCES ON CONCEPTIONS OF HEALTH AND ILLNESS

IN THIS CHAPTER

- Approaches in Defining Health and Illness
- Understanding Health in Different Contexts: A Brief Comparative Analysis
- Gender Influences on Health Behaviors and Conceptions of Health and Illness
- Health Beliefs Versus Desires: Implications for Health Communication
- Cultural Competence and Implications for Health Communication
- Key Concepts
- For Discussion and Practice

"In 1976, as the United States celebrated its Bicentennial, the US Congress passed the American Folklife Preservation Act (Public Law 94–201). In writing the legislation, Congress had to define folklife. Here is what the law says: 'American folklife' means the traditional expressive culture shared within the various groups in the United States: familial, ethnic, occupational, religious, regional;

expressive culture includes a wide range of creative and symbolic forms such as custom, belief, technical skill, language, literature, art, architecture, music, play, dance, drama, ritual, pageantry, handicraft; these expressions are mainly learned orally, by imitation, or in performance, and are generally maintained without benefit of formal instruction or institutional direction" (Hufford, 1991).

Traditional expressions of any culture influence everyday decisions both big and small. They are reflected in the choice of the cake people have for their children's birthday and also in major decisions related to child rearing. They influence the slang children and doctors or handymen use to address their peers or others (Hufford, 1991). They are recalled when grandparents come to visit through tales and stories they transmit to the next generation. They are verbal and nonverbal clues that affect how information on any topic is received, accepted, and elaborated.

These traditions, habits, and beliefs also influence ideas of health and illness among different groups. The reality is that conceptions of health and illness are related to people's upbringing as well as their cultural, religious, ethnic, and gender-related values and beliefs, to name just a few. In health communication, these values and beliefs assume a critical importance in the design and implementation of programs that can reach across cultural boundaries and produce behavioral and social results.

Through a comparative review of some examples of different religious, ethnic, cultural, age, and gender-related influences on the concepts of health and illness, this chapter establishes the need for research-based communication interventions that always take into account audience-specific beliefs, behaviors, and characteristics.

APPROACHES IN DEFINING HEALTH AND ILLNESS

Defining the meanings of health and illness may appear to be an easy task. After all, in Western countries, people seem to know when they are sick with a cold or other illnesses. Why should it be so complicated? In actuality, health and illness have been defined in different ways across cultures around the world. Most authors agree that individual ideas on health and illness have a tremendous impact on people's attitudes toward healthy behaviors as well as disease prevention and treatment.

Following are two of the many models that over time have been used to define health. Although the models need to be considered in the context of the cultural and geographical attributes of intended audiences, they can still help comprehend the evolution of the definitions of health and illness over time.

MEDICAL MODEL

Under the medical model, health is strictly defined as the lack of disease (Balog, 1978; Boruchovitch and Mednick, 2002) and, more specifically, the absence of physical symptoms and signs associated with illness. This concept mirrors the biomedical model discussed in Chapter Two and takes into account only the physiological nature of health and illness. It was particularly popular among physicians and other health care professionals in the first half of the twentieth century (Boruchovitch and Mednick, 2002).

However, as for the biomedical model, the medical concept of health neglects to consider the influence that other factors, such as psychological or lifestyle issues, have on many diseases. Moreover, it defines health by highlighting illness (Boruchovitch and Mednick, 2002) and therefore does not take into account that often a healthy status is more of a general condition of well-being.

Several studies have shown that people tend to feel "healthy" when they are happy, energetic, and feel invulnerable to disease (Andersen and Lobel, 1995; Campbell, 1975). At times, this applies also to cases in which they are "concurrently ill" (Andersen and Lobel, 1995, p. 132). Healthy people tend to bounce back from illness faster and with better outcomes than unhealthy ones (for example, people who are under a lot of physical or emotional stress), so there is something more to a healthy status than just being disease free.

WORLD HEALTH ORGANIZATION MODEL

One of the key principles of the World Health Organization (WHO) Constitution (1946) is a definition of health, which in the past few decades has changed the perspective of many health care professionals on the concepts of health and illness. "Health is a state of complete physical, mental and social well-being and not merely the absence of disease and infirmity" (p. 2). This concept of health refers to the need for a balanced interaction among different physical, medical, psychological, social, and lifestyle-related factors. Balance, and the need for a balanced life that may help achieve good health, becomes a key principle in this definition, which also somewhat reflects the biopsychosocial model discussed in Chapter Two.

The concept of balance is also echoed in the definition of health in many populations and cultures. For example, health beliefs of traditional Southeast Asians, such as most Chinese people, revolve around the concept of balance between yin and yang, the two life forces (Matsunaga, Yamada, and Macabeo, 1998). Yin is the female force and is described as dark, cold, and wet. Yin illnesses are considered cold and need to be treated with yang (hot) to restore health and the right balance. Hot foods such as chicken or herbal mixtures may be recommended to treat yin illnesses (Rhode Island Department of Health, 2005d). Yang is the male force and is considered "light, hot and dry" (Matsunaga, Yamada, and Macabeo, 1998, p. 49). Yang diseases are considered hot and may be treated with cold foods, such as vegetables (Rhode Island Department of Health, 2005d) or herbs. In traditional Chinese culture, hot and cold do not refer to actual temperature but are used to define and characterize opposite forces (Matsunaga, Yamada, and Macabeo, 1998). Cancer is an example of a yin disease, while an ear infection is considered a yang disease (Rhode Island Department of Health, 2005d).

As another example, drinking a lot of cold fluids, such as water or orange juice, to nurture a bad cold may appear strange in some traditional Hispanic cultures, since illness, treatment, and foods are also viewed in terms of seeking a balance between hot and cold (Rhode Island Department of Health, 2005b), which this time refers to actual temperature. Among Hispanics, hot soups or teas may be viewed as an option to becoming healthy. In the United States, Hispanics include many different groups that differ in terms of cultural beliefs and ethnic and geographical backgrounds. However, many Hispanics also look at health as the result of a balance between the ability to function well in society and within one's family, feelings of happiness and well-being, being clean, and having time to rest and sleep well (Rhode Island Department of Health, 2005b).

Even given this information, it would be false to imply that Hispanics or Chinese are unaware of the medical basis of diseases and the role germs may play in the onset of many illnesses; they are actually aware. However, as with many other cultures, health is viewed as the result of a sense of well-being with oneself and others, which goes beyond being disease free.

One of the limitations of this concept of health is its lack of specificity (Lewis, 1953) and measurable parameters. This may complicate the evaluation of medical, behavioral, and social results. Also, it is important to take into account that while conditions such as obesity, diabetes, and depression are more heavily influenced by a number of social and individual factors, a sudden stroke or a head trauma needs immediate and urgent medical intervention that initially is limited to addressing medical causes and symptoms. This intervention focuses on restoring health by addressing only physical symptoms, which is the key assumption of the medical model.

UNDERSTANDING HEALTH IN DIFFERENT CONTEXTS: A BRIEF COMPARATIVE ANALYSIS

The definition of *healthy* varies from culture to culture and region to region. Ethnic, religious, socioeconomic, and age-related factors influence perceptions about health and healthy behaviors. For example, in some countries where malnutrition and poverty may be predominant, a large body size is considered a sign of a healthy lifestyle since it is associated with wealth and enough food (Mokhtar and others, 2001). In many Western countries, however, people often regard heavy weight as a sign of an unhealthy lifestyle (for example, lack of exercise or poor eating habits).

Religious and spiritual factors are also relevant in medicine since they influence beliefs about the nature of illness as well as their ability to cope with disease or adhere to recommended treatments. Several questionnaires and standard models, such as the Royal Free Interview for Religious and Spiritual Beliefs, have been developed and translated in many languages to assess religious and spiritual ideas and their potential influence on patients' behaviors and outcomes. Among other things, the Royal Free Interview is designed to investigate the extent to which people attribute sickness to God's will or rely on religious beliefs and practices to cope with the stress of an illness (Pernice and others, 2005).

In assessing the impact of religion and spirituality on ideas of health and illness, it is important to distinguish between the two terms since they refer to different levels of involvement in organized religious practices. *Religion* is usually defined as a series of spiritual practices and behaviors within an organized religious structure (for example, the Catholic church), which in some cases may also recommend or inspire specific health behaviors; *spirituality* is a larger concept that includes people's values, questions about the meaning of life, and, potentially, some level of involvement in organized religious activities (Mueller, Plevak, and Rummans, 2001; Emblen, 1992; Pernice and others, 2005). Both can play a key role in the way disease is perceived and addressed in different cultures. In fact, religion and spirituality include traditions and values that may affect people's understanding of the causes of illness, compliance to treatment and physician recommendations, or feelings of optimism or fatalism about disease outcomes, to name just a few examples. Religious beliefs have been reported to overrule clinical recommendations in influencing patients' decisions (Coward and Sidhu, 2000). This points to the need for a culturally competent approach to disease prevention and management in which intended audiences' religious or spiritual assumptions should be respected and understood.

Age is another contributing factor in defining health and healthy behaviors. For example, in Canada, awareness of the importance of adequate nutritional habits in relation to health tends to increase with age. When choosing food to eat, older Canadians "place more emphasis on nutrition" than younger Canadians (Health Canada, 2002). As another example, some authors have shown that even within a sample representing different ethnic backgrounds, a significant number of older people in the United States are fatalistic about the cause of many diseases, feel powerless about treatment, and tend to consider disease "a normal part of aging" (Goodwin, Black, and Satish, 1999). In general, concepts of health and illness change over time and often become increasingly more complex with older age.

Finally, access to recent advances in technology has also contributed to defining what people think it means to be healthy. For those who have regular access to it, the Internet has contributed to the merging of cultural perspectives and the understanding of many diseases. Similarly, radio and television have brought into many homes across the world images of models and lifestyles from different countries and cultures that over time can be assimilated or emulated by a given culture. However, it would be naive to expect that people will not incorporate their traditional beliefs and social values in redefining health as a result of new information and models. For any given culture, new ideas of health and illness tend to be the result of a carefully balanced combination of pre-existing and new concepts.

Health communicators should be aware that programs designed to achieve awareness of a specific health issue and its solutions may also have an impact on existing concepts of health and illness because of people's exposure to new models and beliefs. This potential impact should be considered early in program design as well as monitored and evaluated over time. Cross-cultural communication efforts should always be envisioned as an opportunity to integrate cultures and not to convince people of the rightness of a single culture. Adequate resources and tools should be developed to support people who initially adhere to new concepts and behaviors, so they can be encouraged in their new beliefs by their social and family circles. Consider the following story that exemplifies how miscommunication about the ideas of health and illness and the consequential clash of two different cultures may produce disastrous results (Fadiman, 1997):

> Lia Lee was a three-month-old Hmong child with epilepsy. Her doctors prescribed a complex regimen of medication designed to control her seizures. However, her parents felt that the epilepsy was a result of Lia "losing her soul" and did not give her medication as indicated because of the complexity of the drug therapy and the adverse side effects. Instead, they did everything logical in terms of their Hmong beliefs to help her. They took her to a clan leader and shaman, sacrificed animals and bought expensive amulets to guide her soul's return. Lia's doctors felt her parents were endangering her life by not giving her the medication so they called Child Protective Services and Lia was placed in foster care. Lia was a victim of a misunderstanding between these two cultures that were both

intent on saving her. The results were disastrous: a close family was separated and Hmong community faith in Western doctors was shaken [American Medical Student Association, 2005].

Table 3.1 provides a comparative overview of ideas of health and illness among different populations and groups. This table offers a useful perspective on the many variations of these two fundamental concepts that need to be considered in researching and approaching a new audience. The information in the table includes only selected facts, which come from published data and reviews in this field and may not apply to all people in the groups being featured. In fact, people in these groups may have individual conceptions that are shaped not only by sociocultural factors but also by their family upbringing, gender, educational level, and life experiences. Moreover, many other audience- or issue-specific factors that are not highlighted here may influence conceptions of health and illness and should be analyzed on a case-by-case basis.

GENDER INFLUENCES ON HEALTH BEHAVIORS AND CONCEPTIONS OF HEALTH AND ILLNESS

Gender refers to the role and responsibilities that men and women respectively assume in their society and family. It is distinguished from *sex,* which is a biological trait (Zaman and Underwood, 2003). Although these two terms are often used interchangeably, only *gender* refers to cultural values that are associated with a given sex.

In many cultures, gender roles and responsibilities tend to be different. Conceptions of health and illness often reflect this diversity. However, in approaching gender communication, it is important to refrain from applying gender-related stereotypes. The right approach is to research how gender attributes have evolved over time in a given culture and have influenced health care–related decisions and definitions.

In many settings, women's ideas of health and illness have been influenced by their role as wives and mothers in providing health care for the rest of the family. This role has also traditionally influenced the epidemiology and control of many diseases (Vlassoff

TABLE 3.1. A COMPARATIVE OVERVIEW OF IDEAS OF HEALTH AND ILLNESS

	Good Health	Illness Is
Populations/ ethnic group		
African Americans (United States)	The result of "keeping spiritual harmony between mind, body and soul" (University of Michigan Health System, 2005)	The consequence of natural causes, inadequate diet, too much wind or cold (University of Michigan Health System, 2005)
	"Feelings of well being" and the capacity "to fulfill one's role" in society without excessive pain or stress (Rhode Island Department of Health, 2005a)	God's punishment for bad conduct (University of Michigan Health System, 2005)
Vietnamese (country of origin and United States)	The proper balance between *am* and *duong* opposing forces, which are the same as yin and yang in Chinese culture (Matsunaga, Yamada, and Macabeo, 1998; Rhode Island Department of Health, 2005d)	An indication that "the body is out of balance" (Rhode Island Department of Health, 2005d)
Koreans (country of origin and United States)	A balance between organic and inorganic elements, mind and body (Matsunaga, Yamada, and Macabeo, 1998; Pang, 1980)	Imbalance among the many elements that make a person (Matsunaga, Yamada, and Macabeo, 1998)
Hispanics (United States)	A feeling of *bienestar* (well-being), which is related to achieving balance in the emotional, physical, and social spheres; a	An imbalance among emotional, physical and social factors; an unevenness between hot and cold in the body (Rhode Island

TABLE 3.1. A COMPARATIVE OVERVIEW OF IDEAS OF HEALTH AND ILLNESS, CONT'D.

	Good Health	*Illness Is*
	balance between hot and cold body humors (Rhode Island Department of Health, 2005b)	Department of Health, 2005b)
Native Americans (United States)	A cycle, which symbolizes perfection and equality; a balancing act among mind, body, spirit, and nature (Rhode Island Department of Health, 2005c)	
Religious groups		
Catholics		A reflection of fallen nature and something evil; a result of the sin of Adam (Ukrainian Catholic Church in Australia, New Zealand and Oceania, 2006)
Muslims	A state of dynamic equilibrium (Al-Khayat, 1997)	A punishment; a way of washing sins away (CancerBACKUP, 2006)
Hindus and Sikhs	The result of good karma ("the cyclical process of life and rebirth," Sheikh, 1999, p. 600), which is the total effect of a person's actions and determines the person's destiny (Sheikh, 1999; CancerBACKUP, 2006)	A punishment for wrongdoings in the current and previous lives (CancerBACKUP, 2006)
Age groups		
Children (Brazil)	"Positive feelings" (Boruchovitch and Mednick, 1997)	"Negative feelings associated with being ill;" "Not being healthy" (Boruchovitch and Mednick, 1997)

Table 3.1. A Comparative Overview of Ideas of Health and Illness, Cont'd.

	Good Health	Illness Is
Elderly (Mexico)	Something to be grateful to God for; dependent on the situations one lives (Zunker, Rutt, and Meza, 2005)	Normal at their age; due to lack of knowledge about how to keep healthy during youth (Zunker, Rutt, and Meza, 2005)
Elderly (United States)		A normal part of aging (Goodwin, Black, and Satish, 1999)

and Manderson, 1998). For example, Finerman (1989) reports that in rural Ecuador, women may be reluctant to defer medical care to professionals or other people outside their home. They are motivated by their need to protect their privileged and well-respected role as the family's caretaker, which could be questioned by outside interventions. The preservation of a woman's role as a primary caretaker has an important impact on the way diseases are managed, controlled, and prevented.

Gender also affects women's access to health information, financial resources for treatment interventions, and ways to respond to disease in comparison with men (Vlassoff and Manderson, 1998). Moreover, in the case of diseases that are highly stigmatized, such as AIDS or tuberculosis, women tend to be marginalized more than men by family and social circles.

In addition, in many cultures, the imbalance of power between men and women has created the need for developing different role models and recommended behaviors that are specific to each gender (Zaman and Underwood, 2003). For example, there are gender-related differences in talking with adolescents about sex and risky behaviors. Teaching girls about being assertive and demanding that their partners use condoms to prevent sexually transmitted diseases (STDs) is an additional but fundamental gender-specific element of most STD awareness efforts intended for adolescent girls.

As for concepts of health and illness, changes in gender-related roles and responsibilities may be one of the effects of a health communication program on a particular health issue (Zaman and Underwood, 2003). Therefore, gender attributes in the health care setting need to be understood, monitored, and evaluated over time in relation to the influence that health communication programs may have on them. These changes could potentially influence gender-related concepts of health and illness and become one of the many examples of how different elements of the health communication environment are interconnected.

HEALTH BELIEFS VERSUS DESIRES: IMPLICATIONS FOR HEALTH COMMUNICATION

Meeting and managing expectations is a critical attribute of most professional and personal interactions in result-oriented societies such as Western cultures. However, achieving what has been promised is important in all cultures.

In the health care field, when one asks others to change behaviors, the promise is usually for better health. But the concept of health and illness varies across cultures and groups. Health beliefs influence how people estimate the likelihood of different outcomes that may be linked to the recommended behavior. If people feel competent about managing their health, they are more likely to feel optimistic about their ability to reverse negative patterns and become healthier. If instead they feel that illness is God's punishment for some past wrongdoing, they may be more pessimistic about their ability to change what they view as their fate, or they may rely on prayer to seek help. Table 3.2 provides a few examples of disease-specific definitions of illness that may affect how people from different cultures view treatment recommendations and potential outcomes. These definitions have been reported in existing literature on the topic.

Beliefs also affect how people rate the desirability of a certain outcome. In evaluating potential outcomes and their appeal, people are influenced by both logical and emotional arguments. It is

TABLE 3.2. EXAMPLES OF DISEASE-SPECIFIC IDEAS OF ILLNESS

Epilepsy is a "loss of soul" (American Medical Student Association, 2005; Fadiman, 1997)—Hmong

Tuberculosis is due to God's curse, evil spirits, or sin (Kapoor, 1996) —Indians

Mental retardation is due to the "spirit of dead horse" (Chan, 1986; Erickson, Devlieger, and Sung, 1999)—Koreans

"Malaria is caused by mosquito bite and when the child walks or spends too much time in the hot sun, his blood becomes hot and this causes malaria" (Ahorlu and others, 1997, p. 492)—Igbo in Nigeria

"Diabetes is permanent in the body leading to terrible, pessimistic and hard future resulting in loss of independence" (Rednova, 2005) —Asians

"Schizophrenia is split personality or multiple personality. People with schizophrenia are violent and dangerous" (Health Canada and Schizophrenia Society of Canada, 1991)—North America

important to understand and rate the level of priority and desirability placed on potential consequences of recommended behaviors.

Take the example of Julie, a fifty-two-year-old woman who is severely overweight. At her annual checkup, her physician finds out that she has type 2 diabetes, which is frequently associated with obesity and characterized by high blood sugar (glucose) levels. So far, Julie did not have any of the major symptoms of diabetes, with the exception of feeling tired and having a few episodes of blurred vision. She has attributed these symptoms to the long hours she spends working in a local manufacturing company and to recent personal events that "make her feel she wants to sleep more." Therefore, when her physician recommends that she lose weight because of the potential long-term effects of diabetes, which include eye complications, kidney disease, and an increased risk for heart attack, stroke and poor circulation problems (American Diabetes Association, 2005), she does not see the need to follow these instructions. She has no interest in minimizing the potential impact of her diabetes because she does not have any obvious symptoms.

Diabetes prevention and control is only one of the many benefits of weight loss in obese or severely overweight patients. Others are the potential reduction of the psychological effects of obesity, which is a highly stigmatized condition and often limits opportunities in education, employment, personal relationships, and other areas (Wang, Brownell, and Wadden, 2004), and a lower risk for many other conditions associated with obesity, including some forms of cancer, alterations in pulmonary function, hypertension, and cardiovascular disease (Bray, 2004).

Well-planned health communication programs should consider all of these potential outcomes and evaluate their level of importance to intended audiences. In order to convince people to prioritize weight loss (as in Julie's case), communicators and health care providers should identify the most desirable outcomes to the patient. This should become the entry message of all interactions and communication efforts, which creates a receptive environment to introduce and discuss the benefits of other potential outcomes.

Regardless of the context in which they take place (for example, the physician's office or a public forum), communication interactions and related health practices should be both effective and efficient. *Effective* refers to the ability to achieve desired outcomes (for example, in Julie's case, diabetes control or reduction of psychological effect). *Efficient* refers to the ability of achieving these outcomes with minimal time and cost (both economic and emotional).

Of equal importance are people's expectations about the overall quality of the experience. Factors that may influence the quality of the experience are the level of difficulty of complying with recommended activities (for example, limiting consumption of sweets), the kind of support received by friends and family, and many others that are audience or individual specific. Potentially negative consequences of weight loss should also be considered in order to assess the overall appeal of the recommended behavior and its outcomes.

Many experiences have emphasized the importance of understanding and managing health beliefs and desires. As Babrow (1991) reports on the topic of smoking cessation, the probability of achieving expected outcomes as well as the value placed on positive (for example, "improve health, quit successfully, save money") and negative (for example, potential "weight gain, stress, loss of time") consequences of smoking cessation strongly relate to the intention of smokers to participate in programs that would help them quit (Babrow, 1991, p. 102).

Health communication programs can highlight the cause-and-effect relationship between desirable outcomes and recommended behaviors. They can also contribute to the development of tools and resources that will recommend easy-to-achieve steps for recommended behaviors and set realistic expectations. Finally, as Babrow (1991) suggests, communication messages "might inculcate optimism, hope or faith," depending on the health beliefs of intended audiences.

CULTURAL COMPETENCE AND IMPLICATIONS FOR HEALTH COMMUNICATION

Cultural competence has been defined as "the capacity to function effectively as an individual and an organization within the context of the cultural beliefs, behaviors and needs presented by consumers and their communities" (U.S. Department of Health and Human Services, 2006b). Culturally appropriate care, defined as the ability of health care professionals to provide medical care within a socially and culturally acceptable framework that may vary from patient to patient, can lead to enhanced patient outcomes (Frable, Wallace, and Ellison, 2004). In health communication and, more broadly, public health, the importance of cultural competence has been increasingly recognized.

Recent consensus among public health and health communication experts and organizations has highlighted the role culture plays in health outcomes and behaviors, as well as in increasing the effectiveness of health communication interventions (Kreuter and McClure, 2004; Institute of Medicine, 2002, 2003). Well-designed and well-executed health communication programs should rely on an in-depth understanding of intended audiences and be tailored to their needs and beliefs. This implies a true knowledge of cultural values in the many subgroups that may be included in a given audience.

In fact, while shared values and other cultural expressions are often related to age, race, religion, gender, and geographical boundaries, it is likely that even within the same racial or age group, there may be different subgroups with specific cultural connotations or different stages in terms of their understanding and involvement in a certain health issue. For example, it would be naive to believe that a single smoking cessation program could be designed for teenagers who live in the inner city or affluent neighborhoods of a metropolitan area and have different smoking-related habits and beliefs. Some of the program's key elements may be the same, but others should address the unique characteristics of these different subgroups.

Audience segmentation, which is defined as the practice of dividing large groups and populations in smaller groups (segments) that have homogeneous characteristics, is a well-established process in health communication as well as in some related disciplines such as commercial and social marketing. While a detailed discussion of audience segmentation is included in Chapter Ten, readers should start thinking about the potential uniqueness of the cultural, behavioral, psychological, demographic, socioeconomic, and geographical characteristics and risk factors of different audience segments and try to apply them to a recent health situation they encountered. For example, do you think it would be the same to help a friend to quit smoking regardless of whether he or she is aware of the potential risk for many complications and diseases associated with smoking? What about the approach you would take to help a friend who is surrounded by peers who regard smoking as cool versus the kind of support you would provide to someone who feels guilty about not being able to quit and lives with people who disapprove of smoking? There are many variables in approaching audience segmentation, and culture is one of them (Kreuter and McClure, 2004).

The concept of cultural competence establishes the need for targeted communication interventions, which normally use a multifaceted approach to address the concerns and characteristics of all members of a specific audience segment (Kreuter and Skinner, 2000; Slater, 1996; Kreuter and McClure, 2004). Cultural competence is key to a program's success and is strictly related to how information is received, processed, and evaluated by intended audiences. It also points to the importance of tailoring language and cultural references to the specific audience, customizing message delivery to different learning styles, and using credible messengers. (For additional discussion on the role that culture and culture competence should play in message development and delivery, as well as in the selection of appropriate communication channels and spokespeople, see Chapter Twelve.)

KEY CONCEPTS

- Conceptions of health and illness are influenced by cultural beliefs, race, ethnicity, age, gender, socioeconomic conditions, and geographical boundaries, among other factors.
- Gender influences not only ideas of health and illness but also access to health information, financial resources for treatment interventions, and ways to respond to disease. In many cultures, it may also determine differences in the level of social marginalization experienced by patients of different genders who suffer from highly stigmatized diseases such as AIDS or tuberculosis.
- Health communication interventions should analyze and take into account different ideas of health and illness in order to be effective in reaching out to intended audiences.
- Tensions between health beliefs and desires influence people's willingness to adopt and sustain health behaviors. Health communication can highlight the cause-and-effect relationship between recommended behaviors and desirable outcomes.
- Cultural competence is critical in health communication.
- Major implications of cultural competence in health communication are related to the need for audience segmentation as well as the development and selection of audience-specific messages, channels, and messengers.

FOR DISCUSSION AND PRACTICE

1. What is your reaction to the selection in this chapter about Lia Lee, a Hmong child? What (if anything) do you think should have happened differently?
2. When can you say that you feel in good health? Do any family or cultural beliefs affect your ideas of health and illness? Does

your family or ethnic group have any special way to deal with illness? Can you think of an experience in which your health was affected by physical as well as mental and social factors?

3. Describe a personal experience with cross-cultural communications—for example, a health-related encounter with a health care provider from a different cultural or ethnic background or participation in research studies or programs that involved different groups or populations.

4. In health communication, what are the major implications of the potential tension between patients' health beliefs and desires? Can you provide a practical example or personal experience that illustrates how culturally and audience-competent communications can help address such issues?

PART TWO

HEALTH COMMUNICATION APPROACHES AND ACTION AREAS

CHAPTER FOUR

INTERPERSONAL COMMUNICATIONS

IN THIS CHAPTER

- The Dynamics of Interpersonal Behavior
- Social and Cognitive Processes of Interpersonal Communications
- The Power of Personal Selling and Counseling
- Communication as a Core Clinical Competency
- Technology-Mediated Communications
- Key Concepts
- For Discussion and Practice

In 1999, Harry Depew, the 2000 Family Physician of the Year of the American Academy of Family Physicians (AAFP), began his comments to the AAFP Congress of Delegates by first addressing the audience in sign language: "If you were a hearing person in a deaf world, where you could not understand sign language, how would you feel communicating with your doctor?" Then he asked out loud (AAFP, 1999). His question refers to a specific communication need and area of interpersonal communications (provider-patient communications). Still, the feelings of isolation and frustration that may be elicited by the situation Depew describes are likely quite similar to those we may feel in all instances in which health information, or other kinds of information, is misunderstood or blocked out because we cannot relate to the person who is speaking.

Interpersonal communications is an important action area of health communication programs aimed at behavioral (World

Health Organization, 2003) or social change. It includes provider-patient communications, as well as counseling and personal selling (the one-on-one engagement of intended audiences in their own homes, offices, or places of work and leisure), which are two activities that find applicability in many different phases and aspects of the communication process.

This chapter reviews some of the key factors in the dynamics of interpersonal behavior and communication. It also focuses on practical aspects of counseling, personal selling, and provider-patient communications, which are all key areas of interpersonal communications. In doing so, it highlights the importance of considering all encounters as an opportunity for a two-way exchange of information, as well as the potential beginning of a long-lasting partnership.

THE DYNAMICS OF INTERPERSONAL BEHAVIOR

Interpersonal behavior is influenced by several cultural factors. Although each individual has his or her own style of interacting with others, social conventions as well as traditions and values in a given group or community play an important role in how behavior and communication take place and are interpreted and perceived.

All interactions comprise both verbal and nonverbal signs and symbols that contribute to the meanings of behavior and communication actions. Social psychologists tend to consider *signs* to be involuntary behaviors, such as blushing in response to feelings of embarrassment. *Symbols* are defined as voluntary acts, such as using verbal expressions to describe one's feelings (Krauss and Fussell, 1996). According to these definitions, saying "I am embarrassed" is a symbol, while blushing is a sign.

Symbols are the result of social conventions and agreement. For example, the significance of the word *embarrassed* is well known and shared by all English-language users (Krauss and Fussell, 1996). Therefore, using it in this context is supported by social norms and conventions.

A number of so-called signs may be controlled and therefore assume a symbolic value (Krauss and Fussell, 1996). For example, facial expressions can be controlled and modified to induce others to believe what we want them to believe and disguise what we are really feeling (Kraut, 1979). Most people can recall situations in which they met a colleague or attended a business party immediately after a painful disagreement with a loved one. Chances are that facial expressions were controlled to disguise all feelings related to the recent disagreement. As this example demonstrates, it is difficult to strictly apply the theoretical distinction between signs and symbols (Krauss and Fussell, 1996). Still, this distinction can provide a useful framework to explain some of the components of interpersonal behavior and communication.

It is also critical to take into account the impact of culture on the interpretation of signs and symbols. Culture starts influencing meanings quite early in life. In fact, the process of socialization that begins within the family and aims at preparing children for their adult role is influenced by social norms and cultural factors of a given population or group (Moment and Zaleznik, 1964). How a child will address teachers and elderly members of his or her family and community depends on the educational level, cultural values, age, and traditions of the parents, as well as their social environment.

Differences in power and social status also affect the dynamics of interpersonal behavior and the potential intimacy or level of formality of relationships (Hwa-Froelich and Vigil, 2004; Hofstede, 1984, 2001). In some cultures, people are assigned a higher social status in relation to their age, economic wealth, education, profession, or birth order (Hwa-Froelich and Vigil, 2004). For example, in the Chinese language, the eldest sister is addressed with a special word that conveys respect (Hwa-Froelich and Vigil, 2004).

Signs and symbols often assume different meanings in different cultures. Posture, social cues, and facial and idiomatic expressions all influence interpersonal relationships. In interpreting people's behavior, it is important to be aware of cultural differences that may have a powerful effect on the dynamics of interpersonal behavior. Lack of understanding of these differences often undermines the impact of well-meant communication efforts.

In the health care field, understanding how cultural variables and interpretations affect interpersonal behavior has a positive influence on communication that may lead to better patient outcomes, increased patient compliance to treatment, or a better chance for disease control in a given group or population, to name just a few potential positive effects. Table 4.1 compares examples of different aspects of culture that may influence interpersonal relationships and communication during a health care related encounter.

TABLE 4.1. COMPARING CULTURAL NORMS AND VALUES

Aspects of Culture	U.S. Health Care Culture	Other Cultures
Sense of self and space	Informal	Formal
	Handshake	Hugs, bows, handshakes
Communication and language	Explicit, direct communication	Implicit, indirect communication
	Emphasis on content; meaning found in words	Emphasis on context; meaning found around words
Dress and appearance	"Dress for success" ideal	Dress seen as a sign of position, wealth, and prestige
	Wide range in accepted dress	
		Religious rules
	More casual	More formal
Food and eating habits	Eating as a necessity; fast food	Dining as a social experience
		Religious rules
Time and time consciousness	Linear and exact time consciousness	Elastic and relative time consciousness
	Value on promptness	Time spent on enjoyment of relationships
	Time equals money	
Relationship, family, friends	Focus on nuclear family	Focus on extended family
	Responsibility for self	Loyalty and responsibility to family
	Value on youth; age seen as handicap	
		Age given status and respect
Values and norms	Individual orientation	Group orientation
	Independence	Conformity
	Preference for direct confrontation of conflict	Preference for harmony
	Emphasis on task	Emphasis on relationships

TABLE 4.1. COMPARING CULTURAL NORMS AND VALUES, CONT'D.

Aspects of Culture	U.S. Health Care Culture	Other Cultures
Beliefs and attitudes	Egalitarian	Hierarchical
	Challenging of authority	Respect for authority and social order
	Gender equity	Different roles for men and women
	Behavior and action affect and determine the future	Fate controls and predetermines the future
Mental processes and learning style	Linear, logical	Lateral, holistic, simultaneous
	Problem-solving focus	
	Internal locus of control	Accepting of life's difficulties
	Individuals control their destiny	External locus of control
		Individuals accept their destiny
Work habits and practices	Reward based on individual achievement	Rewards based on seniority, relationships
	Work has intrinsic value	Work is a necessity of life

SOCIAL AND COGNITIVE PROCESSES OF INTERPERSONAL COMMUNICATIONS

Interpersonal behavior is usually affected by social needs and factors as well as cognitive processes that may vary at the individual level. Both of these factors play a key role in how information is shared, evaluated, processed, and absorbed.

SOCIAL NEEDS AND FACTORS

Change occurs when people are able to share common meanings and understand each other. In health communication, messages affect attitudes only when people understand, process, and remember them (Krauss and Fussell, 1996) and feel motivated to apply them in their everyday life.

In order to be effective, communication needs to respond to an audience's needs. This general principle also applies to interpersonal communications, such as one-on-one teaching, counseling, personal selling, and provider-patient communications.

Several authors explain people's behavior in the interpersonal communication context in terms of the desire to satisfy a specific need (Step and Finucane, 2002; Kellerman and Reynolds, 1990; Roloff, 1987; Schutz, 1966). Rubin, Perse, and Barbato (1988) developed the Interpersonal Communication Motives Scale (ICM) to explain the dynamics and motivation of interpersonal communication. Based on this model, people interact and speak with each other to satisfy specific needs:

- Being part of a social group or including others in one's group
- Appreciating others
- Controlling other people's actions and increasing behavioral compliance
- Being amused and entertained
- Escaping and being distracted from routine activities
- Relaxing and relieving stress

In their analysis, Rubin, Perse, and Barbato (1988) also showed that people tend to be less anxious when their motivation to communicate is to include others or to feel included. Having a good life, which entails overall satisfaction, good health, economic security, and social gratification, among others, also influences the reasons for which people communicate (Barbato and Perse, 1992; Step and Finucane, 2002). People who are experiencing life difficulties tend to communicate for "comfort," while those with a good life "communicate more for pleasure and affection" (Step and Finucane, 2002, p. 95; Barbato and Perse, 1992).

Age and gender also influence motives for interpersonal communications. For example, young people between eighteen and twenty-five years old often use communication as a means for having fun, relaxing, feeling part of a social group, or escaping from routine activities (Javidi and others, 1990; Step and Finucane, 2002). Alternatively, middle-aged or older adults tend to communicate more to express appreciation or feel appreciated (Javidi and others, 1990; Step and Finucane, 2002). There are gender differences in interpersonal communications as well: women seem to communicate more "to express emotions" or appreciation, while men's motivation is primarily control (Step and Finucane, 2002, p. 95; Barbato and Perse, 1992).

Many other elements contribute to the quality and tone of interpersonal interactions. Some obvious factors are common cultural references, similar upbringing, level of intimacy and mutual trust, level of competence about the topic being discussed, openness to new ideas, and individual state of mind.

Most people can relate to the feeling of recognizing themselves in the values and expressions of those who were born in the same part of the world. This is a good predictor of potentially good interpersonal interactions but needs to be complemented by feelings of trust and respect about the other person's competence or level of empathy on the subject being addressed.

Personal experiences can also affect interpersonal communication and influence relationships with those who previously shared one's cultural values and beliefs. For example, a couple from a conservative country where women are not allowed to participate with men in any kind of social event may reevaluate their beliefs and interact differently with their fellow citizens after living in a country where the concept of equality between men and women is widely accepted. When travelers return from such a trip, their interpersonal relationships may be affected by the urge to change beliefs, while before they were based on shared values and the need to confirm them.

This example points to the importance of cultural and social factors in interpersonal interactions and communication. It also suggests that interactions and communication may change over time according to people's beliefs and values. Therefore, communication needs to be sensitive to belief and attitude changes and recognize that these changes are often the result of other interpersonal relationships and communications. It is important to acknowledge the cause-and-effect impact of interpersonal communications and promptly adapt to change.

COGNITIVE PROCESSES

The process of acquiring knowledge by the use of reasoning, intuition, or perception is strictly related to communication and its modalities. Every time people interact with others, they share information. How new or existing information is acknowledged and processed depends on the approach one takes to communication.

For example, psychologists have long pointed out that people's performance in trying to solve a problem is influenced by the way the problem is presented (Glucksberg and Weisberg, 1963; Chiu, Krauss, and Lau, 1998). In the United States, an "I-can-do" attitude toward professional tasks is considered a major asset. Can-do people feel that all tasks are within their reach and competence, and there is no such thing to them as an insurmountable problem. They also tend to transmit their enthusiasm and confidence to subordinates and colleagues. They present problems and situations with an optimistic flair. This is likely to make people feel competent and able to solve problems and may enhance their performance. In contrast, if a problem is presented by highlighting all the worst scenarios and expressing doubts about the possibility of addressing it, chances are that people may feel that whatever they do may not work.

Knowledge and attitude change are also influenced by the way information is presented. Establishing open and trusting communication is often the first step in creating a receptive environment in which information can be perceived as reliable and worthy of consideration. All successful communications and interactions usually require a reasonably good understanding of the other person's

point of view (Brown, 1965). Openness and trust are usually con-
tagious. People can induce the same kind of open and trusting
communications in others just by beginning first (Deutsch, 1973,
2000). Figure 4.1 shows two different scenarios and their potential
impact on knowledge, attitude, and behavior after a mother's conversation with her infant daughter's pediatrician.

FIGURE 4.1. THE POTENTIAL IMPACT OF INTERPERSONAL
COMMUNICATIONS ON BEHAVIOR: A PRACTICAL EXAMPLE

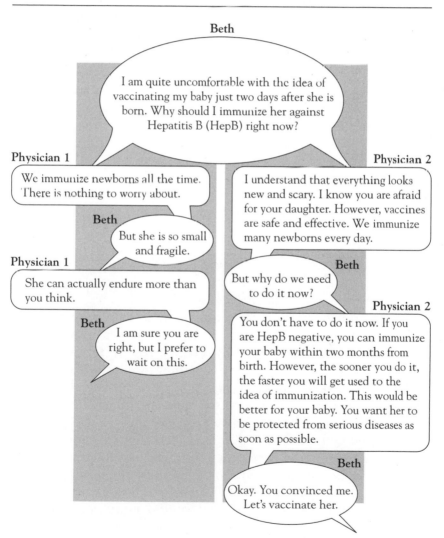

Still, it is important to remember that the sole or singular use of verbal expressions has been shown to have only a temporary impact on attitude change (Chiu, Krauss, and Lau, 1998). Eiser and Pancer (1979) studied the effect of biased language on attitudinal changes by asking study participants to write their views on capital punishment. Some of the subjects were directed to use words in their essays that were pro–capital punishment. Others were told to use words that were anti–capital punishment. Although the attitude of study participants toward capital punishment initially changed to reflect the words they had used in their essays, they had reverted to their original perspectives within six days from when they wrote their papers (Eiser and Pancer, 1979; Chiu, Krauss, and Lau, 1998).

In health communication, it is not enough to define a recommended behavior as "healthy" or "life-saving." In order to determine a more permanent attitude change, all statements need to be supported by evidence (Chiu, Krauss, and Lau, 1998) and translated into tools to facilitate their practical application. This is an important concept in message development in both interpersonal communications and other action areas of health communications. Facts and tools are critical to lend credibility to verbal expressions and motivate people to change.

THE POWER OF PERSONAL SELLING AND COUNSELING

Personal selling is a well-established practice in the commercial sector that also has many applications in public health and health communication. In the commercial sector, it refers to the one-on-one, "door-to-door engagement" (World Health Organization, 2005, p. 27) of potential customers in their own homes, offices, or places of work and leisure. In the health care industry, the figure that comes to mind is the pharmaceutical sales representative who goes to physicians' offices to present a product.

Personal selling is also widely used for nonprofit causes and to spread the word about recommended new health behaviors and practices. In public health and health communication, personal sellers are usually volunteers, social workers, trainers, health professionals, or representatives of development organizations who go door-to-door or attend places where health services are provided. Their role is to engage intended audiences in interpersonal interactions to explain, recommend, and show benefits of a specific health behavior or practice. Often this role is coupled with actual service delivery. It also serves the purpose of answering questions and addressing fears and concerns about recommended health services and practices.

Door-to-door immunization is considered a core strategy of the worldwide polio eradication campaign, for example (Joyner, 2001). WHO, UNICEF, and their partners in the polio eradication effort organize national immunization days in which thousands of volunteers and health professionals travel to remote villages and poor areas in the developing world to set up one-day clinics in schools, markets, and other places where they can reach a large number of people and persuade them to vaccinate their children. In India alone, during National Immunization Day in 1999, "2.5 million volunteers and health professionals traveled by any available means, including by camel and on foot following dry riverbed, carrying the vaccine on ice to their immunization posts" (Joyner, 2001). Another door-to-door campaign aiming to immunize 77 million African children against polio in one year was launched by UNICEF and its partners in 2005 (Li, 2005).

Personal selling does not work in a vacuum. In most cases, personal selling efforts need to be complemented by mass communication programs, such as public relations, community mobilization, and other communication approaches discussed later in this book (see the example in Box 4.1). All of these other activities aim to create social consensus about the importance of responding to the call for action of volunteers, health workers, or school children who will knock on people's doors. Without creating a supportive environment in which people feel motivated to listen to the recommendations of the so-called change agents, most personal selling efforts may fail or produce only minimal results. Still, in the case of polio, door-to-door immunization enables the vaccination of millions of children in areas where war, lack of infrastructures, and poverty would otherwise make vaccine access and delivery impossible (Joyner, 2001). Similarly, personal selling was one of the key success factors in a WHO effort to prevent lymphatic filariasis in several endemic countries (see Box 4.1).

Box 4.1

Personal Selling Case Study

Lymphatic Filariasis
India, Kenya, Nepal, Philippines, Sri Lanka, Zanzibar

Lymphatic Filariasis (LF) is a painful and disfiguring disease caused by thread-like worms that live in the human lymphatic system. LF is transmitted from person to person by mosquitoes. Around 120 million are affected by LF, with more than one billion people at risk of infection.

LF is one of seven diseases targeted for elimination by WHO. The strategy adopted for elimination in 1997 at the World Health Assembly, is to treat entire endemic communities once a year, for 5-6 years, with two co-administered antiparasitic drugs. For the strategy of Mass Drug Administrations to be successful over 70 per cent of the total population should take the prescribed number of LF prevention pills. The other fundamental aspect of the programme is to provide support for those already suffering from LF related disabilities.

Impact

Country	Total population targeted	Coverage rate achieved (% of total population)
India: Tamil Nadu	28 million	74
Kenya	1.2 million	81
Philippines	4.5 million	87
Sri Lanka	9.5 million	86
Zanzibar	1 million	83

The Behavioural Objective
Take your LF pills from your Filaria Prevention Assistants on Filaria Day

COMBI Plans were designed for India (the state of Tamil Nadhu), Kenya, Nepal, Philippines, Sri Lanka and Zanzibar. The campaigns had a sharp, singular focus on the behavioural result expected: the ready acceptance and swallowing of the tablets on a chosen day.

The heart of the entire effort were a group of dedicated individuals (health workers, teachers and volunteers), called Filaria Prevention Assistants, going door-to-door hand delivering a set of tablets to all eligible individuals. They also carried out two preparatory visits to households explaining the elimination programme, showing the tablets, describing what was expected and answering any queries or concerns. The Filaria Prevention Assistants were supported by intense community mobilization, massive advertising, high media coverage and political and religious leadership backing.

Source: World Health Organization. Mediterranean Center for Vulnerability Reduction. "Lymphatic Filariasis." In *COMBI in Action: Country Highlights.* 2004. http://wmc.who.int/pdf/COMBI_in_Action_04.pdf. Retrieved Nov. 2005. Used by permission.

Still, the practice of personal selling is an acquired communication skill that relies on many of the principles of interpersonal communications discussed so far in this chapter, as well as on individual characteristics and strengths. It requires training, awareness of people's needs, strong listening skills, and the ability to engage others, as well as to counter objections by acknowledging the other person's perspective and empathizing with it. It involves the ability to resolve conflicts by brainstorming and finding common ground. In the case of a specific health communication campaign or public health intervention, it requires a level of competence and knowledge on the subject matter that, at the minimum, should be sufficient to elicit trust among intended audiences.

Furthermore, the term *personal selling* can refer to the ability to sell one's image and expertise, a helpful skill in most kinds of consulting activities. This second definition refers primarily to a communication skill, while the first definition is related to a key area of interpersonal communications. These two meanings are strongly connected and interdependent in their practical application.

Personal selling (the ability to sell one's image and expertise but also a skill that is needed in the one-on-one engagement of intended audiences) is dependent on a number of verbal and nonverbal signals that should be recognizable by intended audiences. Among others, these include posture, overall confidence, speech and expressions, dress code (casual versus formal), and the ability to relate to others and express genuine concern. However, signs and symbols are not the same across differing populations and cultures. As previously discussed (see Table 4.1), several cultural and social factors may influence people's ability to sell their image, competence, and expertise among members of different intended audiences, populations, and groups.

In *counseling*, which could be defined as the help provided by a professional on personal, psychological, health, or professional matters, personal selling is a powerful determinant of one's ability to have an impact on the beliefs, attitudes, and behavior of the person who is seeking counsel. This is true for all forms of counseling. In fact, personal selling skills may affect the ability of health communication practitioners to counsel others on communication strategies or engage opinion leaders in prioritizing a given health issue. Personal selling also influences patient-provider relationships and treatment compliance.

Because of their special role in giving advice and shaping other people's professional or personal lives, counselors, whether they are physicians, nurses, psychologists, lawyers, health communication practitioners, or other public health professionals, need to be trusted and respected by their intended audiences. Their audiences (whether they are patients or nonprofit organizations or others) need to have faith in their commitment to a common cause (for example, a patient's well-being or the success of a communication intervention) in order to relate to counselors and follow their advice.

Most important, people need to feel a sense of ownership of the issue on which they are being advised. And how could it be otherwise? Even if health professionals are knowledgeable about a given disease or health problem, it is the patient's life that is directly affected by its symptoms and potential consequences. And what about key stakeholders, such as professional organizations, senior government officials, or top physicians who decide to endorse a health issue after being solicited by health communication practitioners or other public health professionals? Given their busy schedule and conflicting priorities, they are likely to dedicate significant portions of their time to addressing a specific issue only if they feel needed and can make a significant contribution to the problem's solution.

Several cultural nuances may affect these general concepts. In some cultures, patients tend to defer more to their physicians or do not participate as much in treatment and prevention decisions because of their views of illness as God's will or punishment or other cultural beliefs. Nevertheless, in all situations, the role of counselors, including health care providers, is to reach out, bridge cultural differences, and try to transform each encounter into a productive partnership.

Because of the documented impact of provider-patient communications on patient outcomes and overall satisfaction, the rest of this chapter focuses primarily on this important form of interpersonal communications in health care. In doing so, it provides a practical and research-based perspective on how to transform ordinary relationships into successful partnerships that may lead to improved disease outcomes.

COMMUNICATION AS A CORE CLINICAL COMPETENCY

Being sick is among one of the most vulnerable times in people's lives, especially in the case of severe, chronic, or life-threatening diseases. It is also a time in which patients need to understand and feel comfortable with the information their provider shares with them. From a patient's perspective, it is important to feel that their case is a key priority for the health care provider they have selected. From a provider's perspective, conflicting priorities, managed care requirements (see Chapter Two), time barriers, or insufficient communication training may limit the ability to establish trusting and open relationships with patients.

Still, effective communication has been shown to have a positive impact on patient compliance to health recommendations, patient satisfaction, patient retention rates, overall health outcomes, and even a reduced number of malpractice suits (DiMatteo and others, 1993; Garrity, Haynes, Mattson, and Engebretson, 1998; Lipkin, 1996; Lukoscheck, Fazzari, and Marantz, 2003; Belzer, 1999). As Lukoscheck, Fazzari, and Marantz highlighted (2003), the patient-provider encounter offers one of the most important opportunities "to have a major impact on reducing morbidity and mortality of chronic diseases, through personalized information exchange" (p. 209). Box 4.2 provides a health care provider's perspective on the impact of effective communications on patient outcomes and social well-being.

Box 4.2

The Impact of Effective Provider-Patient Communications on Patient Outcomes: A Pediatric Nurse Practitioner's Perspective

Mary Beth Koslap Petraco, CPNP, is the coordinator for child health in the Suffolk County Department of Health Services, New York; chair of the Immunization Special Interest Group of the National Association of Pediatric Nurse Practitioners; and a clinical assistant professor at the State University of New York at Stony Brook. Her thoughts on the importance of provider-patient communications (interview and other personal communications with the author, 2006), which follow, reflect her extensive patient-related experience.

Cultural competence is very important in nursing. U.S. nurses are specifically educated to put aside their cultural bias and work with the patient's cultural beliefs. This is a unique attribute of U.S.-educated nurses and helps establish effective relationships with patients.

Good provider-patient communications are very important in changing patients' attitudes toward disease, helping them use their culture in a positive way, and empowering them to make the changes in their lives that are associated with better health outcomes.

I learned a long time ago that the parents of the children I see know more than I do. When I acknowledge this fact, it's much easier to guide parents to make the changes that are needed for their children, as well as to reinforce the positive things they are already doing.

There are a number of key factors that help establish a good provider-patient relationship. First, give patients respect. Introduce yourself, and explain the role you will play in their care. Don't talk down to them. Use language the patient understands. Acknowledge positive points and accomplishments. Always think of them as people with their unique needs and beliefs.

Nurses are well positioned to establish good provider-patient relationships because of their education and training. Nursing is at the same time an art and a science and is based on the same key steps (assessment, implementation, and evaluation) of effective communication.

Patient-provider encounters should be used not only to determine the physical fitness of the patient and treat potential illnesses but also to assess the overall patient's well-being. For example, when a twelve-year-old Hispanic girl presented with vague stomach complaints that were preventing her from attending school, we discovered that physical symptoms and causes had nothing to do with her condition.

The girl was happy at home and loved her mother, who was a domestic worker and spoke only Spanish. She was also a very good student. Yet recently she had refused to go to school. By talking with her and her mother, we discovered that she had been bullied and threatened of physical assault by a group of children in the school.

We taught both her and her mother to talk to the school counselor, request a Spanish translator, and speak with the families of the other children. We did a role-play with the mother so she would feel comfortable once at school. We also recommended she mention that the police would get involved if this would not stop.

It was priceless to see the smile on the mother's face when she came back to our office a few weeks later for a follow-up visit. It is also priceless to know that the girl is now happy in school and doing very well academically.

Nurses can make a difference in their patients' lives. This is why I think nurses should always advocate for their patients' rights, especially in the case of underserved populations.

In all disease areas, effective communication is part of the cure. So, what is the best way to make it happen and overcome existing barriers to good patient-provider relationships?

One important step is to recognize that communication is a core clinical competence that can help improve effective use of time while helping patients comply with recommended treatment and healthy behaviors, as well as optimize overall patient satisfaction and outcomes. As for other kinds of interpersonal interactions, understanding the patient's cultural values, language preferences, differences in style, and specific meanings attributed to verbal and nonverbal expressions (see Table 4.1) are fundamental in establishing a satisfactory relationship.

It all starts with training. Some studies have shown that a patient's comprehension of health information is highly influenced by physicians' attitudes toward the importance of sharing information with their patients, which is shaped by their experience during medical training (Lukoschek, Fazzari, and Marantz, 2003; Eisenberg, Kitz, and Webber, 1983). For example, after three years of training, most medical residents tend to maintain a participatory attitude toward the decision-making process related to treatment and other recommendations. But after the same time period, surgical residents have switched to a more authoritarian attitude, even if they started with similar views as those of medical residents. This may reflect the hierarchical status and the task-oriented characteristics of surgeons' medical training (Eisenberg, Kitz, and Webber, 1983). Still, it would be unfair to generalize these findings without taking into account personal and cultural factors and experiences.

The example in Box 4.3 shows how different physician attitudes toward communication may result in different outcomes. It also points to the importance of an empathetic and participatory approach to provider-patient communications, which may be better suited to motivate patient compliance and establish true partnerships.

Box 4.3

Impact of Physician Attitudes on Patient Behavior: A True Story

Carmen was a sixty-one-year-old Spanish woman visiting her relatives in the United States. (The name of the patient as well as some other facts have been changed to protect the patient's and physicians' privacy.) During her trip, she was hospitalized for emergency spine surgery. She had been suffering from excruciating back pain that her physicians in Spain had misdiagnosed. While in the United States, her pain had worsened, and it turned out that a major infection had almost destroyed two of her vertebrae and was threatening her ability to walk.

The surgery was successful. However, Carmen felt isolated in a foreign hospital where she could not communicate with physicians and nurses. She spoke no English. Her relatives visited her as often as they could, but they also needed to deal with work and family obligations. They hired an interpreter for a few hours each day so Carmen could communicate with the hospital staff and perhaps feel a little less lonely.

Approximately fifteen days after the surgery, one of Carmen's physicians recommended that she try to stand up and sit on a chair. When he went to visit Carmen, he did not speak to her through the interpreter. He just instructed the nurse to help her and did not show much empathy for Carmen's pain. Carmen tried to get out of bed, but her pain was really bothering her. After the first attempt, she asked her interpreter to tell the physician that she was tired; she needed to rest and might try later.

A few hours later, her internal medicine specialist came by. She has been alerted about the earlier events and had called Carmen's relatives to discuss how to approach this issue. She greeted Carmen warmly and started to speak with her through her interpreter. Carmen talked about her attempt to stand up. She was still in a lot of pain. Despite the words of reassurance by her relatives who had just telephoned her, she was not sure she wants to try again. After all, in most countries, patients who have this kind of surgery, or even less invasive surgery, are confined to bed rest for much longer. Carmen found the request unreasonable.

The internist explained to Carmen that this was a common procedure in the United States and helped improve and accelerate a patient's rehabilitation. She highlighted the benefits of early ambulation. She also showed empathy for Carmen's pain. She mentioned that she would consult the pain specialists to see whether they could do something else to reduce her pain while she tried to regain mobility. Through the interpreter, she made sure that Carmen understood all the information and also asked if she had additional questions.

Carmen decided to try again with the help of the nurse and her interpreter. After a few attempts, she stood up and managed to sit on a chair. The entire team—the physician, the nurse, and the interpreter—encouraged and congratulated her for trying. She was still in a lot of pain, but she was happy about having succeeded. After all, this was a sign that things might go back to normal soon.

The physicians' recommendations proved to be effective. After less than a month after her surgery, Carmen was able to walk with the aid of a cane. Without the skillful communication intervention of the internal medicine specialist, this story might have had a different outcome. Carmen might have taken longer to stand up and perhaps suffered some of the medical consequences that may result from prolonged immobility.

Finally, it is also important to remember that most health care providers care about communicating well with their patients. For most physicians, nurses, and other care providers, helping others is one of the primary reasons they chose their profession. However, lack of communication training or other patient- or physician-related barriers may prevent some of them from being effective in establishing productive partnerships with their patients.

BARRIERS TO EFFECTIVE PROVIDER-PATIENT COMMUNICATIONS

Although many health care providers and public health professionals believe in the importance of optimal provider-patient communications, data suggest that many interactions could be improved. For example, in the United States, studies have shown that the average patient speaks for eighteen to twenty-two seconds before the physician interrupts (Belzer, 1999; American Medical Association, 2005a). Yet additional research shows that "if allowed to speak freely, the average patient would initially speak for less than 2 minutes" (American Medical Association, 2005a). Most important, in this short period of time, the patient would be able to express most of his or her concerns and symptoms (Belzer, 1999). This is likely to translate to a better provider-patient relationship as well as to "less follow-up visits, and shorter, more focused, interactions" (American Medical Association, 2005a).

Time is not the only barrier that could be addressed by effective communication. Most of the patient-related barriers in Table 4.2 could be removed by improved interactions and simplified information. For example, research shows that education level and language barriers may lead to low comprehension of medical information among patients (Lukoschek, Fazzari, and Marantz, 2003), so the use of jargon and complex medical terms negatively affects patients' comprehension. As the American Medical Association (2005b) suggests, most patients, regardless of their education level, prefer health information that "is simple and easy to understand." In fact, most people can relate to the feelings of vulnerability and stress associated with the diagnosis of a chronic or life-threatening disease or the fear that a temporary medical condition may jeopardize imminent events in one's life. In these situations, even well-educated patients may prefer not having to deal

TABLE 4.2. BARRIERS TO EFFECTIVE PROVIDER-PATIENT
COMMUNICATIONS: PATIENT FACTORS

Education level
Health literacy level
Language barriers
Cultural or ethnic differences
Age
Cognitive limitations
Lack of understanding of medical jargon and scientific terms
Disease-related stress
Power imbalance compared to health care providers

with the additional burden of making an effort to understand their provider's suggestions.

Similarly, language and cultural barriers can be addressed by the use of interpreters as well as an increased emphasis on cultural sensitivity and competence during medical training and communication training sessions (both before and after graduation) targeted to physicians and other health care providers. Research shows that patients may attribute different connotations to words that are used interchangeably by health professionals (Lukoschek, Fazzari, and Marantz, 2002; Heurtin-Roberts and Reisin, 1992). For example, African Americans attribute a different meaning to the words *hypertension* and *high blood pressure* (Lukoschek, Fazzari, and Marantz, 2002; Heurtin-Roberts, 1993), and this may affect their compliance to providers' suggestions (Heurtin-Roberts and Reisin, 1992).

As Heurtin-Roberts (1993) reports, the term *hypertension* is often replaced by "*high-pertension,* a chronic folk illness related to the biomedical hypertension and involving blood and nerves" (p. 285). A percentage of African Americans consider hypertension (or high-pertension) different from high blood pressure. High-pertension is regarded as a chronic condition that may become worse with older age and may be related to being "high tempered" (p. 290). Because it is considered a chronic illness, high-pertension is often a way to cope with difficult living conditions and is "one of the few means of controlling the behavioral environment available to the individual" (p. 285).

Some health care providers are quite savvy about cultural differences and other kinds of barriers, while others may not have had an opportunity to focus on them throughout their careers. From the provider's perspective, the demands and long hours of most health care professions are often too burdensome to leave time for pleasantry and more effective communication. Physicians in the primary care or pediatric environment are being required to see an increasing number of patients to satisfy managed care policies and other cost-cutting interventions (see Chapter Two).

In the United States, the number of office visits per year has increased by more than 40 percent, rising from 581 million in 1980 to approximately 838 million in 2003 (Robert Graham Center, 2005). Pediatricians, for example, see an average of 93.6 patients per week (American Academy of Pediatrics, 2005a). In addition, only 30 percent of them feel they have received adequate training in counseling and behavior modification techniques. Most are fulfilled by many elements of their professional life, but more than half feel "stressed trying to balance work and personal responsibilities" (American Academy of Pediatrics, 2005b).

Still, when most health care providers are given an opportunity to attend a communication training session, a most common reaction is pleasant surprise about skills, methods, and facts they may not have considered but that may help save time, improve overall patient satisfaction, and avoid conflicting or stressful patient-related situations. After some initial reluctance and skepticism, most providers enjoy testing their knowledge about communication methodologies as well as their skills as effective communicators. For many of them, hearing that most physicians do not let their patients speak for more than eighteen to twenty-two seconds without interrupting is often a surprise.

TRENDS IN PROVIDER-PATIENT COMMUNICATIONS

For several decades, people in Western countries have witnessed an ongoing shift in provider-patient relationships. Patients have become more involved with their own care and are more educated about health issues. Several patient organizations have worked to reinforce patients' rights and to create networks and tools that contribute to patient education and empowerment. Patient activism and lessons learned from the AIDS crisis, which have shown the importance of patient and public participation in health care decisions and policies, have contributed a new perspective on more traditional patient-provider communications.

Physicians, nurses, and other health care providers have been adapting to, and in many cases encouraging, a new kind of relationship where the power balance weighs less heavily on the physician's side. While many providers have been enjoying and adapting to this new trend, others have been struggling to find the time to accommodate patients' increasing requests and demands. Providers who have made successful transitions have thriving practices (patients like physicians who are good communicators and personable) and have relied on a number of tools developed by their professional associations.

Recent initiatives by the American Medical Association (2005d), the American Association of Family Practitioners (2005), and the Association of American Medical Colleges (1999) highlight the importance of physician-patient communications and aim to equip physicians with skills and tools to communicate effectively with patients and incorporate communication as a core competency at all levels of medical education.

Among them, the AAMC (1999), which represents 125 accredited medical schools in the United States, 16 medical schools in Canada, and over 400 teaching hospitals, has identified several communication-related goals for medical students. Also, the AMA Foundation (2005c) has become a member of the Partnership for Clear Health Communication, which includes several prestigious organizations and industry leaders, in an attempt to address the problem of low health literacy.

Increasingly health care providers are also learning communication skills that may help them break bad news. For example, special communication courses teach oncologists how to talk with cancer patients about their diagnosis, life expectancy, treatment, and other sensitive issues in an empathetic and effective way. Some of these courses use standard communication techniques such as role playing to help providers practice their communication approach with actors who pose as patients (Zuger, 2006).

Moreover, some professional organizations have been focusing on equipping both practitioners and patients with communication skills and tips. Ask Me 3, an initiative of the Partnership for Clear Health Communication, teaches patients to ask their providers three questions that will help them understand their problem and recommended solutions (American Medical Association, 2005b). This approach may help patients stay focused, ask the right questions, and minimize miscommunication with their providers. At the same time, it is a service to physicians and other health care providers since it may lead to shorter and more focused conversations.

Although there is still a lot to do in the area of provider-patient communication, new trends and initiatives in Western countries have established a path for a more participatory attitude to health care. The hope is that this will teach patients to make the best use of encounters with providers and help providers to be more effective at conveying information. In most developing countries, as well as in many traditional cultures where the power balance has not shifted yet, health communication training and other kinds of interventions can help encourage people become more responsible for health care decisions by communicating better with their physicians. In doing so, it is important to remember that models that have worked in Western countries may not work in other regions of the world or among members of different ethnic groups.

TRANSFORMING PATIENT-PROVIDER RELATIONSHIPS INTO PARTNERSHIPS

By definition, partnerships require that all partners are equally committed to pursuing a common cause and are aware of their role. In the provider-patient relationship, the common cause is the patient's health.

Health communication can help improve provider-patient relationships by raising awareness of common communication issues as well as roles and responsibilities in achieving good health outcomes. Training in communication methodology and message development may help health care providers sharpen their communication skills and address patients' questions and concerns in a more effective way. It may also help physicians conduct conversations in a way that patients will stay on topic and feel that their provider is truly concerned about their health.

Ideally, communication training for health care providers should focus on these topics:

- A brief overview on communication methodologies and how to affect behavioral change
- How communication skills can help make effective use of time
- Benefits of effective communication
- Common barriers and how to address them
- Differences in cultural-, ethnic-, age-, and gender health-related beliefs and attitudes
- Practical tips and examples
- Interactive session in which health care providers practice and test their communication skills in different potential scenarios

Some practical tips that may help providers establish good and trusting relationships with their patients are common to all human interactions:

- Greet patients properly and according to their cultural and ethnic preferences. For example, calling patients by their first name is appropriate in many Western countries and can help break down barriers but is not advisable when addressing Korean patients, who prefer to be called by their full name (Matsunaga, Yamada, and Macabeo, 1998).
- Put patients at ease by smiling, asking about the patient's family, and establishing good eye contact (if culturally appropriate).
- Do not make patients feel that the next patient may be more important by looking at the watch or at the door (Belzer, 1999).
- Show empathy about patients' concerns and needs.
- Listen, and avoid interrupting.
- Help patients stay focused on their medical issues.
- Recognize nonverbal clues.
- Reinforce key messages and recommendations by providing written materials and scheduling follow-up visits or contacts.

Focusing on only the communication skills of health care providers may not be sufficient to achieve an effective patient-provider partnership. As patients' participation in health decisions increases, communication tools and events targeted to patients may help them do their share in establishing a true partnership with their providers. Primarily, training can help patients in several ways:

- Asking the right questions.
- Staying focused.
- Becoming familiar with common medical terms.
- Understanding how to differentiate between credible and noncredible informational sources (on the Internet as well as in other settings).
- Dealing with conflicts or other kinds of impediments that may prevent them from following or trusting a provider's recommendations.
- Showing respect for the provider's time and experience.

Communication specialists can help address issues in provider-patient relationships by helping professional associations, patient groups, and individual health care providers understand the issues at stake, as well as improve overall communication skills. They can also help influence policies and medical curricula to recognize the central role that effective communication can have on health outcomes.

TECHNOLOGY-MEDIATED COMMUNICATIONS

A discussion about interpersonal communications would not be complete without acknowledging the impact that the advent of the Internet, video technology, telephone, and other media has had on interpersonal relationships over several decades. Increasingly, many interactions are mediated by technology and take place using e-mail, voice mail, videoconferencing, or other media channels. This may shape the quality and implications of communication by depriving it of nonverbal expressions (for example, facial expressions, gestures) and other influences (for example, the potential impact of different venues—formal versus informal venues—on health care or business conversations) that are normally common in face-to-face encounters.

Still, as several authors report, even when people rely on electronic media, they continue to engage in the process of *grounding*, which refers to the ability to find, understand, and share common meanings (Brennan and Lockridge, 2006; Brennan, 1990, 2004; Clark and Brennan, 1991; Clark and Schaefer, 1989; Clark and

Wilkes-Gibbs, 1986; Schober and Clark, 1989). Take the example of an e-mail in which a mother asks a close friend to pick up her child from school. If the e-mail states only, "Could you please pick up my child from school?" the request may not be clear unless the recipient already knows the school's address, the dismissal time, the names of the child and the teacher, as well as where he or she should bring the child. These additional facts will allow the recipient to evaluate and eventually rule out the existence of potential conflicts (for example, previous work commitments) or other impediments. Still, the mother would have to wait for her friend's reply. This dynamic is quite similar to what occurs in face-to-face encounters. As other authors highlight, the interpersonal exchange in both cases has two phases: the presentation phase, when the mother asks her friend for help and describes the task's requirements, and the acceptance phase, which implies the need for the friend's reply to confirm he or she understood and accepted the task (Brennan and Lockridge, 2006; Clark and Schaefer, 1989).

In health care, technology-mediated communications have provided a private forum to discuss sensitive matters, connect with others who may have experienced similar health issues, network, and learn about new medical solutions, among others. They have also affected provider-patient relationships. For example, some physicians may complain about the number of unnecessary questions and concerns that patients raise because of noncredible medical facts found on the Internet. Yet the Internet and other technology advances have improved the ability of patients and the general public to participate in personal and public health decisions.

In the case of life-threatening conditions such as HIV/AIDS, the use of the Internet has increased people's ability to deal with their illness. Primarily, use of the Internet appears to have influenced the coping skills of people living with HIV by promoting individual empowerment, increasing social support, and helping them help others (Reeves, 2000).

The influence of media technology on interpersonal communications and other aspects of health communication varies from population to population and group to group. It is related to media access as well as specific media uses and preferences among members of intended audiences. It is obviously more widespread in developed countries than in many countries in the developing world, where more conventional ways of communications (for example, word of mouth) may still predominate, especially in remote areas.

Still, when using any form of technology to communicate about health matters, it is important to remember and apply all general principles and values that pertain to interpersonal communications. Gender, age, and cultural, ethnic, and geographical factors as well as literacy levels still influence technology-mediated communications and should be considered. This is about using one of the many kinds of media to have a heart-to-heart discussion about health and health behaviors.

KEY CONCEPTS

- Interpersonal communications is an important action area of health communication.
- Interpersonal behavior and communications are highly influenced by cultural-, social-, age-, and gender-related aspects, as well as literacy levels and individual factors and attitudes.
- The dynamics of interpersonal communication are determined by signs (for example, involuntary acts) and symbols (for example, use of verbal expressions) that may differ among cultures and groups.
- Examples of interpersonal communications are personal selling, counseling, and provider-patient communications.
- Personal selling refers to (1) one-on-one engagement of intended audiences in their own homes, offices, or places of work and leisure and (2) the ability to sell one's image and expertise, an important skill in most consulting activities. It is an acquired communication skill that requires training but is also dependent on individual, social, and cultural factors. The two definitions are strongly connected and interdependent in their practical application.
- Personal selling interventions may not be very effective in the absence of other communication activities (for example, public relations, community mobilization) that would help create a receptive environment for door-to-door interventions and the message they carry.

- In counseling, which could be defined as the help provided by a professional on personal, psychological, health, or professional matters, personal selling is a powerful determinant of one's ability to have an impact on the beliefs, attitudes, and behavior of the person who is seeking counsel.
- Provider-patient communications is an important area of interpersonal communications and has been shown to affect patient satisfaction, retention, and overall health outcomes.
- Effective communication in the provider-patient setting depends on several patient- and physician-related factors, as well as external factors (for example, time constraints, managed care requirements).
- Communication specialists can help improve provider-patient communications. They can help health care providers and patients understand the issues at stake and improve their communication skills. They can also work with professional associations, patient groups, and individual health care providers to help them influence policies and university curricula, including communication as a core clinical competency.
- Technology advances have had a tremendous impact on interpersonal communications. Many interpersonal communications are now mediated by technology and take place using e-mail, videoconferencing, telephone, and other media.
- Technology-mediated communications are influenced by many of the same factors that rule interpersonal communications, such as literacy levels and cultural, ethnic, age, gender, and individual factors.

For Discussion and Practice

1. Describe the most common verbal and nonverbal clues that, according to your culture, age group, gender, family values, personal preferences, or others, may affect your satisfaction with health-related encounters and communications and prompt you or your peers to comply with the health care provider recommendations. For example, how do you like to be greeted by your physician? Is there any specific personal or cultural value or belief that you need to have acknowledged in order to trust and comply with the health information being

presented to you? Is there any nonverbal clue that you may find confusing or offensive?

2. Maria is a forty-one-year-old Caucasian woman who is expecting her first baby. Eight weeks into the pregnancy, it becomes clear that she is likely to have a miscarriage. She really wants the baby and may be very upset at the idea of a miscarriage, especially because she fears she may not become pregnant again. Think of how her physician should break the bad news in a way that would acknowledge Maria's feelings and set realistic expectations. Use role playing to simulate the actual discussion, and try to envision some of Maria's potential questions. Evaluate the pros and cons of potential physician approaches and attitudes toward communication on this matter.

3. In this chapter, personal selling is defined as one-on-one door-to-door engagement of intended audiences and the ability to sell one's image and expertise. Discuss practical examples from your professional or personal experience or recent readings that illustrate these two definitions.

4. Review Figure 4.1 and use five to ten adjectives to describe the style and communication approaches of physicians 1 and 2. Then discuss key factors that in your opinion influenced the mother's decision in both scenarios.

CHAPTER FIVE

PUBLIC RELATIONS AND PUBLIC ADVOCACY

IN THIS CHAPTER

- Public Relations Defined: Theory and Practice
- The Power of Mass Media in Health Care Decisions
- Key Elements of Public Relations Programs
- PR Evaluation Parameters
- When Public Relations Becomes Public Advocacy
- Key Concepts
- For Discussion and Practice

"Years ago, Americans grabbed toast and coffee for breakfast. Public relations pioneer Edward Bernays changed that" (Spiegel, 2005). Bernays, whom many regard as the historical father of public relations, referred to many of the theories of his uncle, Sigmund Freud, in developing a public relations campaign to help convince Americans that "bacon and eggs was the true all American breakfast" (Spiegel, 2005; Museum of Public Relations, 2005) and that it was ultimately healthier. Bernays's campaign in the mid-1920s was successful at changing the public's mind (Museum of Public Relations, 2005). Although eggs and bacon have been somewhat eclipsed by new habits, such as eating cold cereals or not eating breakfast at all (ABC News, 2005), they remain a very popular breakfast: only one in ten Americans usually eat toast or some other kind of bread or pastry (ABC News, 2005).

Outside the breakfast setting, public relations strategies and activities are normally used to create interest among multiple publics about an idea, a product, a specific behavior, a company, an institution, or a nonprofit organization. Ethical public relations relies on reputable facts and figures and has found many applications as part of health communication interventions in the commercial, nonprofit, and public health sectors.

This chapter establishes public relations as one of the action areas of health communication and reviews some key aspects of its theory and practice. It also provides practical suggestions on key success factors of a public relations campaign. Finally, it touches on the role of public relations in advocacy and government relations.

PUBLIC RELATIONS DEFINED: THEORY AND PRACTICE

Public relations (PR) is defined as "the art and science of establishing and promoting a favorable relationship with the public" (*American Heritage Dictionary of the English Language,* 2004). The word *relationship* is fundamental to all definitions of PR, as well as their practical applications. As with other action areas of health communication, PR is a relationship-based discipline. Similarly to the entire field of health communication, health care PR is based on an in-depth understanding of its publics, as well as their needs, wants, and desires. This overall concept applies to all functions of PR listed and defined in Table 5.1: public affairs, community relations, issues or crisis management, media relations, and marketing PR.

PUBLIC RELATIONS THEORY

The theoretical basis of PR has been influenced not only by Bernays's relationship with Sigmund Freud, the father of psychoanalysis, but also by many other observations and models. Nevertheless, some of Bernays's theoretical assumptions still apply to the modern practice of PR. If you want people to do what you want, "you don't hook into what they say. You try to find out what they really want" (National Public Radio, 2005), according to Bernays. This concept recognizes the importance of psychological, emotional, and subconscious factors in human behavior, one of the main ideas Freud developed (National Public Radio, 2005; Museum of Public Relations, 2005).

TABLE 5.1. Public Relations Functions in Health Care

Public affairs	A strategic approach to promote public discussion and, eventually, agreement on health policies or administrative procedures that may be practiced by a given organization or its key stakeholders and intended audiences.
Community relations	An area of PR practice through which practitioners and organizations establish, cultivate, and strive to maintain mutually beneficial relationships with the communities (defined as groups with common values, causes, and needs) that can affect or are affected by their actions. Community relations is one of the many aspects of constituency relations and building (see Chapter Eight) and a component of all other health communication areas.
Issues management	A multifaceted and "formal management process to anticipate and take appropriate action on emerging trends, concerns, or issues likely to affect an organization and its stakeholders" (Issue Management Council, 2005).
Crisis management	A proactive approach based on the advance development of contingency plans and activities to anticipate, avert, and deal with potential crises. It often includes a strong focus on the use of the mass media to help organizations assure their publics that a solution is being implemented and a specific concern or issue is being addressed.
Media relations	A proactive and reactive approach that aims at interacting with key health journalists and makes "use of the media in a planned way" (Economic and Social Research Council, 2005a).
Marketing public relations	An area of PR that focuses on developing strategic programs and relationships that would support endorsement and use of the organization's health products and services among its key stakeholders and publics.

Some of the most recent theories in PR also highlight the relevance of psychological aspects of human personality in moving intended audiences through the three desirable effects of PR interventions: "attention, acceptance and action" (Smith, 1993, p. 193). For example, some authors advocate the use of the psychological type theory in public relations practice (Smith, 1993). This theory has been primarily used in education, religion, and business to understand and predict "patterns of human interaction" (p. 177). According to Smith, if applied in PR, it could help practitioners tailor their messages to intended audiences by taking into account their personal psychological type and learning preferences. As Table 5.2 shows, Smith (1993) identified four primary types:

ST: Sensitive/thinking
SF: Sensitive/feeling
NT: Intuitive/thinking
NF: Intuitive/feeling

Each of these types has distinguished characteristics and learning habits (listed in Table 5.2) that influence their decision-making process, as well as the way they may react to different ways that information is presented (for example, factual information versus information that appeals primarily to emotions).

Although the psychological type theory may be difficult to apply rigorously to actual PR practice (in fact, data on psychological types exist only for select audiences and may be too expensive to collect in a timely and statistically significant manner), keeping in mind the influence of both "reason and sentiment" (Smith, 1993, p. 195) on people's beliefs and behavior is quite common among PR practitioners. Understanding people's learning styles and other preferences is part of the process of preparing for the development of a PR program.

Similarly, the notion of multiple publics and the need to address them differently in response to their characteristics, needs, desires, and issue-specific beliefs is common practice in PR. It is also one of the main assumptions of field dynamics models and methods, that, in their application to PR, attempt to explain the relationship between an organization and its different publics, as

Table 5.2. Characteristics of Types Relevant to Public Relations

	ST	SF	NT	NF
People who prefer . . .	Sensing and thinking	Sensing and feeling	Intuition and thinking	Intuition and feeling
Focus on . . .	Facts: What is . . .	Facts: What is . . .	Possibility: What could be	Possibility: What could be
Make decisions based on . . .	Impersonal analysis; reason	Personal warmth; emotion	Personal warmth; reason	Impersonal analysis; emotion
Tend toward . . .	Practical and pragmatic	Sympathetic and friendly	Logical and ingenious	Enthusiastic and insightful
Adept at . . .	Applying facts and experience	Meeting daily needs of people	Developing theoretical concepts	Recognizing aspirations of people
Sensitive to . . .	Cause and effect	Feelings of others	Technique and theory	Possibility for people

Note: ST: Sensitive/Thinking; SF: Sensitive/Feeling; NT: Intuitive/Thinking; NF: Intuitive/Feeling.

Source: Smith, R. (1993). Psychological Type and Public Relations: Theory, Research and Applications. *Journal of Public Relations Research* 5(3), 177–199. © Lawrence Erlbaum Associates. Used by permission.

well as the mutual interaction among such publics. For example, one method describes and compares this interaction in terms of "dominance-submissiveness, friendly-unfriendly, and group versus personal orientation" (Springston, Keyton, Leichty, and Metzger, 1992, p. 81). In practice, when there is public debate about an organization, an idea, a product, or a behavior, it is quite common to find a variety of opinions, levels of involvement (for example, leaders versus followers), and interest and attitudes among multiple audiences. PR interventions often tip the preexisting balance and prompt a shift in the attitudes and opinions of multiple audiences. As a result, it may also change the dynamics of the relationship among such audiences.

Within this perspective, PR is considered "the management function that establishes and maintains mutually beneficial relationships between an organization and the publics on whom its success or failure depends" (Cutlip, Center, and Broom, 1994, p. 2). The concept of PR as a relationship management discipline has emerged as a fundamental part of its theoretical basis (Ledingham, 2003) and finds application in actual PR practice. As Center and Jackson observe (1995), "the proper term for the desired outcomes of public relations practice is public relationships. An organization with effective public relations will attain positive public relationships" (p. 2).

The value of PR practitioners to the general public and the organizations they serve is often determined by the extent and closeness of their contacts with the media and community representatives, as well as other key stakeholders. In this way, PR strategies and activities become a fundamental tool of larger health communication and public health interventions by means of expanding the reach of health messages, as well as using the power of mutually beneficial relationships to advance the discussion and solution of a given health issue. Several other authors or organizations also include PR among communication's key action areas (World Health Organization, 2003) or recognize, among other fields, the role or influence of PR in health communication (Springston and Lariscy, 2001).

PUBLIC RELATIONS PRACTICE

While the practice of public relations is less than a hundred years old, PR is now employed by a broad variety of organizations beyond companies that sell products, including universities, foundations, nonprofit organizations, schools, hospitals, and associations. In fact, the official definition of the Public Relations Society of America (PRSA) highlights both the widespread use of PR by different types of organizations and the existence of multiple publics from which these organizations "must earn consent and support. . . . Public relations helps an organization and its publics adapt mutually to each other," notes the PRSA (2005a). In most cases, it also helps organizations and their publics discuss and eventually come to an agreement on ideas, recommended behaviors, products, or services. In this way, it becomes an essential area of health communication.

Over the past few decades, PR growth has been related to the diversification of the mass media and its increasing influence on society. While still relying primarily on print and broadcast media, PR has expanded its reach using the Internet and other technologies.

In the commercial world, PR helps create market share and se-cure product endorsement and use. In the public health world, it helps create a receptive public environment that could motivate people to change their behavior. In doing so, it provides the pub-lic with widespread access to information and helps build support for recommended health behaviors.

Nonprofit and commercial efforts to feature a specific disease area or health issue sometimes complement each other. For ex-ample, in promoting a product through the mass media, compa-nies often discuss other important facts, such as awareness about a disease, disease incidence, or risk factors. If the information is based on reputable sources and scientifically relevant data, these efforts may contribute to the disease awareness endeavors of many nonprofit and government organizations in the same field. In some cases (see Box 5.1), corporations may help tackle a general public health problem by providing resources, funds, and pro-grams to elicit interest in the subject.

Box 5.1

Johnson & Johnson's Campaign for Nursing's Future Initiative

Recognizing that the United States was experiencing the most severe nursing shortage in history, Johnson & Johnson, a multinational health care company, launched the Johnson & Johnson Campaign for Nurs-ing's Future in 2002. This is a multiyear, nationwide effort to enhance the image of the nursing profession, recruit new nurses, and retain nurses currently in the system.

Campaign elements have included: a *national television, print and interactive advertising campaign* in English and Spanish cele-brating nursing professionals and their contributions to health care; a multifaceted and highly visible *public relations campaign* with press releases, video news releases and satellite radio tours available to hun-dreds of media outlets across the country; *recruitment materials* in-cluding brochures, pins, posters and videos in English and Spanish distributed free of charge to hospitals, high schools, nursing schools, and nursing organizations; *fundraising* efforts for student scholarships, faculty fellowships, and grants to nursing schools to expand their program capacity; *celebrations at regional nursing events* to create enthusiasm and feelings of empowerment among local nursing communities; a Website (www.discovernursing.com) about the benefits of a nursing career featuring searchable links to hundreds of nursing scholarships, and more than 1,000 accredited nursing educational programs; and activities to *create and fund retention programs* designed to improve the nursing work environment. Numerous organizations, including the White House, with the Ron Brown Award for Corporate Leadership, the American Hospital Association, the American Organization of Nurse Executives, the National Student Nurses Association, the American Nurses Association and NurseWeek, have honored Johnson & Johnson for this campaign and their overall contribution to addressing the current nursing shortage.

Key Outcomes

- Forty-six percent of 18–24 year olds who participated in a 2002 Harris Poll survey recalled the campaign.
- Sixty-two percent had discussed a nursing career for themselves or a friend.
- Twenty-four percent of the respondents in the above group said the campaign was a factor in their consideration.
- The discovernursing.com Website traffic has tallied over 3,000,000 unique visitors, spending an average of 12–15 minutes exploring the site.
- Surveys show that recruitment materials are being used by 97 percent of high schools and 73 percent of nursing schools.
- Eighty-four percent of nursing schools that received the materials reported an increase in applications and enrollment for the Fall 2004 semester.
- The Campaign has raised over $8 million (to date) at regional fundraising events. These funds have been used to provide scholarships to thousands of nursing students and nurse educators and have been complemented by over 100 Johnson & Johnson grants to area nursing schools to help them expand their program capacity and, therefore, accept more students.
- The American Association of Colleges of Nursing reported that Baccalaureate nursing school enrollments have seen double-digit increases every year since the launch of the Campaign in 2002.

Key Success Factors

- Relevance of the issue to Johnson & Johnson's key publics as well as the community at large, and organizational competence to address it
- Strong relationship-building effort in support of the campaign with organizations including health care systems, nursing schools and professional associations around the country
- Multi-media strategy with consistent messages in broadcast, print, publicity, special events, printed materials, videos and the Internet

---

While the issue of partnerships with commercial entities will be discussed in Chapters Eight and Twelve as part of the broader subject of partnerships in health communication, it is worth mentioning here that many reputable nonprofit and government organizations, including the U.S. National Cancer Institute (National Cancer Institute and National Institutes of Health, 2002), consider collaborations or partnerships with for-profit entities. In doing so, many of them have developed strict guidelines and criteria that help them protect the public interest and avoid endorsing specific products or services (see Chapter Eight).

PR practice must be held to high ethical standards. The ongoing debate on PR ethics and related dos and don'ts is legitimate and should never be abandoned. However, while it is fair to assume that the main motivation of any industry is profit, it would be unfair to think that all companies would go to any length to sell their products.

The power of the mass media, on which PR relies, can be abused if facts are misrepresented or inflated. However, in the battle for free media coverage, this is a risk that the general public may encounter with a variety of organizations (even those with the best intentions) if they become too enamored with an idea or the opportunity to raise their own profile and visibility. Because of the nature of their profession, PR practitioners need to meet the challenges of serving their client's interests (whether their client is a business, a nonprofit, or a government organization) while preserving an honest and ethical relationship with the publics they cultivate and address. Most professional societies in this field, including the PRSA (2005b), have a comprehensive code of ethics for their members.

Table 5.3 lists some of the key characteristics of ethical PR programs. Many of them are common sense but always should be considered in designing and implementing a PR campaign.

In addition to promoting public discussion of ideas, services, or behaviors, PR also contributes to increasing the visibility of nonprofit organizations, commercial entities, and other kinds of institutions, as well as their mission, activities, and spokespeople. This is a fundamental function of PR that helps establish organizations and their experts as leaders in a field. Together with other kinds of activities, PR helps them gain the favorable reputation and the public respect that are needed to have an impact on behavioral and social change, as well as to encourage others to join the debate on a health issue and its potential solutions.

As an example of PR activities reaching out to multiple publics, Box 5.2 shows the Media and Public Relations page of the Web site of the Schepens Eye Research Institute, an affiliate of Harvard Medical School. The page includes information that helps position the institute as a resource for the media on information on eye diseases and related research and treatment news. By providing resources on the institute's history, mission, and activities, as well as

TABLE 5.3. KEY CHARACTERISTICS OF ETHICAL PUBLIC RELATIONS PROGRAMS

Based on research

Feature reputable and scientifically relevant facts and figures

Strive to maintain an honest and direct relationship with the publics they address

Adhere to general ethical principles such as identifying sources, conflicts of interest, and grant disclosures

Seek to establish trusting and long-term relationships between organizations and their publics and therefore discourage unethical approaches that may harm relationships

Include standard procedures to promptly correct potential mistakes and misinformation

Encourage free information exchange

Preserve the public interest

the background and expertise of its faculty and spokespeople, the page appeals to journalists in search of story ideas on the subject. In addition, it appeals to many different audiences (for example, health care providers, professional organizations, patient groups) that may have an interest in this field and may want to engage in collaborations or just participate in the public debate on eye disease research and treatment.

Box 5.2

Using the Internet as a Key Public Relations Channel: The Schepens Eye Research Institute

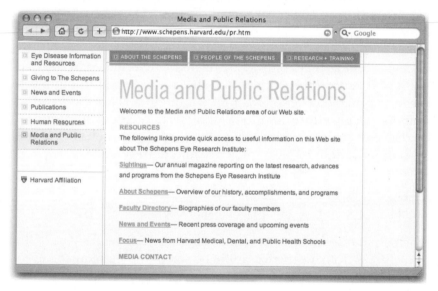

Source: The Schepens Eye Research Institute, "Media and Public Relations" (http://www.theschepens.org/pr.htm). Copyright © 2003, The Schepens Eye Research Institute. Retrieved in November 2005. Used by permission.

PR VERSUS ADVERTISING: THE DIFFERENCES

Media coverage stemming from PR campaigns is free of charge, but placing a story requires an in-depth understanding of journalists' and audiences' preferences among PR practitioners and the organizations they represent. Faced with countless choices for story ideas, journalists select what they cover primarily on the basis of its newsworthiness, which is what they think their audiences may find interesting (Fog, 1999; Gans, 1980; Erickson, Devlieger, and Sung, 1987). Other parameters include level of comfort or knowledge about the topic, the way the information is framed and presented to them, and the relationship they have with their sources, such as PR practitioners, organizations, and politicians. In this highly competitive environment, achieving national media coverage is a major endeavor.

Different from advertising, PR is a less controlled but more credible way to approach the media. In advertising, organizations pay for the print or broadcast space to place their ads, so the media have no editorial power on the ad content. The ad content is immediately recognized and identified with a specific health organization by the media's audiences. In PR, the media placement is free of charge, but its final tone and content are determined by the journalist who authors the story. In the absence of breakthrough news, achieving media coverage using PR strategies is not easy and requires strategic efforts and tools, long-term relationships with the media, and a true understanding of the concept of newsworthiness. Most important, it requires patience and perseverance.

THE POWER OF MASS MEDIA IN HEALTH CARE DECISIONS

No one can dispute the increasing power of mass media. Part of this power stems from the media's influence on public opinion and everyday decisions. Often the general public view the mass media as an objective source of information. Another important factor is related to the media's relationships with important decision makers and stakeholders around the world, including governments and multilateral organizations as well as the nonprofit and business sectors. In addition to the entertainment appeal of the media, both of these factors have contributed to the increasing power of the mass media.

Since mass media are the main channel of mass communication in Western society, competition for media coverage is quite fierce. People rely on the media as their main source of news and are increasingly conditioned in their health, political, or life choices by what they hear or read (Fog, 1999).

For many successful companies, one of their major accomplishments, other than the services or goods they manufacture and sell, is the success of their advertising and media coverage efforts, which help strengthen their reputation and increase their visibility. In public health, the media can influence people's perception of disease severity, their views about the potential risk of contracting the disease, or their feelings about the need for prevention or treatment. Media coverage can also affect what people eat or do in their leisure time. It can help reduce the stigma associated with many diseases or break the cycle of misinformation and silence about health conditions that are underdiagnosed, undertreated, or underreported. It can help convince policymakers to develop new prevention or treatment policies.

In summary, especially in the United States and most of Europe, where there is a widespread media culture, mass media can have an enormous impact on people's health behaviors. In fact, in the average U.S. home, "the time per day that TV is on is 7 hours and 40 minutes" (TV-Turnoff Network, 2005). People do not see their best friends that often, so the media may become more influential than actual people.

Mass media campaigns have proven to be effective in helping to increase immunization rates (Porter and others, 2000; Paunio and others, 1991), vaccination knowledge (McDivitt, Zimicki, and Hornik, 1997), cervical cancer screening among Hispanic women (Ramirez and others, 1999), awareness of the risks associated with smoking (Murray, Prokhorov, and Harty, 1994), and use of tobacco (Centers for Disease Control, 1994b). The list of media influence (positive or negative) on health beliefs and behavior is enormous.

Most important, mass media have been defining the concept of health and fitness by bringing into everyone's homes seductive images of men and women, such as healthy and fit celebrities, with whom average people would like to identify. Sometimes these images are used for the right purpose (for example, encouraging people to exercise or remember about their annual medical checkup), but other times they promote unhealthy behaviors such as smoking. The power of mass media is such that not everyone can understand what is really behind a seductive image and make the right health decision.

Vulnerability to the power of the mass media and some of the unhealthy behaviors the media may consciously or subconsciously promote is related to many factors, including educational level, prior knowledge or experience on the subject, age, socioeconomic conditions, personal experience, and psychological status. For example, in recognizing the vulnerability of young adults and adolescents to media messages that encourage smoking, the U.S. government in 1998 limited forms of advertisement or PR activities that would directly target this age group (Centers for Disease Control, 1999; Advertising Law Resource Center, 2006) with positive messages on smoking. Similarly, in many countries, direct-to-consumer advertising is prohibited for prescription drugs and other kinds of products that are used for the treatment or prevention of serious diseases (DES Action Canada, 2006; Mintzes and Baraldi, 2006; Mintzes and others, 2002).

This brings us back to the discussion on the ethics of PR as well as the importance of following the code of ethics highlighted by many professional societies and keeping in mind the suggestions in Table 5.3. Fortunately, most PR practitioners think that preserving the ethics of their actions is in the best interest of their own practice, as well as the publics and organizations they serve.

DOS AND DON'TS OF MEDIA RELATIONS

Interacting with the media is an acquired skill. Because of limited time and conflicting priorities, journalists do not like to be approached by people who sound incompetent about the story they are trying to place or show little awareness of the media industry and its rules. In an attempt to help junior PR practitioners approach the media in the way the media want to be approached, several professional societies, including the Public Relations Society of America, organize workshops and lunch meetings in which journalists speak about their daily routine, their preferred communication channels (for example, e-mail, telephone, or fax), and the kind of health issues and stories they may be interested in covering. Since PR is increasingly recognized as an important skill in public health, as well as a key area of health communications, one of the sessions of the 2005 annual meeting of the American Public Health Association focused on media advocacy and featured journalists from broadcast and print media who discussed the dos and don'ts of media and press relations with public health professionals.

In approaching the media, it is essential to remember that they are just another audience, so it is important to know them well. Because of their influence on many of the publics of PR and larger health communication interventions, knowing them and understanding how to spur their interest in a story and its core messages is even more critical than with many other audiences.

The average U.S. reporter now receives approximately two hundred e-mails each day, and some receive as many as five hundred per day (101PublicRelations, 2005). They have time to read only a small portion of them, and usually it is the first few lines. The *media pitch,* defined as a brief summary statement, letter, or e-mail message that explains why the information is new, relevant to the journalist's target audience, and worth covering, should be the focus of these first few lines. Only stories that stand out for their newsworthiness and relevance to the publication's audience actually are published; each reporter files no more than one to three stories on any given day.

Using the mass media to publicize the core messages and activities of a larger health communication or public health intervention can help expand the reach of the program to different audiences and publics. It can also help create a critical mass in support of the recommended health behavior or social change. However, getting there, and seeing a story published, is a story in itself. Once the first stories are published, it is still important to secure ongoing attention from multiple media to reach new audiences or reinforce the message over time. Table 5.4 highlights some of the dos and don'ts of media relations. All of them are based on PR practice. Others may apply to specific situations, countries, reporters, or media channels.

WHAT MAKES A STORY NEWSWORTHY

The concept of newsworthiness is strictly related to the preferences, needs, and interests of the target audience of a given publication or media outlet. For example, it is not a surprise that most parenting magazines in the United States and Europe dedicate a lot of space to stories on babies or toddlers and their sleeping habits. Sleep deprivation is a common problem among new parents as well as parents of toddlers who struggle to teach their children how to

TABLE 5.4. DOS AND DON'TS OF MEDIA RELATIONS

Do	Don't
Identify the names and interests of journalists who usually cover health generally or specific health topics.	Waste reporters' time by pitching them randomly regardless of their specific interests.
Establish long-term relationships.	Use jargon or technical terms in writing press releases and speaking with reporters (ESRC, 2005b).
Be aware of reporters' deadlines and respond in a timely fashion.	
Be polite, accurate, and helpful.	Agree to disclose information off the record unless you have a special relationship with a reporter. You are always at risk of seeing that information in print.
Understand why reporters are calling. Are they seeking to quote you, or do they want only a background briefing (ESRC, 2005b)?	
Make yourself available for a few days after issuing a press release.	Call repeatedly or leave multiple voice messages on the same topic.
Make sure all partners in your program are aware of their media-related roles and responsibilities (ESRC, 2005b).	
Media-train key spokespeople.	
Learn when reporters are on deadline, and don't call at that time.	
Read the news. It is the best way to understand reporters.	

go to sleep on their own and stay asleep for the entire night. Parenting magazines and other consumer publications perceive the topic as something that sells the magazine to their audience. In fact, in 2005 alone, there were at least seventy-four articles on "getting your baby to sleep" or related topics in different kinds of consumer publications (LexisNexis, 2006).

Sometimes newsworthy topics for specific publications can be found in the publication name. For example, the *Chapel Hill News* looks primarily for stories that appeal to the residents of Chapel Hill, North Carolina. *Infectious Diseases News* includes breaking news, editorials, and feature articles that appeal primarily to infectious disease specialists but also to other health care providers (for example, family physicians, pediatricians, and internal medicine specialists) who are involved in preventing and managing infectious diseases among their patients. The type of media (print, radio, television, or online publications) influences the concept of newsworthiness as well.

Understanding the relevance of a story to the media's target audiences is only the first step in defining whether the story may be newsworthy. Many other criteria need to be met to maximize the chances for media coverage of an organization's data, information, and messages—for example:

- The story's timeliness: it just happened or is about to happen.
- The existence of new data or information from clinical trials, opinion surveys, and other kinds of studies and their potential impact on the media's intended publics.
- The presentation of these new data or information at a major professional, community, or interdisciplinary meeting or their publication in a prestigious peer-reviewed journal, which would legitimize the public impact and relevance of the information.
- Reputable spokespeople, such as opinion leaders (for example, top physicians, researchers, and community leaders), top executives, or celebrities who appeal to the media's target audiences.
- A new angle to a story of current interest or to an issue that has not been covered for a while. Reading the news is the best way to find new media hooks.
- Human interest stories, such as the testimonial of a mother who decided not to immunize her child who then died or almost died of a vaccine-preventable disease.
- The announcement of a new large program or event targeted to the media's intended audiences and either providing a unique health-related service or conveying big names in the field.
- The use of appropriate media tools.

The following PR tools are the ones most commonly used.

- *Press release:* A written announcement of an event, program, or other newsworthy items for distribution to the media. It includes information on the details of the event, program, or news item; the organization that issues the press release; facts and data on the topic being featured; telephone and e-mail of a media contact person; and the name and credentials of an expert to interview.
- *Media alert:* A one-page announcement including information on the what, when, where, and who of a specific event and the telephone number and e-mail address of a media contact. It is used for media distribution to announce press conferences, speakers' availability for telephone interviews, and program kick-off events, for example.
- *Op-ed article:* A signed article expressing a personal opinion and the viewpoint of a specific group or organization. It is usually published on the page opposite the editorial page and is targeted to one publication. It is not sent to multiple publications simultaneously.
- *Public service announcement:* Noncommercial advertising for distribution to radio, broadcast, or print media that includes information and a call to action for the public good. The format varies to accommodate the characteristics of print, radio, and broadcast media. It can also be sent to multiple media outlets for free and unrestricted use.
- *Radio news release:* The radio version of the press release, sent to radio stations for free use, and lasting forty-five to sixty seconds. It includes a sound bite from one of the PR program's spokespeople.
- *Video news release:* A video segment designed in the style of a news report and distributed to local and national television and cable networks for free and unrestricted use. It is rarely used in the United States but remains somewhat common in some European countries. Media outlets often use only portions of the release. It is provided for free and unrestricted use.
- *B-roll:* A series of video shots on a specific topic, packaged in the format of unedited material (footage) and distributed to local and national televisions and cable networks. It is commonly used in the United States to pitch a story to local TV news shows.

- *Mat release:* A ready-to-use feature story, usually including a photograph or some artwork, for distribution to community newspapers and other local and smaller publications for free and unrestricted use.

    Selecting the right tools for target media is not an optional step. Since all of these tools are designed, among others, to facilitate the reporter's job and make it easy to cover the story, using the wrong tool sends a negative message to the media about the source's knowledge of the media industry and, potentially, his or her level of competence on the issue at hand. (Table 5.5 identifies the mass media channels and most common PR tools used to address each of them specifically).

KEY ELEMENTS OF PUBLIC RELATIONS PROGRAMS

PR plans and key success factors borrow heavily from other action areas of health communication and in general from the overall field. Although the **tactics** (those activities, materials, and events that are strategically connected with other elements of health communication planning) are different, all of these approaches exist to meet the overall goal of a health communication program.

TABLE 5.5. MASS MEDIA CHANNELS AND RELATED PUBLIC RELATIONS TOOLS

Media	Tools
Print media (for example, national newspapers, magazines)	Press releases, op-ed articles, letter-to-editor, print public service announcement, media alerts
Radio (local and national radio stations)	Radio news release, radio public service announcement, media alerts, live interview with expert (by telephone or in a studio)
Broadcast (national and local TV stations)	Press release, video news release, B-roll, public service announcement, media alerts
Local publications/ community newspapers	Mat release
Online publications	Press release, media alerts, opinion piece, public service announcement

PR strategies and activities cannot be developed in the absence of a careful analysis of the existing situation and needs. In fact, they should respond to the wants and desires of all intended constituencies and make it easy for them to understand and apply the information that is passed along through the media. For this purpose, it is important to create and identify multiple messages and media channels that will reach each intended audience (for example, the general public, opinion leaders, physicians, or policymakers). The level of complexity and the connotation of key messages as well as the types of publications and media outlets that need to be selected are quite different if the intervention targets policymakers instead of the general public. This approach also draws heavily on marketing and social marketing principles.

PR programs should take into account the needs and characteristics of the type of media being targeted. In some developing countries, it is still possible to engage the media in partnerships and coalitions. In the United States and most of the rest of the Western world, the media are just another audience and should be treated as such. Moreover, the PR component of a health communication program should be designed by keeping in mind the overall program goals and the other results the program is attempting to achieve.

Finally, methods of evaluation should be defined in advance and be related to the overall health communication intervention. As for other areas of health communication, it is important to remember that in most cases, PR interventions alone are not sufficient to achieve health communication goals and objectives. Most commonly, a multifaceted approach that complements other public health interventions and also relies on interpersonal communications, professional communications, and other strategic areas is likely to produce faster and more durable results.

Building public will and commitment to a health issue is a complex process. Integrating the use of the mass media with community involvement at the national or grassroots levels is likely to produce long-term results by creating the social and community support needed to effect and sustain behavioral and social change.

Moreover, instead of providing a quick fix and satisfying short-term wants and desires of intended audiences, a multifaceted approach is more effective at connecting existing values and beliefs systems with the recommended behavior or social change. In other words, one of the key functions of PR, community relations, should serve to engage community leaders and organizations to contribute in ways that are supportive of their key values and core mission.

PR EVALUATION PARAMETERS

Although PR results should be evaluated as part of the larger behavioral and social outcomes of the health communication program for which strategies and activities are designed, a few specific parameters are commonly used in PR to measure quantitative and qualitative results. (A complete discussion of evaluation parameters and methodologies of health communication interventions is included in Chapters Twelve and Thirteen. The methodologies discussed here more specifically apply only to PR and reflect current practice.)

As for all other areas of health communication, the evaluation and measurement of the PR component of a program should be related to the specific and measurable PR goals and objectives defined at the onset of the program (Institute for Public Relations, 1997, 2003). In other words, what was the PR component of the program trying to accomplish? What are or were the specific objectives of each strategy or activity? Which of them were accomplished?

The Institute for Public Relations (1997, 2003) defines three categories to measure PR programs:

- *PR outputs:* Short-term and process-oriented measurements, such as the number of stories published by the media, the number of times a specific spokesperson is quoted, the tone and content of the media coverage, and the number of Internet hits received by an online article.
- *PR outtakes:* The way the PR program is received by the media and other target audiences as well as overall message recall and retention. For example, did the media find the design and packaging of press materials appealing and easy to use? Was the language used in press releases and other materials received favorably, or did the media have problems understanding and using it? Did the actual message recipients (for example, the media's intended audiences such as consumers or professionals) respond positively to the message? Did the recipients ask for more information by, for example, going to a recommended Web site? Did they write any letters to the editor or commentaries in response to media coverage?

- *PR outcomes:* The evaluation and measurement of changes in the opinions, attitudes, or behaviors of the media's targeted audiences.

PR outputs can be simply measured by "counting, tracking and observing" (Institute for Public Relations, 1997, 2003, p. 7). In media and press relations efforts, a common parameter to measure PR outputs is the number of media impressions, defined as "the number of people who might have the opportunity to be exposed to a story that has appeared in the media" (Institute for Public Relations, 2002, p. 13). It is related to the total circulation (for example, number of copies sold by a newspaper or number of viewers of a TV news program) of a given publication or broadcast media outlet (Institute for Public Relations, 2002). For example, the *New York Times* has an audited circulation of approximately 1.2 million (daily issues) to 1.7 million (Sunday issue) readers (New York Times Company, 2005). Therefore, a story in the *Times* will generate 1.2 million to 1.7 million media impressions, depending on whether it is published on a weekday or on a Sunday.

PR outcomes and to some extent PR outtakes (for example, for the part concerning the evaluation of message recall and retention by intended audiences) can be measured only through extensive pre- and postintervention studies (Institute for Public Relations, 1997, 2003) and are difficult and expensive to assess. Common methodologies for evaluating PR outcomes as well as some types of PR outtakes are similar to those generally used in health communication. (These are discussed in Chapters Twelve and Thirteen.) The contribution of the PR component of a health communication intervention should be measured as part of the overall evaluation of such intervention in relation to its impact on social and behavioral change and the attainment of its public health or organizational goal.

WHEN PUBLIC RELATIONS BECOMES PUBLIC ADVOCACY

The American Heart Association (2006a) defines *public advocacy* as "the act of influencing decision makers and promoting changes to laws and other government policies to advance the mission of a particular organization or group of people." Similarly, many other organizations use public advocacy strategies—which also rely on the use of the mass media—to advance their agenda or preserve the interest of their key constituencies. Several of them have developed guides or specific training sessions to advance the public advocacy skills of their key constituencies as well as other organizations in the same field (for example, Society for Neuroscience, 2006; American Heart Association, 2006a).

Public advocacy strategies and tactics are also used to influence companies and other publics to change their policies or manufacturing practices. An example of public advocacy efforts targeted to the commercial sector is the HIV treatment access campaign by Doctors Without Borders and many other international organizations (Calmy, 2004; World Health Organization and Joint United Nations Programme on HIV/AIDS, UNAIDS, 2005) that have been advocating for a price reduction of essential HIV medications when sold in the developing world. While treatment access is actually dependent on many other factors in addition to price (see Chapter Two), their efforts were successful in engaging several pharmaceutical companies in the public debate as well as in an attempt to find appropriate solutions. Similarly, recent consumer awareness of the potentially negative health effects of transfat acids has motivated many companies in the food industry to develop transfat-free products (MSNBC, 2006; FoodNavigatorUSA, 2006a, 2006b; Unilever, 2006).

Public advocacy relies on multiple tools and activities, including community or town hall meetings and one-on-one encounters with policy and decision makers. However, a fundamental component of public advocacy efforts is the use of the mass media. More recently, public advocacy that heavily relies on the strategic use of the mass media is also called *media advocacy*.

For example, at the time this book is being written, the State of New Jersey is considering legislation that, if approved, would grant rights to adopted children to seek medical and personal information about their birth parents. This legislation is considered essential by several advocate groups as well as adoptees, who fear that lack of access to their medical and family history may jeopardize their health. Several op-ed pieces and letters to the editor, among the most common mass media vehicles used in public advocacy, have appeared in prominent local and national newspapers (Barbieri, 2005). All of them feature personal stories or testimonials of adoptees or highlight the official position of adoption and advocate groups.

Because of the power of the mass media to influence public opinion, local or national publications, community newsletters, broadcast media, and the Internet can all be useful channels to advance public commitment to and awareness of a health issue or policy. They can help create the critical mass that is needed to motivate legislators or other decision makers to endorse the policy being advocated by their publics. Public relations thus becomes public advocacy when it seeks to influence health policies, laws, and practices.

Public advocacy is very similar and uses the same tools as public affairs, a key PR function. However, in public advocacy, organizations and their constituencies go beyond promoting a public debate of policies and practices and demand the endorsement of specific policies or changes on existing practices and legislations. In order to appear legitimate in the eyes of decision makers, such demands need to be evidence based and gain the support of large percentages of a given group or population.

As a consequence, PR is also a fundamental component of government relations because of its ability to influence legislators and other key decision makers. As Paletz (1999) describes, congressional leaders and their staff review a variety of local and national newspapers, Web sites, journals, magazines, and other print and broadcast media outlets to monitor public response to legislative and policy matters. The tone and content of media coverage often shape their decisions and perspectives on a given issue. Still, change does not occur overnight; only long-term and sustainable PR efforts can produce results.

KEY CONCEPTS

- Public relations is one of the action areas of health communication and an essential component of many health communication programs. It "helps an organization and its publics adapt mutually to each other" (Public Relations Society of America, 2005a).
- PR strategies and activities can help create interest about an idea, a behavior, a product, or an organization among multiple publics.
- As is true for the entire field of health communication, PR is a relationship-based discipline and practice.

- Key PR functions are public affairs, community relations, issues management, crisis management, media relations, and marketing PR.
- Key theoretical constructs of PR are recognizing the importance of psychological, emotional, and subconscious factors in human behavior; understanding and addressing multiple publics in the light of their unique characteristics as well as their mutual relationships and interaction; and understanding its role in relationship management.
- Because of the significant power of the mass media on public opinion and the potential risk for manipulation and misrepresentation, PR ethics should be always held to the highest standards. Professional codes of ethics as well as key characteristics of ethical PR programs should be considered in developing PR programs.
- The success of media-based campaigns depends on the story's newsworthiness as well as key elements of media and press relations.
- PR alone is not as effective in affecting the public and encouraging behavioral and social change as larger and multifaceted interventions that rely on other action areas of health communication, use community-based strategies and activities, and complement existing or future public health programs.
- Overall outcomes of PR programs should be evaluated in the context of the health communication intervention for which they have been designed. Still, it is important to understand and take into account qualitative and quantitative parameters that specifically apply to PR.
- PR becomes public advocacy when organizations and their constituencies use PR strategies and activities to advocate for specific policies, practices, and laws that may affect a specific group or society. As a consequence, PR is often an essential component of government relations.

FOR DISCUSSION AND PRACTICE

1. You are pitching consumer publications (for example, women's magazines, local and national newspapers, online publications) with a story that aims at raising awareness of the importance of regular mammograms for breast cancer prevention in women

over forty years of age. List some potential elements and angles for your story in order to attract reporters' attention and secure media coverage.

2. This chapter lists some of the key factors in designing ethical PR programs and also refers to existing guidelines. Share your reaction to each of these characteristics (see Table 5.3). Can you recall any example to which they may apply? Can you think of opposite examples? Is there anything else you would do to preserve public interest and the ethics of PR while designing the PR component of a health communication program?

3. When does PR become public advocacy? Provide examples of health-related public advocacy campaigns that you have noticed in recent news articles or broadcast programs.

CHAPTER SIX

COMMUNITY MOBILIZATION

IN THIS CHAPTER

- A Bottom-Up Approach to Community Mobilization
- Community Mobilization as a Social Process
- Implications for Community Mobilization Programs of Social Marketing and Other Theoretical and Practical Perspectives
- Impact of Community Mobilization on Health-Related Knowledge and Practices
- Key Steps of Community Mobilization Programs
- Key Concepts
- For Discussion and Practice

"Ask Canadians what the name ParticipACTION conjures up, and the majority of adults will easily recall the 60-year-old Swede" (Costas-Bradstreet, 2004, p. S25) "Is it true that the average 30-year-old Canadian is only as fit as the average 60-year-old Swede?" (Canadian Public Health Association, 2005) was one of the many questions addressed by the early public service announcements of a health communication program that ran for over thirty years and was established by ParticipACTION, a nonprofit organization.

Public service announcements were the main tool of Particip-ACTION in the early days of its implementation. Once the program's name had been established and Canadians became increasingly aware of the importance of fitness, ParticipACTION also implemented innovative strategies to involve people at the community level. The program "used community mobilization as a way to empower communities and motivate individuals to get more active" (Costas-Bradstreet, 2004, p. S25).

Community mobilization efforts originally focused on the city of Saskatoon in central Canada. Soon the enthusiasm generated by ParticipACTION community events, including "Walk a Block a Day" and other mass participation activities, spread to several levels of Canadian society, including other cities and regions, as well as provincial, territorial, and national governments (Costas-Bradstreet, 2004).

In 1992 alone, ParticipACTION trained fifty community animators who "generated 21,000 registered community events involving over 1 million volunteer leaders" (Costas-Bradstreet, 2004, p. S26). Over the years, the program attracted volunteers from all segments of society, including health professionals, the media, business communities, ordinary people, and government officials. It also developed partnerships with the federal government, professional societies (for example, Ontario Physical and Health Education Association, College of Family Physicians), the commercial sector (for example, the Ontario Milk Marketing Board, Merck Frosst Canada), and major health organizations, such as the Canadian Public Health Association (Costas-Bradstreet, 2004). All partners contributed with funds, activities, and other resources that expanded the program's reach.

The long-term impact of this program, which closed its doors in 2002, remains to be seen. The growing prevalence of obesity in Canada (Canadian Public Health Association, 2005) seems to point to the need for future and sustained efforts in this direction. Still, many of the success stories and lessons learned from ParticipACTION and other similar programs around the world demonstrate the importance of community mobilization as a fundamental strategy of health communication and, more broadly, public health interventions.

This chapter establishes community mobilization as a key area of health communication. It also reviews some of the current theoretical assumptions and topics in relation to this approach. Finally, it provides practical guidance on the key ingredients of community mobilization programs and the need for considering this approach as part of a multifaceted and multidisciplinary intervention.

A Bottom-Up Approach to Community Mobilization

Definitions often provide a useful framework for understanding the platform and the key assumptions of any given approach. In the case of community mobilization, the importance of community participation and self-reliance is emphasized in its theoretical definition and practical applications.

In fact, *community mobilization* is often defined as "empowering individuals to find their own solutions, whether or not the problem is solved" (Fishbein, Goldberg, and Middlestadt, 1997, p. 294). Although this definition does not and should not absolve community mobilization strategies from the pressure and responsibility of producing results, it clearly indicates that local leaders and ordinary people are the key participants in this approach. At the same time, it places in their hands the potential for involving other levels of society (for example, governments, professional organizations) in the solutions they have found. In this way, community mobilization is a bottom-up approach because it tends to rely on people's power to involve the upper hierarchical levels of society.

For example, one of the main success factors of Particip-ACTION was its community-driven approach, which helped secure "long-term government and sponsor support" (Costas-Bradstreet, 2004, p. S25). Similar conclusions were drawn in regard to a community mobilization project in Cameroon that aimed at increasing knowledge and use of family planning methods and reproductive health services (Babalola and others, 2001). Babalola and others highlight that once innovations were spread throughout local associations (called *Njangi*), they continued "to spread throughout the larger community, making community mobilization an effective tool for large-scale behavioral change communication" (p. 476).

The term **community** can indicate a variety of social, ethnic, cultural, or geographical associations, and it can refer to a school, workplace, city, neighborhood, or organized patient or professional group, or association of peer leaders, to name a few. As another example, *Njangi* are local socioeconomic associations that are quite common in most of Africa and "are formed on a geographic basis, by family structure, or through shared professions" (Babalola and others, 2002, p. 461). Communities always tend to share similar values, beliefs, and overall objectives and priorities. According to UN-AIDS (2005), a community is a "group of people who have shared concerns and will act together in their common interest."

When communities drive public health or health communication interventions, they are not merely consulted. They share power and decisions. Community mobilization may be initiated by leaders within the community or stimulated by external agencies, organizations, or consultants. Still, the role of external organizations, health communication practitioners, and other consultants is to facilitate and follow the mobilization process (Health Communication Partnership, 2006a).

In this context, one of the main objectives of health communication practitioners and other health professionals who may be involved in the community mobilization effort is to provide local leaders and their community with technical assistance to accomplish a number of goals:

- Find solutions that build on the community's strengths and fit well within its overall context (Fishbein and others, 1997; Costas-Bradstreet, 2004).
- Facilitate partnerships with other segments of society (Costas-Bradstreet, 2004).
- Become aware of potential obstacles and ways to overcome them.
- Resolve conflicts among community members, and create a consensus on potential solutions.
- Establish a process for community involvement, including the development of communication messages, materials, and activities, which can ultimately lead to social and behavioral change.
- Point to resources and approaches that may facilitate long-term sustainability of all programs and health solutions.
- Design a rigorous evaluation process so that the community can check on its own progress and accommodate changing needs.
- Keep the community focused on what it wants to accomplish.

COMMUNITY MOBILIZATION AS A SOCIAL PROCESS

The impact of community mobilization is greater when different communities interact with each other and create a social force for change. This concept is incorporated in the idea of *social mobilization*. Although some of the premises of social mobilization may be different from those of community mobilization, the two terms are closely related and are used here interchangeably. *Social mobilization* has been defined "as the process of bringing together multisectoral community partners to raise awareness, demand, and progress for the initiative's goals, processes and outcomes" (Patel, 2005, p. 53). This definition is in agreement with the key elements of community mobilization as discussed in this chapter.

In the context of health communication, community mobilization tends to be disease specific and addresses behavioral issues that may help reduce the morbidity and mortality of a given condition. Still, there are a number of cases in which community mobilization is a component of health communication programs that complement larger public health interventions and aim at guaranteeing or expanding community access to health services and products or addressing social issues. In fact, community mobilization may entail and refer to different kinds of actions, from people marching to demonstrate their discontent about the paucity of research funds dedicated to a specific disease area to community members communicating with others about the importance of disease prevention and leading the behavior change process.

Mobilizing local leaders and their communities is a long process that may vary according to the community's makeup and needs. However, several success factors can be extrapolated from existing experiences and programs and apply generally to this kind of effort:

- Evidence-based information, which is critical to attract attention to a health issue and convince people to prioritize it within a community. Moreover, it can help communities identify strategies and approaches that are likely to involve their members as well as other communities in the health behavior change process.

- A behavior-centered mind-set. In other words, what is the community mobilization effort asking people to do?
- The inclusion of all influential audiences in the planning and implementation of the community mobilization process.
- The quality of the technical assistance and training provided to local leaders and their communities by health communication practitioners and other key health professionals. Outside support and technical assistance are critical to sustaining the effort over the long term (UNAIDS, 2005).
- The potential for community ownership and program sustainability.
- The existence of complementary interventions (for example, mass media campaigns, capacity building training, widespread access to services) that reinforce the community-based communication efforts and encourage its members' adherence to the process of change.

Most of the above factors are common to the overall field of health communication and public health. Still, it is worth mentioning them here because of their critical importance in community mobilization programs.

Finally, facilitating a community-driven intervention requires good listening skills, a firm belief in the "value of collective action" (Costas-Bradstreet, 2004, p. S29), enthusiasm for the health cause, and a strong ability to transmit it. It also requires the application of many of the skills and theories previously discussed in relation to interpersonal communications.

IMPLICATIONS FOR COMMUNITY MOBILIZATION PROGRAMS OF SOCIAL MARKETING AND OTHER THEORETICAL AND PRACTICAL PERSPECTIVES

Over time, community mobilization has been influenced by social marketing from both a theoretical and practical perspective. Yet it is a different approach for behavioral and social change that perfectly fits the current emphasis on participatory strategies to communication.

Although community mobilization often uses social marketing strategies (see Chapter Two) as well as participatory research (either market or audience related), "these terms are not synonymous" (Health Communication Partnership, 2006a). Community mobilization goes beyond participatory research, which involves intended audiences in the design, implementation, and analysis of research protocols and data related to the health issue and its audiences. Also, community mobilization is a different approach from social marketing.

Fishbein, Goldberg, and Middlestadt (1997) point to the definitions of social marketing and community mobilization in order to highlight their differences. Social marketing is designed to "influence the behavior of target audiences to improve their personal welfare and that of the society of which they are part" (Fishbein and others, 1997, p. 294; Andreasen, 1995, p. 7). Community mobilization seeks to promote community empowerment by developing skills that can be used beyond addressing the specific problem or health issue (Fishbein, Goldberg, and Middlestadt, 1997). It works toward a long-term change in community skills that can be replicated within different communities and segments of society as well as in addressing other kinds of health issues.

In planning a community mobilization effort, community participants are likely to analyze the situation by trying to define the best way for the community to address the health issue. Social marketers are likely to think about the behavior that needs to be influenced and the strategies to accomplish that (Fishbein, Goldberg, and Middlestadt, 1997).

However, even in a participatory and community-driven approach, defining potential behavioral and social outcomes helps community participants frame the health issue in a way that will respond to community needs and effectively address it. "A behavioral science orientation can help design interventions aimed at influencing behavioral determinants" (Fishbein, Goldberg, and Middlestadt, 1997, p. 298).

In fact, the influence of marketing models in community mobilization efforts may help community members define and pursue the changes they want to address using a systematic approach. As in other areas of health communication, marketing's major implication for community mobilization is its research-based and structured approach to planning. Still, the emphasis of community mobilization efforts should be primarily on building the capacity of the community to address its own problems.

Too often, it is possible to observe in the developing world the vacuum that is left when capacity building is not one of the key priorities of community mobilization as well as larger health communication or public health interventions. As soon as the outsiders leave, communities are left to manage programs and priorities they are not prepared to address. Many times circumstances revert to the original situation shortly after international agencies leave. This is exactly what well-designed and well-implemented community mobilization programs should try to avoid in both the developing and developed worlds. The recent emphasis on behavioral and social outcomes as well as increased audience participation in communication efforts is well positioned to accomplish that.

For example, models such as the community action cycle draw on several social change theories and are designed to help communities "acquire the skills and resources to plan, implement and evaluate health-related actions and policies" (Lavery and others, 2005, p. 611). Under the community action cycle, outcomes are defined in terms of changes in "social norms, policies, culture, and the supporting environment" (Health Communication Partnership, 2006a). Instead, under COMBI, the World Health Organization (2003) model for communication for behavioral impact, community mobilization efforts, which are also participatory and aim at building community skills, emphasize the importance of behavioral change as a key program outcome even when the program ultimately aims at social change.

Whether the emphasis is on behavioral or social outcomes should be determined by the unique characteristics of the health issue being addressed, as well as those of the specific communities and audiences and their existing health and social behaviors (see Chapter One). It is critical to remember that social change occurs only as a result of gradual behavioral changes at different levels of society. Therefore, these changes should be measured and considered key program outcomes. Ideally, all interventions should aim at creating permanent changes in social rules and community structure. This is also in agreement with some of the key premises of the larger public health field of community health. In fact, "the movement called community health means more than just access to healthcare. It's strong families, good schools, safe neighborhoods, caring adults, and economic opportunities" (Emanoil, 2002, p. 16).

In most cases, the connection between health or social issues and behavior is quite evident. For example there are many severe diseases and health topics for which changes in individual, group, or community behavior can effectively address disease incidence as well as morbidity and mortality rates and other important disease-related issues.

Box 6.1 offers a case study showing the correlation between behavior and disease burden and highlights how community mobilization can effectively address that. In reviewing this case study, readers should take into account that this intervention was aimed at reducing the impact of a sudden health crisis. Strategies used in this case may be different from more extensive interventions that would address and sustain a health behavior. Nevertheless, the case study provides a helpful example of the direct correlation between behavior and health outcomes.

Box 6.1

Social Mobilization to Fight Ebola in Yambio, Southern Sudan

Controlling communicable diseases demands not only medical expertise but also social education. To meet this goal, WHO has adopted a type of social mobilization known as communication for behavioural impact (COMBI) that focuses on influencing behaviour at both the individual and community level. This strategy was implemented in Yambio, from late May to June 2004, during an outbreak of Ebola haemorrhagic fever that resulted in 17 confirmed cases, including 7 deaths.

In late May, WHO's social mobilization experts, from the WHO Mediterranean Centre for Vulnerability Reduction (Tunis, Tunisia), were included among the international WHO-coordinated Ebola response team. Upon arrival in Yambio, their first task was to determine what changes in behaviour were necessary to contain the Ebola outbreak.

The social mobilization team was immediately confronted with numerous misconceptions about the outbreak. For example, many people in Yambio were unconvinced that there was actually an Ebola outbreak, while others believed that blood and skin samples were being removed from patients and sold. There was also an unsubstantiated fear of the isolation ward, wariness of the surveillance teams and irrational behaviour. For example, some people refused to leave home between 17:00 and 19:00, believing this would reduce their risk of contracting Ebola.

To counter these misconceptions, the social mobilization team, which included pastors, teachers and community development workers (who wore uniforms to increase credibility), spoke to villagers daily at their homes, market places, restaurants, churches and schools. Simple measures were emphasized, such as asking sick individuals to contact the Ebola team within 24 hours of the onset of symptoms, recommending to people that they avoid direct contact with sick individuals and suggesting that the community refrain from traditional practices of sleeping next to or touching dead bodies for the duration of the outbreak.

A key element of the team's strategy was the distribution of informational pamphlets, which answered basic Ebola questions, as well as dispelling common rumours. Recognizing the stigma that accompanies Ebola, the social mobilization team also worked to explain the need for the isolation ward at Yambio Hospital, and included pictures of the ward in the pamphlet, to show the local population that the fence around the ward was short enough for patients to see and talk to their family and friends from a safe distance.

By placing communities at the centre of the social mobilization programme, the rapid containment of the Ebola outbreak in Yambio can largely be attributed to the efforts of local people themselves.

As WHO and partners gain more experience in identifying and responding to Ebola outbreaks, social mobilization will undoubtedly continue to play an important role in the successful containment of future outbreaks.

Source: World Health Organization, Mediterranean Center for Vulnerability Reduction. "Social Mobilization to Fight Ebola in Yambio, Southern Sudan." Action Against Infection, 2004 ©. http://wmc.who.int/pdf/Action_Against_Infection.pdf. Used by permission.

Community (or social) mobilization has been positioned by several authors and organizations as a key component of global health communication, especially in the context of behavior and social change models (World Health Organization, 2003; Health Communication Partnership, 2006b; Patel, 2005; Rengenathan and others, 2005). For example, in Namibia, one of the core elements of the Health Communication Partnership (2006c) communication program is a community mobilization effort aimed at increasing HIV community awareness as well as the use of HIV preventive measures and competent health services.

Still, community mobilization is not an all-inclusive tool to address community health issues. Its likelihood for success is related to the use of a multifaceted approach in which other tools and areas of communication are used to reinforce the community change process. Multiple channels (for example, mass media, theater, interpersonal communication channels) should be used to deliver a consistent and clear message in order to create the kind of support needed for behavioral or social change within a community. Most important, community mobilization efforts should complement other relevant public health interventions.

IMPACT OF COMMUNITY MOBILIZATION ON HEALTH-RELATED KNOWLEDGE AND PRACTICES

As for other areas of health communication, community mobilization efforts aim to influence health behavior. This section reviews some of the key aspects and potential outcomes of the process of influencing health-related knowledge and practices through community mobilization interventions.

RELIANCE ON COMMUNITY MEMBERS

Communicating ideas about health and behavior as well as social issues related to health outcomes is a long and difficult process. Using a peer-to-peer approach, such as relying on credible community members, to diffuse new ideas and prompt action may shorten this process (Babalola, 2001).

Because of the involvement and leadership of community members in the different phases of program planning, implementation, and scaling up, community mobilization can be a time-saving and effective approach to influence health-related knowledge and practices. When external organizations, health communicators, and other kinds of facilitators approach a community, they should always identify, engage, and train local leaders who have an interest in speaking at community meetings and carrying on the mobilization process. This may pass through many different stages, which include but are not limited to communication and disease-specific training.

Sometimes people who are well suited to become community leaders because of personal characteristics and social status lack the knowledge and understanding of the health problem's relevance within the community or need to go through a process of change themselves. Sometimes leaders already exist within a community and are ready to facilitate the process of change but may need technical assistance in the planning and implementation of the process. Other times people become leaders because of life events or the exposure to different communication tools and activities that influence their core beliefs and attitudes prompt a personal change and make them want to help others. The example in Box 6.2 shows the different phases of the process of personal growth, disease awareness, and commitment to the prevention of sexually transmitted diseases (STDs) that a young man in Kenya experienced after attending a few community theater sessions on the topic and engaging in a series of discussions with the health communication staff and the local coordinators from the Program for Appropriate Technology in Health, an international health organization that had developed the theater sessions.

Box 6.2

How Bingwa Changed His Ways

At age twenty-four, Bingwa (not his real name) represents the typical Kenyan out-of-school youth: unemployed and hot-blooded, but generally hopeful and lively. He had been a regular attendee of the community theater sessions organized by Program for Appropriate

Technology in Health (PATH), an international nonprofit organization, in collaboration with the local Rojo-Rojo troupe in Mumias, in Kenya's Western province.

Between January and September 2002, Bingwa's life evolved dramatically. This very average young man—married, father of a fifteen-month-old son, sexually active outside his marriage but insulated by a sense that he was not at risk of any infection—became one of the first youths to be stimulated by Magnet Theatre to navigate a course to new personal behavior that has made him a community role model. He volunteered to go for voluntary counseling and testing (VCT), learned for himself that he was not infected, and took serious steps to reduce his sexual risk by taking charge of his personal life.

Bingwa made a living by taking care of his uncle's four rental houses and eked out his income by selling Coca-Cola and odds and ends from a kiosk. His buddies would hang around at the kiosk, talking about politics, football, jobs, and girls. Bingwa, married and with a child, was economically better off than his friends, and indeed the de facto group leader. There was a time, in his bachelor days, when his house used to be known as The Butchery in recognition of the fact that the young men in the estate would bring girls over for sex there. Bingwa was always happy to make his house available and disappear for a while.

Bingwa's first questions came on a Friday in January 2002, at the end of a session of community theater by the Rojo-Rojo Magnet Theatre troupe. PATH's theater coordinator, Madiang, was looking forward to the weekend and was packing up after a Magnet Theatre show.

Bingwa approached Madiang, and after a few moments of small talk, asked, "Say, is an STI [sexually transmitted infection] the same as AIDS?"

Madiang answered in the negative. But Bingwa became pensive and launched a second question: "Okay then, if they are not the same, does an STI later become AIDS if it is not treated?"

Madiang explained to Bingwa the difference between STI and HIV, and that HIV is just one of various STIs. After citing some examples of other STIs, he offered an explanation on how some STIs can pave the way to infection with HIV.

Bingwa now asked, rather hesitantly, "So which STIs are treatable?"

As they spoke, Madiang was trying to understand why Bingwa was asking these questions. He came to several assumptions: Bingwa could be infected with an STI; he might be seeking treatment for that STI; he could be concerned about his HIV status. He possibly engaged in multipartner or unprotected sex.

Ironically, Bingwa believed that he was not at risk for HIV at that time, even though he was regularly having unprotected sex with multiple partners outside his marriage. Bingwa wrongly believed that one could get HIV only from a sex worker.

Three weeks later, Bingwa had more questions, this time about VCT, which had been the topic of the play. *What was VCT? Does the test also check for the other STIs? Must someone undergo the counseling in order to be tested?*

In truth, Bingwa had already heard about VCT but did not understand it well. He confessed that it was at the Magnet Theatre discussions that he had begun wondering if he might be a candidate for VCT. The enactments had led him to start reflecting on his former life. He had become convinced that he was probably infected with an STI and that it was only a matter of time before this issue came to light. VCT seemed to him an opportunity to check his STI status.

These questions also seem to have been a turning point in Bingwa's life. It was after asking these questions that he "sat back alone in the kiosk and really looked at his life." Every answer he received only confirmed his fear that he was already infected. It was around this point that he decided, in his words, to "stop engaging in sex, even with my wife. I was afraid!" Bingwa had never met anyone who had gone for VCT and even doubted whether anyone actually did.

Not long after, Bingwa decided to go for VCT. He spoke to Madiang in private for nearly one-and-a-half hours and asked him more questions than he ever had before. He would listen to the answers keenly, be quiet for a while, and then launch another question. Two days later, Bingwa became one of the first young men to go for VCT as a result of his exposure to the Magnet Theatre process.

Bingwa's life has not been the same since he went for VCT. He has already spoken out on a popular Kenyan radio serial drama produced by PATH, *Kati Yetu*, strongly urging others to go for VCT and reflect on their sexual lives and behaviors. Standing in front of his peers in a Magnet Theater session, Bingwa pledged that he would no longer engage in multipartner sex. As of that year's end, Bingwa affirmed that he had had neither extramarital nor unprotected sex. That was six months after he adopted a new behavior. Today Bingwa has become a role model in his community and has helped innumerable numbers of his peers to also go for VCT. He is often asked to share his experience and the benefits of VCT, information he is always willing to give out.

And his house is no longer called "The Butchery."

Source: Program for Appropriate Technology in Health, "How Bingwa Changed His Ways." Unpublished case study, 2005. Copyright © 2005, Program for Appropriate Technology in Health. www.path.org. The material in this case study may be freely used for educational or noncommercial purposes, provided that the material is accompanied by this acknowledgment line. All rights reserved. Used by permission.

ADVANCING KNOWLEDGE AND CHANGING PRACTICES

Regardless of how leaders decide to become engaged in the community mobilization process, this approach has proven to be effective in prompting changes in people's health knowledge and practices. For example, one of the most important lessons learned in the past few decades is that "a fully mobilized and supportive environment is a crucial element of effective HIV prevention" (Amoah, 2001, p. 1).

In the United States, gay activists have played a fundamental role in controlling the AIDS epidemic. By speaking up, they have helped break the cycle of misinformation, shame, and stigma that is still an issue in too much of society but was even more relevant in the early years of the epidemic and risked paralyzing any form of progress. AIDS activists not only have ensured that "HIV prevention, treatment and care stayed a global, national and local priority" (Gay Men's Health Crisis, 2006) but have influenced disease awareness, drug approval regulations, work-related policies, prevention and treatment strategies, and access to medications, to name a few. In doing so, the gay community, which started the overall AIDS activism movement in the United States, has involved different segments of society and contributed to show that AIDS is not only a gay disease. Box 6.3 presents a timeline of AIDS events that summarizes some of the most important stages and results of this community mobilization process. The example also highlights that many of the policy and social changes were triggered by knowledge and behavioral changes at the legislative, general public, or scientific community levels.

Box 6.3

Gay Men's Health Crisis HIV/AIDS Timeline

1981   CDC reports Kaposi's sarcoma in healthy gay men.
         NY Times announces "rare cancer" in 41 gay men.
         Eighty men gather in NY to address "gay cancer" and
            raise money for research.
         CDC declares the new disease an epidemic.

1982   GMHC (Gay Men's Health Crisis) is officially established.
         An answering machine, which acts as the world's first
            AIDS hotline, receives over 100 calls the first night.
         GMHC holds its second AIDS fundraiser; produces and distributes 50,000 free copies of its first newsletter to doctors, hospitals, clinics, and the Library of Congress and creates Buddy Program to assist PWAs (persons with AIDS).
         CDC changes the name from "gay cancer" to AIDS.

1983   PWAs form National Association of People with AIDS (NAPWA).
         GMHC funds litigation of first AIDS discrimination suit.
         NY state (NYS) Department of Health AIDS Institute established.

1984   CDC requests GMHC's help to plan public conferences on AIDS.
         GMHC publishes its first safer sex guidelines.
         The human immunodeficiency virus (HIV) is isolated in France and later in the U.S.

1985   Revelation that Rock Hudson, a U.S. TV and movie star, has AIDS, makes the disease a household word.
         FDA approves first test to screen for antibodies to HIV.

The American Association of Blood Banks and the Red
   Cross begin screening blood for HIV antibodies and
   rejecting gay donors.
GMHC's art auction is world's first million-dollar AIDS
   fundraiser.
First international conference on AIDS held in Atlanta,
   Georgia.
CDC estimates 1 million HIV-infected people worldwide.
U.S. military starts mandatory HIV testing.
First conference to discuss AIDS in communities of color
   held in NYC.

1986   NYC's first anonymous testing site opens.
GMHC's client base now includes heterosexual men and
   women, hemophiliacs, intravenous drug users, and
   children.
U.S. Surgeon General calls for AIDS education for children
   of all ages.
GMHC holds first AIDS Walk in New York.
Several states pass bills to ban PWAs from food-handling
   and educational jobs, making it a crime to transmit HIV,
   and force testing of prostitutes.

1987   AZT, the first drug approved to fight HIV, is marketed.
President Reagan uses the word "AIDS" in public for the
   first time.
CDC expands the definition of AIDS.
The United States shuts its doors to HIV-infected immi-
   grants and travelers.
Political attacks against GMHC and educational efforts on
   safer sex that "encourage or promote homosexual sexual
   activity."

1988   Condom use is shown to be effective in HIV prevention.
The first World AIDS Day held on December 1.
Surgeon General mails 107 million copies of "Understand-
   ing AIDS" to every American household.
The United States bans discrimination against federal work-
   ers with HIV.

1989   GMHC leads successful effort to draft and pass New York
   state's AIDS-Related Information Bill, ensuring
   confidentiality.

GMHC and other AIDS organizations protest against U.S. immigration policies.

1990   AIDS activist Ryan White's death points to need for urgent funding legislation.

The Ryan White Comprehensive AIDS Resources Emergency (CARE) Act passes, authorizing $881 million in emergency relief.

Americans with Disabilities Act (ADA) signed to protect people with disabilities, including people with HIV, from discrimination.

The first book to talk about long-term survivors of AIDS is published.

The first GMHC Dance-a-thon raises over $1 million.

U.S. AIDS deaths pass the 100,000 mark.

1991   Earvin "Magic" Johnson announces he is HIV-positive, becoming the first celebrity to admit contracting HIV via heterosexual sex.

Condoms become available in NYC high schools after months of debate.

A Roper poll commissioned by GMHC finds that a majority of Americans believe that more explicit AIDS education is needed.

1992   In response to mounting activism and protest, FDA starts "accelerated approval" to get drugs to PWAs faster.

A federal court strikes down proposed "offensiveness" restrictions on AIDS education materials.

First time that a U.S. president is elected on a campaign platform that also contains HIV and AIDS issues.

1993   CDC expands the definition of AIDS. New AIDS diagnoses expected to increase by as much as 100 percent as a result of the change.

Over 13,800 PWAs have been clients of GMHC at this point.

The CDC, NIH, and FDA jointly declare that condoms are "highly effective" for prevention of HIV infection.

1994   GMHC begins a NYC subway campaign aimed at gay, lesbian, and heterosexual young adults.

WHO estimates 19.5 million HIV-infected people worldwide.

1995   CDC announces that AIDS is the leading cause of death among Americans aged 25 to 44.

The FDA approves the first in a new class of drugs called protease inhibitors.

1996   The FDA approves the sale of first home HIV test kit.
GMHC launches its first prevention campaign for HIV-negative men.
The FDA approves HIV viral load test, used to track HIV progression and efficacy of combination therapy.
Cover stories hailing AIDS breakthroughs and the "end" of the epidemic start appearing in major U.S. publications.

1997   The first human trials of an AIDS vaccine begin.
WHO estimates 30.6 million HIV-infected people worldwide.
GMHC begins providing on-site HIV testing and counseling services.

1998   GMHC launches the largest survey of gay and bisexual men, "Beyond 2000 Sexual Health Survey."
New York state HIV Reporting and Partner Notification Act signed, requiring that cases of HIV (not just AIDS) be reported to the Department of Health.
A GMHC study reports that an estimated 69,000 people in New York state have HIV but remain unaware.

1999   First large-scale study of young gay men finds that large numbers have been infected in the last two years, many among black men.

2000   As the result of years of lobbying by HIV/AIDS organizations, New York state passes legislation decriminalizing sale and possession of syringes without prescription.
The CDC reports that black and Latino men now account for more AIDS cases among gay men than white men.
The GMHC AIDS Hotline becomes accessible via e-mail.

2001   Twentieth year of AIDS epidemic.
In response to the arrest of participants in needle exchange program, federal court rules that police may not interfere with public health initiatives that combat disease through education and prevention.
UN General Assembly adopts global blueprint for action on HIV/AIDS and calls for creation of $7 to $10 billion global fund for the developing world.
Abstinence-only HIV prevention programs begin to be promoted by U.S. government.

2002   The FDA approves a new rapid HIV testing device.

GMHC joins activists to protest U.S. underfunding of domestic and global AIDS programs.

GMHC begins offering on-site hepatitis C testing and launches new initiative looking at gay men's health in broader context.

2003   GMHC holds Eighteenth Annual New York AIDS Walk.

U.S. bill authorizing up to $15 billion for global AIDS, TB, and malaria treatment and prevention for twelve African and two Caribbean countries is signed.

Activists express doubts about provision that assigns abstinence-only programs a third of USAID's prevention funding.

Source: The Gay Men's Health Crisis HIV/AIDS Timeline. Copyright © 2006, Gay Men's Health Crisis (GMHC). Used by permission.

As another example, in India and Armenia, a community mobilization effort that was implemented within a multichannel behavior change strategy, was shown to improve knowledge and practices in many areas of childhood diseases management, including "improvements in births attended by skilled practitioners, exclusive breastfeeding, immunization, and HIV/AIDS awareness and prevention knowledge" (Baranick and Ricca, 2005).

The list of disease areas and health issues where community mobilization has made or could make a difference is endless. By empowering people to take their lives and health in their own hands, community mobilization can produce long-lasting results in health behaviors and practices as part of a multidisciplinary and multifaceted approach.

KEY STEPS OF COMMUNITY MOBILIZATION PROGRAMS

There are several models and frameworks that describe the key steps of community mobilization. Although some of the stages they describe may be different or use interchangeable terms, a few general criteria are common to all of them or reflect practical experience:

- The importance of understanding the community's key characteristics, structure, values, needs, attitudes, social norms, health behaviors, and priorities
- A cross-cultural communication approach through which health communicators and other community mobilizers should refrain from any form of cultural bias in exchanging information about health systems, beliefs, and behaviors, as well as other kinds of topics
- The need for engaging community members at the onset of the intervention, including during the community assessment or participatory research phase (and whenever possible, prior to that)
- A research-based planning process that should respond and evolve according to community needs and priorities
- An emphasis on capacity building and community autonomy
- A rigorous evaluation process that needs to be mutually agreed on by all community members and leaders, identifies behavioral or social outcomes as key evaluation parameters, and includes a number of other evaluation measurements to monitor the process at different stages
- The ability for the process to be replicated during the scaling-up phase (in which the program is expanded to reach other communities and regions) as well as to address similar issues within the community

Following are a few examples of models for community mobilization that incorporate all these criteria in different phases or by using slightly different terminologies. Methodologies used for most of these steps are common to the planning and implementation process of the overall field of health communication and are described in further detail in Part Three of this book.

COMMON TERMS AND STEPS IN COMMUNITY MOBILIZATION

Community mobilization is a long-term process that relies on a variety of sequential yet interdependent steps and activities. Some of the most common terms and phases of community mobilization are described next, starting with how to select and engage community organizations and leaders.

Selection of Community Organizations and Leaders

Before conducting any community mobilization effort, health communicators and other community mobilizers need to identify communities that may have an interest in participating in such effort. These key criteria should be considered:

- The community has expressed a preliminary interest in participating and places a high priority on the specific health issue.
- There are high rates of disease incidence, morbidity, and mortality within the community.
- Specific community characteristics can be used as a model for replication of the effort.
- The health issue is relevant to the community's health and development.
- There are relevant special needs or issues.

Engaging and training community leaders in defining the key elements and initial steps of the intervention is critical and should be part of the initial community engagement process.

This phase should be informed by preliminary formative research, including analysis of secondary data (literature, articles, and other information compiled by others) as well as stakeholders' interviews, which will inform health communicators about how to approach the community regarding the specific health issue. At this stage, key stakeholders may include representatives of local nongovernmental organizations (NGOs), companies, international health agencies, local churches, women's groups, government, and everyone who can provide initial information on the community's key characteristics, structure, and issues as well as existing interventions in the same health area. Formative research can also be instrumental in identifying potential community leaders.

Preliminary research findings and analysis should be shared with community members formally and informally. For example, as part of a joint malaria prevention effort in Angola by UNICEF and the local ministry of health, preliminary research findings were shared first with a team of government officers and then with a larger group representing local NGOs, companies, universities, and other key stakeholders (Schiavo, 1998, 2000). This gave an opportunity to all participants to brainstorm about the findings, pri-

oritize their relevance within the community, and develop preliminary strategies for a community outreach effort aimed at enhancing
malaria awareness as well as the use of insecticide-treated mosquito
nets for malaria protection (Schiavo and Robson, 1999). At the same
time, this helped recruit and train community members for the participatory research effort and other phases of the program.

Participatory Research

Participatory research, also referred to as *community-driven assessment* and *participatory needs assessment* (Centers for Disease Control,
2006a), is a collaborative research effort that involves community
members, researchers, community mobilizers, and interested agencies and organizations. It is a two-way dialogue that starts with the
people and through which the community understands and identifies key issues, priorities, and potential actions. Participatory research should inform and guide all phases of the community
mobilization effort.

The U.S. Agency for Healthcare Research and Quality (AHRQ)
defines participatory research as "an approach to health and environmental research meant to increase the value of studies for both
researchers and the community being studied" (Viswanathan and
others, 2004, p. 1). Participatory research uses traditional research
methodologies such as focus groups and one-on-one or group
interviews.

While the community should be involved in designing the research protocol and questions as well as recruiting research participants and analyzing research findings, experience shows that
"participation levels vary" and depend on many factors, related to
both the community and the health communication and research
team (Mercer, Potter, and Green, 2002). Also, the concept of participation may mean different things to different people and
institutions.

Ideally, the community should be the main protagonist of this
process. This phase should represent an opportunity to exchange
information; understand community preferences, concerns, and
priorities; and identify culturally appropriate communication activities, channels, messages, and spokespeople, as well as the behavioral or social outcomes that need to be achieved through the
intervention.

Community Group Meetings

Community group meetings involve larger segments of the community in addition to the original members who have been recruited for the participatory research phase. They can be existing meetings (for example, monthly administrative meetings of a women's group, hospital or other kind of community) that are used to inform and engage community members in the community mobilization efforts. They can also be specifically organized for other reasons:

- Sharing participatory research findings and securing feedback from a larger number of community members
- Informing about the health issue, its relevance to the community, and potential behavioral or social changes that have been identified during formative or participatory research, and then securing feedback and suggestions on all elements
- Advancing understanding of the community's priorities and needs
- Promoting an ongoing dialogue among community members on the health issue and its potential solutions
- Motivating and engaging additional volunteers or community leaders to participate in the community mobilization effort
- Identifying roles and responsibilities of community members for program implementation
- Addressing other community- or issue-specific topics

Ideally, community leaders should conduct these meetings with the help, when necessary, of health communicators and other facilitators. Sometimes if local leaders are not ready or adequately trained to conduct such meetings, the community mobilization external team should take the lead, but only after discussing and agreeing on core messages and meeting strategies with relevant community leaders.

Partnership Meetings

Once the community has identified its key priorities and actions, partnership meetings can be held to define and start establishing collaborations among community members, agencies, and organizations that have participated so far in the process or to introduce them to potential new partners and organizations. These kinds of meetings should attempt to achieve several goals—for example:

- Defining the roles and responsibilities of all different partners
- Advancing agreement on standard procedures and specific contributions to the community mobilization effort
- Developing strategies and action plans
- Defining and mutually agreeing on evaluation parameters
- Discussing lessons learned
- Providing an update on progress

A discussion on establishing and maintaining partnerships is included in Chapter Eight of this book.

Development of Communication Approaches, Activities, Tools, and Spokespeople

Community mobilization is complemented by or relies on many different communication approaches and tools, such as theater, traditional media, brochures, home visits, workshops, and rallies. (A detailed discussion about the development of communication messages and tools is included in Part Three of this book as part of the overall health communication planning and implementation process.)

Nevertheless, it is important to note here that all strategies and action plans need to include community-based tools (for example, existing meetings and communication vehicles) and methodologies, address community priorities and needs, and support behavioral or social outcomes. Most important, communication tools and messages need to be developed and delivered by and for the people.

COMMUNITY ACTION CYCLE OR MODEL

Several versions of the community action model have evolved over time. Some of them include evaluation as one of the key steps (Health Communication Partnership, 2006a) while others consider evaluation a separate step from the overall cycle (Lavery and others, 2005). Some also include a scaling-up phase (Health

Communication Partnership, 2006a), while others describe scaling up as a separate process. Including evaluation and scaling up as part of the overall planning and implementation cycle may signal the importance of these steps to inform and guide follow-up interventions, as well as the replication of the same intervention in other communities at different times. Nevertheless, fundamental premises of this model remain the same and include community participation, emphasis on social outcomes, capacity building, and the importance of an ongoing dialogue among community members in relation to health issues (Health Communication Partnership, 2006a; Lavery and others, 2005).

Under this model, health communicators and other facilitators assist the community in "creating an environment in which the individuals can empower themselves to address their own and their community health issues" (Health Communication Partnership, 2006a). One of the versions for this model includes the following key steps (Health Communication Partnership, 2006a):

- "Organize the community for action" by identifying community leaders who have an interest in becoming engaged in the process, training them, and facilitating the discussion about issues that are important to the community.
- "Explore health issues and set priorities" using participatory research.
- "Plan together" to establish the community actions that need to be implemented to support social change and address the specific health issue. Actions need to be achievable, sustainable, and have the potential "to persuade groups, organizations or agencies to make policy changes" (Lavery and others, 2005, p. 615). They may include different kinds of activities such as lobbying with local governments, stakeholder presentations about a specific health issue, or organizing a health fair.
- "Act together" in the implementation of the actions previously defined.
- "Evaluate together" through a process of participatory evaluation in which all community members and program partners compare actual outcomes with the presumed social outcomes defined at the onset of the program.

The major difference of this model compared with other participatory models used by the World Health Organization (2003), the Centers for Disease Control (2006b, about the CDC's syphilis elimination effort), or other key organizations is its emphasis on social outcomes instead of behavioral outcomes. When the specific health situation as well as the community characteristics and level of preparedness allow for it, this model is well suited to address health disparities (Lavery and others, 2005) and other broader social issues related to health. Still, it is always important to remember that social change begins and ends with a series of individual, group, and community behavioral changes within multiple sectors of society.

KEY CONCEPTS

- Community mobilization is a key area of health communication that seeks to empower communities to make the changes needed for better health outcomes. It often starts with ordinary people and attempts to engage all different levels of society.
- Community mobilization describes different kinds of actions, from people marching to demonstrate their discontent about the paucity of research funds dedicated to a specific disease area to community members communicating with others about the importance of disease prevention and leading the health behavior change process.
- In this chapter, the terms *community mobilization* and *social mobilization* are used interchangeably. One of the key premises of the definitions and case studies used in this chapter is that the potential impact of community mobilization is greater when several communities come together and create a force for social change.
- As part of health communication interventions, community mobilization tends to be disease focused but often also addresses broader health and social issues and complements other health communication and public health efforts.
- Community skills building as well as community participation and autonomy are fundamental aspects of community mobilization.
- The role of health communicators and others who may facilitate the community mobilization process should not take away

from community autonomy and power. So-called community mobilizers should act only as consultants and technical experts in accompanying the process of community reflection and empowerment on relevant health issues.

- The effectiveness of community mobilization interventions increases when they are part of larger health communication programs and complement existing public health initiatives and strategies.
- Community mobilization has been influenced by several theoretical and practical models, including social marketing and participatory research. Nevertheless, these terms are not synonymous.
- Several models describe key steps of community mobilization efforts. All of them focus on behavioral or social outcomes and share many common characteristics.

FOR DISCUSSION AND PRACTICE

1. Discuss your reaction to the Bingwa case study in Box 6.2. List all factors that in your opinion contributed to Bingwa's change and rank them in order of importance. Use role-play to imagine a potential conversation on the same topic (STDs and their prevention) you may have with your peers or someone like Bingwa.

2. Do you have any personal or professional experience with community mobilization? Did you ever participate in a community-based meeting or event? If yes, describe and apply key concepts from this chapter to your description whenever they are relevant.

3. Can you think of an example in which a series of behavioral changes led to a health-related social change as the result of community engagement and mobilization? Describe the sequence of events as well as the specific changes that occurred at different levels of the community or society. You can refer to examples that recently appeared in the news or to personal experiences. In the absence of specific examples, think of a desirable social change (for example, a new health policy in a specific health area or removal of the stigma associated with a specific disease), and identify the behaviors that may lead to social change.

CHAPTER SEVEN

PROFESSIONAL MEDICAL COMMUNICATIONS

IN THIS CHAPTER

- Communicating with Health Care Providers: A Peer-to-Peer Approach
- Theoretical Assumptions in Professional Medical Communications
- How to Influence Health Care Provider Behavior: A Theoretical Overview
- Key Elements of Professional Medical Communications Programs
- Overview of Key Communication Channels and Activities
- Key Concepts
- For Discussion and Practice

Health care systems and, consequently, the practice of medicine have changed tremendously in the past few decades. For example, Fischer (2001) reports finding among the personal memorabilia of his father-in-law, a surgeon in Sioux City, Iowa, and a governor of the American College of Surgeons, a number of records showing that many of his patients did not actually pay him. Instead, "in-kind contributions of chickens, potatoes, knickknacks, etc., served sometimes as 'payment' for the care he delivered uncomplainingly for the better part of his 91 years" (pp. 71–72).

My own great-grandfather, who was a general practitioner in a small town in southern Italy, led a very different life from today's physicians and other health care providers. He died at the age of 102. One can speculate that good genes, a good diet, his passion for his work and long walks, and a relatively stress-free lifestyle all contributed to his long life. There are not many health care providers in this era of technological advances, malpractice suits, increased medical specialization, insurance-based health care, and other cost-cutting interventions who can say they lead a stress-free life.

Today, physicians and all other health care providers are faced with a number of additional day-to-day demands and tasks:

- Containing costs and being aware of the cost-effectiveness of the procedures and medications they recommend
- Keeping up with technology advances and the rapid evolution of medical standards and practices
- Being prepared to answer complex medical questions by increasingly informed patients
- Competing with other practices for patient retention
- Completing significant paperwork to satisfy billing and health insurance requirements

Professional communications can help health care providers meet their challenges with peer-to-peer information and tools that contribute to the effectiveness of their medical practices and, ultimately, better health outcomes for their patients. The importance of this communication area is directly correlated to the need to ensure that "medical practice reflects state-of-the-art scientific knowledge" (Solomon, 1995 p. 28). This is also the rationale for the recent emphasis on behavioral and institutional change models that may encourage physicians and other health care providers to adopt new behaviors and practices (Solomon, 1995).

This chapter defines medical professional communications and describes theoretical assumptions that influence this communication area. It also highlights key elements and commonly used activities and tools of professional communications programs. Finally, it establishes the context for professional communications and emphasizes how this approach can complement other strategies and areas of health communication and public health in general.

Communicating with Health Care Providers: A Peer-to-Peer Approach

Scientific exchange was recognized as both a need and an opportunity in the early history of medicine and other health care fields such as psychology and nursing. In most contexts and situations, peer-to-peer scientific exchange aims at advancing medical practices and advocating for the application of new standards of care. An everyday example of scientific exchange is the role of mentors, such as senior physicians and head nurses, who train or advise younger health care practitioners on different areas.

The concept of scientific exchange can be traced to Hippocrates, the ancient Greek physician who is considered the father of modern medicine (Pikoulis, Waasdorp, Leppaniemi, and Burris, 1998). Hippocrates, a prolific writer of his ideas and findings, "recommended that physicians record their findings and their medicinal methods, so that these records may be passed down and employed by other physicians" (Crystalinks, 2006; Winau, 1994).

Professional medical communication has evolved from the concept of scientific exchange as a peer-to-peer communication approach directed to physicians, nurses, physician assistants, and all other health care providers, as shown in Table 7.1. Professional medical communication can be defined as the application of health communication theories, models, and practices to programs that seek to influence the behavior and the social context of these professionals directly responsible for administering health care. In other words, it is the process of planning, executing, and evaluating communication programs intended for health care providers.

In professional communications, the concept of *peer* describes professionals with similar education, training, and overall capacity. Some peers who are recognized by their community as thought leaders in a field or on a health issue tend to take the lead in communicating with other physicians or nurses about new information in their area of competence. Other times, professional associations and other organizations, which may be responsible for setting new standards of care or keeping their membership up to date on recent medical and scientific progress, act as peer leaders in a communication effort.

TABLE 7.1. KEY AUDIENCES OF PROFESSIONAL MEDICAL COMMUNICATIONS

Physicians

Physician assistants

Medical directors

Nurses

   Nurse practitioners

   School nurses

   Visiting nurses

   Camp nurses

Therapists

   Speech therapists

   Physical therapists

   Other therapists

Dentists

Nutritionists

Dietitians

Thought leaders

Other health care providers

Although physicians and other health care providers are just another audience of health communication and should be treated as such, some differences exist. In fact, professional communications relies on several specific tools and activities as well as specialized skills (for example, excellent science writing skills and the ability to speak in complex medical terms), which are not always used in addressing the needs of other audiences. This is why professional communications is considered a separate area of health communication in this book.

This also reflects the actual practice of health communications. In fact, health communicators who facilitate the development of professional communications programs need to be able to relate to physicians and other health care providers using their own terms. This requires an in-depth technical understanding of the health issue and a much higher level of knowledge about the peer-reviewed literature related to it. Similarly, science writers are often specialized members of the health communication team.

Professional medical communications is often an important component of health communication programs. This approach is instrumental in a number of ways:

- Promoting the adoption of best practices
- Establishing new concepts and standards of care
- Raising provider awareness of recent medical discoveries, beliefs, parameters, and policies
- Changing or establishing new medical priorities
- Advancing health policy changes by engaging thought leaders and professional organizations in advocating such changes

Finally, professional medical communications are an important component of multifaceted interventions that ultimately seek a behavioral or social change at the patient or public level. In fact, they are instrumental in creating a receptive environment for patient demands and increased use of health services.

Take the fictitious example of José, a Puerto Rican man who reads in the local newspaper about the higher risk for oral cancer among Puerto Ricans versus other ethnic groups (Hayes and others, 1999; Parkin and others, 1997). At his next appointment, he asks his dentist whether he regularly performs oral cancer screening. If his dentist is not aware of the higher risk among Puerto Ricans or does not consider oral cancer screening one of the priorities of his practice, he may dismiss José's request and reassure him that he has nothing to worry about. In this case, any intervention directly targeted to José and other Puerto Ricans may not be effective if it is not supported by efforts that involve dentists and other primary care physicians in prioritizing and performing oral cancer screening at routine visits.

Similarly, the mother of a nine-year-old boy who still wets the bed at night as the result of primary nocturnal enuresis (PNE), a common medical condition that is still highly misdiagnosed and misunderstood in the United States (Hodge-Gray and Caldamone, 1998), may be rebuffed by her son's pediatrician when she asks for help. The pediatrician may believe that wetting the bed is a behavioral problem, which has been shown to be irrelevant in the etiology and treatment of PNE (Cendron, 1999). This may lead to additional years of suffering and humiliation for the boy, who would be limited in his ability to participate and enjoy common childhood activities such as summer camps and sleepovers (Hodge-Gray and Caldamone, 1998). The recurrence of this health problem will also continue to have a negative effect on family interactions and stress levels (Cendron, 1999).

These two examples confirm that professional medical communications efforts should be based, like all other communication interventions, on a true understanding of the audience's common beliefs, attitudes, practices, and needs. They should focus on changing the behavior of health care providers and, when necessary, the social norms and policies of the professional community to which they belong. Finally, they should engage health care providers in the design, implementation, and evaluation of such programs and elicit among them feelings of ownership and leadership in the solution of the health issue.

THEORETICAL ASSUMPTIONS IN PROFESSIONAL MEDICAL COMMUNICATIONS

Planning and implementing professional communications interventions is not so different from planning interventions intended for other audiences. "Whether directed to physicians or others, there is a standard method for designing interventions that includes the selection of an appropriate target audience, program goals, and messages as well as methods for delivery, implementation and evaluation" (Solomon, 1995, p. S28).

As in other areas of health communication, an important factor in the potential success of professional communications efforts is the participation and involvement of health care providers as well as the key institutions that represent or exert an influence on them. This process helps engage and train key opinion leaders in similar ways to those described in the chapter on community mobilization (see Chapter Six). After all, the medical and scientific community is still a community.

Sometimes taking an institutional approach to physician behavior change may help produce faster results (Solomon, 1995; Solomon and others, 1991). When reputable professional organizations take the lead in changing the beliefs, priorities, and practices of their memberships or employees (for example, in the case of a hospital), they implicitly acknowledge and influence what Solomon (1995) calls the "social nature of decision-making" (p. S30).

While all shifts in policies and practices are gradual and require a systematic and step-by-step approach, chances are that attempting to change an institutional policy may help implement the kind of peer pressure that is sought at the individual health care provider level. Still, in order to change the policy of an institution or organization, a series of behavioral changes is needed at the different hierarchical levels of the institution. Sometimes it is an ordinary member who believes in the need for change and starts modifying his or her practice as well as discussing the changes with colleagues and other members of the organization, all the way to the top. At other times, the behavioral and institutional changes start with the vision and leadership of top management, which becomes convinced because of professional communications programs, direct experience, or new scientific discovery of the need for new policies and practices.

Regardless of the original approach to behavioral change, the overall aim of professional medical communications efforts is to make sure that the largest number of individual physicians and health care providers endorses and implements practices that result in the best patient outcomes. It all starts with the awareness that scientific and medical discovery is just one step in improving patient outcomes. Despite such progress, the practice of medicine in most countries varies from region to region, practice to practice, and physician to physician (Burstall, 1991; Woods and Kiely, 2000).

In the United States, there are still common and widespread gaps in the quality of care patients receive (Institute of Medicine, 2001), which may be explained by differences in the use of state-of-the-art technologies or recommended medical practices as well as managed care restrictions (see Chapter Two). For example, "a review of 48 MEDLINE studies about US quality of care showed that 50% of recommended preventive care, 40% of recommended chronic care, and 30% of recommended acute care was not provided, whereas 20% to 30% of the care given was not recommended and so ranged from unnecessary to possibly harmful" (Grol, 2002, p. 245; Schuster, McGlynn, and Brook, 1998).

Closing the gaps and improving the overall quality of care is a step-by-step process that includes many of the stages highlighted by the behavioral and social change theories discussed in Chapter Two and requires a systematic audience-centered approach. As Grol (2002) highlights, several studies and experiences have shown that knowledge and more traditional educational activities are not sufficient to change physician behavior. "Activities and measures at different levels (individual, team, hospital, practice and the wider environment) are required to be successful" (p. 246). This is one of the fundamental and more general assumptions of well-designed and well-implemented health communication programs.

All theories and models that more generally apply to health communication are also relevant to professional medical communications. As in other areas of health communication, theories and models should be selected because of their relevance to the specific health problem and customized to meet the needs of physicians and other health care providers. Still, there are a few more specific considerations and theoretical assumptions that may help explain why health care providers do what they do and how to influence provider change.

HOW TO INFLUENCE HEALTH CARE PROVIDER BEHAVIOR: A THEORETICAL OVERVIEW

Health care providers should be considered just another audience. In designing communication interventions intended for them, their professional role as well as the key factors that influence providers' behavior should be analyzed in the same way health communicators would do with any other audience.

While there is a general lack of agreement on the theoretical basis for physician behavior or, more in general, health care provider behavior, many authors do agree about the relevance of behavioral and social change theories (Grimshaw, Eccles, Walker, and Thomas, 2002; Grol, 2002). Most of these theories were examined in Chapter Two and should be considered part of a toolbox that would also be used to guide the design of professional medical communications. Behavioral, institutional, and social outcomes of each professional intervention should be defined early in the process and used to measure the potential success of the professional communications effort.

Another emerging theoretical perspective is the importance of finding the right balance between individual and organizational or community-based interventions (Grol, 2002). For example, Slotnick and Shershneva (2002) suggest that physicians learn in communities of practice, which they define as "a group of people who share interests in an aspect of human endeavor and who participate in collective learning activities that both educate and create bonds among those involved" (p. 198).

Well-designed professional medical communications use a strategic blend of activities and channels that aims at involving individual providers and professional organizations to which they belong. In planning the behavioral change process, health communicators and other professionals should ask at what levels the intervention should occur and which kinds of actions are expected at each level. "Usually, actions focusing on individuals should be complemented by those directed at teams, organizations and the wider environment" (Grol, 2002, p. 248).

Sporadic and single communication activities almost never produce long-term results. Professional communications should be viewed as a process that is integrated by many other interventions, such as public relations, government relations, and physician communication training.

Prior to designing any activities, it is important to understand providers' beliefs, attitudes, current behavior, and potential peer pressure about the health issue or practice being addressed. Of equal importance is the need to assess their level of comfort with the medical topic.

The analysis should consider more general social factors that influence providers' behavior and practices. These may include both personal factors, such as the overall level of satisfaction with their profession, and practice-related factors, such as medical priorities established within their practices, level of collaborations with other medical specialties or health care providers, policies and social norms that prevail in their communities, or managed care or other cost-related restrictions. The same analysis should be conducted about organizations or professionals who influence health care provider behavior and practices: professional organizations, insurance companies, medical schools, and hospitals, for example. Finally, serious consideration should be given to potential obstacles to the implementation of new practices as well as the strategies to remove them. Multifaceted interventions that also focus on addressing potential barriers tend to be more effective (Grimshaw, Eccles, Walker, and Thomas, 2002) and produce sustainable behavior change.

Table 7.2 lists some of the common obstacles to behavioral change among health care providers. This list is not all-inclusive and, in some cases, would need to be modified in relation to the specific health issue or provider's specialty.

KEY ELEMENTS OF PROFESSIONAL MEDICAL COMMUNICATIONS PROGRAMS

One of the most important elements of professional communication programs is their multidisciplinary and multifaceted nature. Only interventions that rely on a sustained effort as well as on multiple tools and activities have the potential to become effective elements for provider change.

A list of some of the key characteristics of professional communications programs, which are discussed in further detail in this section, follows. Interestingly, many of them also reflect the key ele-

TABLE 7.2. KEY OBSTACLES TO CLINICIAN CHANGE

Gaps in knowledge or specific skills

Time constraints

Conflicting priorities

Information overload

Insufficient facilities or medical equipment

Lack of financial incentives

Managed care restrictions or other cost-cutting interventions

Sources: Grimshaw, Eccles, Walker, and Thomas (2002); Spickard and others (2001).

ments of best medical practices. In other words, best practices in professional communications planning often mirror the same key considerations that the health care and scientific community consider in establishing best medical practices. The asterisks in the list below indicate that these are also key elements of best clinical practices according to Steenholdt (2006):

- Evidence based*
- Audience specific
- Behavior centered
- Patient centered*
- Practical*
- Inclusive of easy-to-implement recommendations and tools
- Multifaceted
- Consistent*

EVIDENCE BASED

Health care providers are accustomed to basing their decisions on statistically significant data, scientific information, and professional guidelines. Large-scale clinical trials, new scientific discoveries, and clinical experience, which often lead to the development of organizational or disease-specific guidelines, provide evidence to support the need for a new medical practice or behavior.

Professional communications interventions should take into account the data-driven mind-set of physicians and other health care providers and rely on reputable scientific evidence to advance the adoption of the best medical practices.

AUDIENCE SPECIFIC

As in all other areas of health communication, professional communications efforts should be tailored to specific medical specialties and health care providers. In fact, the level to which different providers may need to apply new medical recommendations and practices can vary in relation to their level of competence and responsibility for a specific aspect of care.

For example, detailed information on how to reconstitute a vaccine from its powder formulation as well as storage conditions and vaccine appearance is particularly relevant for nurse practitioners, who are usually responsible for the actual administration of vaccines. However, since nurses are also on the front line with patients in addressing questions about the safety and efficacy of vaccines, information on new vaccines and their characteristics should be as comprehensive as that discussed with physicians. In this way, provider-patient communications will be consistent and accurate, and all members of the health care team will be adequately equipped to influence patient outcomes and decisions.

BEHAVIOR CENTERED

As always in health communication, behavioral outcomes should be clear at the onset of program planning. In other words, program planners should ask themselves what they want physicians or other health care providers to do. All interventions should be designed to encourage such behaviors and changes in practices.

PATIENT CENTERED

The patient is often at the center of health communication interventions. This is especially true in professional communications, where the ability of health care providers to digest and apply new medical and scientific information to day-to-day care may have a fundamental impact on health outcomes. As a consequence, professional communications strategies, activities, and tools should always strive to remind health care providers of the connection between the information being presented and potential patient outcomes.

Whenever possible, information about specific diseases or new medical practices should be integrated with the discussion and modeling of approaches to improve provider-patient communication on that specific topic. This is particularly relevant in the case of chronic illnesses or other medical issues that have a long-term physical or psychological burden on the patient.

PRACTICAL

Professional communications should always begin with asking, "So what?" Health care providers should leave all encounters and readings that are part of the professional communications program with a clear understanding of how the material applies to their day-to-day practice. Painter and Lemkau (1992) make a similar observation in relation to the organization of didactic materials for psychologist-led activities targeted to physicians.

For example, in developing a workshop on malaria, professional communicators should first emphasize practical approaches about the disease diagnosis and treatment and only later address the debate about the efficacy of different strategies for malaria prevention—for example, use of insecticide-treated mosquito nets versus house spraying or use of chloroquine (American Association for the Advancement of Science, 2006; Centers for Disease Control, 2006d; World Health Organization, 2006b).

EASY TO IMPLEMENT

Time barriers, conflicting priorities, managed care restrictions (see Chapter Two), and other obstacles often limit providers' ability to change and implement new practices. Therefore, professional communications should strive to make it easy to sustain the adoption of such practices. As Grol (2002) writes, "Particularly important here is that the change activities are embedded within day-to-day activities as much as possible and that the change will not be seen as extra work" (p. 249). This could be achieved by developing disease-specific or practice-specific activities and tool kits that health care providers can use as a reference or with their patients.

For example, as part of a communication effort to improve recognition and management of mild traumatic brain injury (MTBI), a condition that in the United States affects 1.1 million people and still is underdiagnosed and undertreated, the Centers for Disease Control (2006e) has developed a physician tool kit that includes "easy-to-use clinical information, patient information in English and Spanish [which physicians can distribute to their patients to complement or initiate in-office discussions], scientific literature, and a CD-ROM." The kit is aimed not only at improving the diagnosis and treatment of MTBI but also at providing physicians with the tools to communicate with patients and the community at large on how to prevent MTBI. The kit is complemented by other initiatives targeted to the general public, state departments of health, and special audiences (for example, athletes' coaches) that aim at increasing awareness and prevention of MTBI. In this way, physician change is also supported by attempts to change health behaviors in the patient communities that physicians attend to.

Multifaceted

A multifaceted approach has been proven to be more effective than single and sporadic activities. Table 7.3 provides an analysis of thirty-six systematic reviews and compares different approaches in relation to their effect on changing clinical performance (Grol, 1997, 2002). As part of this analysis, the table shows that single approaches have limited or mixed effects, while multifaceted interventions are mostly very effective.

As another example, when the U.S. National Foundation for Infectious Diseases (NFID) took over the leadership in advocating for policy and practice changes related to pediatric immunization against flu (see Box 7.1), it used a multifaceted approach that encouraged

TABLE 7.3. COMMUNICATION APPROACHES AND TOOLS AND
THEIR EFFECTS: ANALYSIS OF THIRTY-SIX SYSTEMATIC REVIEWS

Approaches and Tools	Number of Reviews	Effect of Studies
Educational materials, journals, mailed information	Nine	Limited effects
Continuing medical education courses, conferences	Four	Limited effects
Interactive educational meetings, small group education	Four	Few studies; mostly effective
Educational outreach visits, facilitation, and support	Eight	Particularly effective for prescribing and prevention
Feedback on performance	Seven	Mixed effects
Use of opinion leaders	Three	Mixed effects
Combined and multifaceted interventions with education	Sixteen	Mostly (very) effective

Source: Adapted from Grol, R. "Changing Physicians' Competence and Performance: Finding the Balance between the Individual and the Organization." *Journal of Continuing Education in the Health Professions,* 2002, 22, 244–251. Used by permission.

and supported the Centers for Disease Control recommendation for pediatric immunization as well as a widespread use of this practice.

Box 7.1

National Foundation for Infectious Diseases
Flu Fight for Kids: Case Study

Research shows children under 2 years of age are hospitalized due to influenza infection at the same high rate as persons 65 years and older. In 2002, the Centers for Disease Control and Prevention (CDC) issued a new policy to encourage influenza vaccination of all children 6 to 23 months of age. Extensive research and communication with key pediatric influenza thoughtleaders, policy makers and practicing physicians showed most physicians supported pediatric influenza immunization, but needed to overcome infrastructure barriers in their practices to implement annual flu vaccination programs. In addition, thoughtleaders and physicians identified several perceived barriers to 6- to 23-month-old influenza immunization.

In 2002, the National Foundation for Infectious Diseases launched the *Flu Fight for Kids* initiative to stimulate discussion on the topic and to create a climate of receptivity for routine annual influenza vaccination of infants and children 6 to 23 months of age. Thoughtleaders and policy makers needed to be convinced that immunization of 6- to 23-month-old children was feasible. At the same time, parents needed to become aware of their children's risk for flu and ask their health care providers to vaccinate their children.

Key Actions

2002 Roundtable Meeting/Consensus Document

NFID convened a roundtable meeting with the participation of experts from many sectors, including public health, private practice, nursing and infectious diseases. This was instrumental to reach a consensus about the severity of pediatric influenza and highlight best practice models to help pediatric practices implement annual vaccination programs. A comprehensive consensus report, *Increasing Influenza Immunization Rates in Infants and Children: Putting Recommendations Into Practice*, summarized the meeting proceedings. The report outlines barriers to influenza vaccination, as well as strategies to overcome them. It also provides "best practice models" for achieving optimal influenza vaccination rates. The document was widely distributed and presented to the CDC's Advisory Committee on Immunization Practices (ACIP) as a resource to demonstrate that annual influenza vaccination programs can be implemented in physician practices.

Media Outreach

Trade and consumer media outreach were conducted to communicate to the medical community, as well as parents, the serious nature of influenza illness among children 6 to 23 months of age. Outreach also focused on strategies for immunizing this population within pediatric practices throughout the *Flu Fight for Kids* initiative. Key placements were secured in leading consumer and trade media throughout the campaign, including *USA Today, AAP News, Parents* and *Child*.

Satellite Symposium at American Academy of Pediatrics (AAP) Annual Meeting

NFID sponsored a continuing medical education (CME) satellite symposium highlighting the proceedings from the roundtable meeting and report at the American Academy of Pediatrics annual meeting in November 2003. Hundreds of physicians attended the program on-site and several hundred more participated in an online CME program, which was made available following the event. The CME program provided information to help pediatricians prepare their practice for routine influenza vaccination of all children 6 to 23 months of age.

CDC Issues Full Pediatric Recommendation

During the campaign, two key meetings of the CDC's ACIP took place in June and October of 2003. Before both meetings, NFID invited key thoughtleaders to highlight the strategies from the roundtable meeting and consensus report. At the October meeting, NFID enrolled a practicing pediatrician to address the panel about his successful vaccination program.

Results—First Year of Routine Recommendation

On October 15, 2003, the CDC's advisory committee unanimously voted to recommend influenza vaccination for 6 to 23 months of age, beginning in fall 2004. NFID's steady, year long outreach to thoughtleaders, physicians, policymakers and parents contributed to early adoption of the recommendations. Data from the first year of the full recommendation (2004–05 influenza season) reported the new vaccination recommendations for all children 6 to 23 months of age resulted in a higher than expected 48 percent coverage rate. This is the most rapid uptake of any routine pediatric vaccine to date.

Continuing its efforts to help physicians implement the new recommendations and improve immunization rates in the population, NFID developed a comprehensive resource kit, *Kids Need Flu Vaccine, Too!* The kit helps healthcare providers establish in-practice influenza vaccination programs. The kit was issued in 2004 and updated with additional educational materials in 2005. Key objectives of the resource kit are supported by the American Academy of Pediatrics (AAP) and the National Influenza Vaccine Summit, which is co-sponsored by the American Medical Association and the CDC.

Source: National Foundation for Infectious Diseases, "Flu Fight for Kids," unpublished case study, 2005. Copyright © 2005. National Foundation for Infectious Diseases. Used by permission.

CONSISTENT

Communication messages should be consistent throughout the stages of the professional communications intervention. They should also be consistent with recent medical discoveries, best practices, and clinical guidelines.

Message consistency is a fundamental concept in communication and helps establish a clear path to change. Conflicting recommendations and messages may confuse intended audiences, hinder their willingness to change, and affect their overall perception about the quality of the communication program.

OVERVIEW OF KEY COMMUNICATION CHANNELS AND ACTIVITIES

Physicians and other health care providers have traditionally relied on peer-reviewed publications to communicate with their communities about scientific and medical discoveries as well as clinical

practices. This remains an important evidence-based tool for credible scientific exchange about research findings. However,
Grimshaw, Eccles, Walker, and Thomas (2002) identify a number
of limitations by relying solely on this approach as well as its impact on translating new evidence to actual medical practice: (1)
the limited time physicians dedicate to reading, which according
to several polls is on average not more than one hour per week;
(2) the fact that many physicians lack specific training to evaluate
the quality of published research; and (3) the existence of several
barriers to the application of evidence-based information to actual clinical practice. Well-designed and well-implemented professional communications programs rely on multiple channels and
activities that do the following:

• Complement peer-reviewed publications.
• Present information in an easy-to-digest and practical format.
• Prioritize and highlight the weight of different research find-
  ings in relation to actual clinical practice.
• Point to specific guidelines and best practices.
• Provide guidance and tools to overcome existing barriers to
  the adoption of new clinical practices and behaviors.

Table 7.4 sets out tools, activities, and channels that are traditionally used in professional communications. All of them—and
many others—should be considered in identifying the strategic
elements of issue-specific and audience-centered professional communications programs. Among them, peer-reviewed or trade publication articles are normally written by opinion leaders and
scientific advisers who are close to an organization's mission or are
actually members of their scientific board of advisers. In fact, it is
common practice for nonprofit and other private organizations to
ask their scientific leaders to be directly involved in publicizing the
data or ideas developed or advocated by such an organization.
Other times, the organization simply keeps track in a publication
plan of all forthcoming articles on a specific topic and makes sure
to extend the reach of the publication through other professional
communication channels and activities.

Another important point is that serious consideration should
be given to active approaches, such as interactive workshops and
opinion leaders meetings, which should be designed to fit in the

TABLE 7.4. KEY COMMUNICATIONS TOOLS AND CHANNELS
IN PROFESSIONAL COMMUNICATIONS

Communications venues and channels	Annual meetings, professional conferences
	Regional meetings, professional chapter meetings
	Institutional meetings (for example, hospital or patient conferences)
	Special events (roundtables, symposia, lecture series)
	World Wide Web
	Professional and trade media
	Special communication tools
Key tools	
Print	Monograph: a document, book, or leaflet that is complete in itself and contains multiple articles or sections
	White paper: a type of monograph that is based on the discussion at a thought leader roundtable or working group
	Consensus document: a type of white paper to establish consensus on a health issue or practice, with conclusions voted on by all members of the working group or closed roundtable
	Call-to-action document: a type of consensus document that calls for specific actions to be implemented by different audiences in the medical and professional community; may help shape new health policies or practices.
	Journal supplement: a compilation of scientific articles or meetings proceedings, usually packaged with the primary journal for distribution
	Trade publication article: an article being published by a thought leader or professional organization on publications that target specific professional audiences,

Table 7.4. Key Communications Tools and Channels
in Professional Communications, Cont'd.

	including op-ed pieces and letters to the editors. Standard editorial process; not peer reviewed.
	Peer-reviewed journal article: peer-reviewed article on original research data or new ideas on existing research
Online	Web sites
	E-alerts: issued by professional organizations to their membership and key constituencies to alert them to new medical practices, publications, events, and other information of interest
	Online discussions, live seminars, symposia, educational programs
	Electronic versions of print tools
	Audio and video programs
Audio and video programs	Training videos
	Spin-off of a primary program (for example, audiotaped conference, videotaped symposium)
	Videos to support topic- and audience-specific presentations at conferences and meetings
Easy-to-implement tools	Tool kits: print or electronic versions of materials that clinicians can use for a variety of issue-specific reasons: communication with patients, diagnostic tool, training sessions for all members of the clinical team, as a reminder of the importance of a new medical practice; may include brochures, fact sheets, videos, CD-ROM

busy schedule of clinicians. Interactive approaches are more likely to be effective even if they are more expensive (Grimshaw, Eccles, Walker, and Thomas, 2002; Spickard and others, 2001). Practical experience has always confirmed this view.

Finally, professional communications activities and tools should respond to program strategies and be designed to transform "roadblocks into stepping stones" (Painter and Lemkau, 1992, p. 183) toward clinician change and, ultimately, better patient outcomes.

KEY CONCEPTS

- Professional medical communications is the application of health communication theories, models, and practices to programs that seek to influence the behavior and the social context of health professionals who are directly responsible for administering health care.
- Professional communications is a peer-to-peer approach directly related to the need to ensure that clinical practice always reflects the state-of-the-art scientific evidence.
- Because of the influence of health care providers on patients' outcomes and decisions, professional medical communications is a very important area of health communication. Often it is also a critical component of larger health communication programs that seek to encourage behavioral changes at the patient or public level or advocate for a medical policy or practice change.
- Although physicians and other health care providers are just another audience and should be considered as such, there are several specific skills (for example, advanced scientific writing ability) and tools that are used primarily or solely in professional communications. This creates the need for considering professional communications as a separate area of health communication.
- Although there is no consensus on theories and models for clinician change, recent emphasis has been placed on the importance of behavioral and social change theories as well as many other constructs that are already part of the health communication theoretical tool box (see Chapter Two).

- As in other areas of health communications, behavioral and social outcomes should be defined in advance and used to evaluate the intervention's effectiveness. Ultimately professional communications programs should aim to facilitate and encourage the adoption of best practices that may result in better health outcomes.
- The key characteristics and tools of effective professional communications programs should be considered in planning and implementing such interventions.
- Given the complexity of the health care environment, special consideration should be given to the following observations:
  - Professional communications programs that address existing barriers to clinician change are more likely to be effective.
  - Although more expensive, interactive approaches should be preferred because of their higher potential to motivate behavioral change among health care providers.
  - Multifaceted approaches are usually more effective than single or sporadic approaches in converting state-of-the-art scientific evidence in the adoption of new or best practices by clinicians.
  - Practical experience has validated the importance of using the right combination of individual and group strategies with institutional strategies.

For Discussion and Practice

1. In your opinion, in what circumstances may professional medical communications programs be an essential component of health communication interventions? Use specific examples or anecdotal experiences.
2. What are the key differences between professional medical communications and other areas of health communication? What are the key similarities?
3. How do health care providers' social networks and professional associations influence clinician behavior and practices? What are some implications of the providers' social context in professional medical communications?
4. Review Table 7.2, and rank what in your opinion are the most important obstacles to clinician change. Explain your rank or-

dering, and relate any personal or professional experiences that may support your selection.

5. A national nursing association launches a communication program to raise awareness of the reemergence of an infectious disease as well as recommended approaches to prevent it. Until then, the disease had been underestimated and underdiagnosed. In year one, the program's primary audience encompasses only health care professionals; in year two, the program's reach is extended to patients and the general public. List potential reasons for the association's decision to target only providers in the first year of the program, and discuss pros and cons of this approach.

CHAPTER EIGHT

CONSTITUENCY RELATIONS IN HEALTH COMMUNICATION

IN THIS CHAPTER

- Constituency Relations: A Practice-Based Definition
- Recognizing the Legitimacy of All Constituency Groups
- Constituency Relations: An Effective and Structured Approach
- Key Concepts
- For Discussion and Practice

In most democratic societies, constituency relations is a structured approach that policymakers and elected government officials use "to consult, interact and exchange views and information with the public, so that citizens can express their preferences and provide their support for decisions that affects their lives and livelihood" (United Nations Development Programme, 2006). The general public as well as special groups and communities are the main constituents of policymakers.

At the same time, local government officials are a key constituency for public health. In fact, they influence the actions of local health departments as well as the allocation of funds and human resources to public health intervention and fields. Helping local government officials understand the true meaning of public health, which sometimes they regard only as the provision of specific health services and not as broad-based and community-centered interventions to improve public health outcomes, has been identified as an important role of public health managers. This helps gain visibility for public health (Lind and Finley, 2000) and enhances the chance that funding of public health interventions becomes a priority in a specific state or region.

These examples are only a few among the many contexts of constituency relations in which two different groups (policymakers and the general public, or local government officers and public health officials) can mutually influence each other. Constituency relations is an approach that is used in the public health, nonprofit, and commercial sectors to address a variety of health issues and situations, often in the context of health communication. It applies to different kinds of constituency groups that vary in function concerning the specific health issue or disease area.

This chapter defines constituency relations and establishes its key contexts. It also provides examples on how the practice of constituency relations is relevant to the field of health communication and can be used as an integral approach of all communication action areas. Finally, it highlights examples, key steps, and dos and don'ts of this health communication area.

CONSTITUENCY RELATIONS: A PRACTICE-BASED DEFINITION

Before defining constituency relations, it is important to understand what a constituency is. **Constituents** range from the body of voters who elect a specific policymaker or a political party or the board member of a professional organization to "groups of supporters or patrons" of different causes or groups "served by an organization or institution" (*American Heritage Dictionary of the English Language,* 2004). In health care, they include patients, physicians, and other health care providers, hospital employees, professional and advocacy groups, nonprofit organizations, pharmaceutical companies, public health departments, the general public, and policymakers, to name just a few. These groups mutually influence each other. Depending on the specific health issue, situation, or setting, some of them may be more effective than others in helping to advance public health causes, organizational missions, or corporate goals.

In health communication, *constituency relations* can be defined as the process of convening, exchanging information, and establishing and maintaining strategic relationships with key stakeholders and organizations with the intent of identifying common goals that can contribute to the outcomes of a specific communication program or health-related mission. In fact, "communicating often involves reaching out to the audience first and building a constituency for the message" (Carter, 1994, p. 51). This process of establishing effective relationships and building key constituencies relies on all action areas of health communication (for example, interpersonal communications, public relations). It is also an integral element of all of them and at the same time a communication area of its own. Often constituency relations leads to strategic partnerships and coalitions.

Constituency relations has been used for the past twenty years as a strategic area of communication in the private and commercial sectors. It has been employed to develop alliances "to address public-policy issues" as well as "to extend political or marketing reach" by corporations. In this context, key constituency groups are also called *third-party groups* and include nonprofit, special interest, and advocacy organizations (Burson-Marsteller, 2006). Usually all parties in these relationships have shared goals that often can be achieved through collaboration, partnership, or interaction.

In the corporate world as well as in many health care institutions such as private and public hospitals, constituency relations may be explained by looking at the stakeholder theory (Freeman, 1984). Originally developed to describe which groups in a corporation should receive management attention, the stakeholder theory recognizes that there are internal (for example, employers, investors) as well as external parties (customers, of course, but also political groups and communities) whose needs and wishes should be addressed as part of corporate decisions and initiatives. "A stakeholder in an organization is (by its definition) any group or individual who can affect or is affected by the achievement of the organization's objectives" (Freeman, 1984, p. 25; Scholl, 2001).

Other theoretical influences in the practice of constituency relations can be found in theories and models that look at the interrelation between different individual, group, or community factors, organizations, and levels of society, as well as their influence on health and social behavior (for example, the socioecological model mentioned in Chapter One and the ideation theory covered in Chapter Two). In general, constituency relations is a structured approach that can maximize the value of these connections and unleash the power of relationships to achieve health or social goals. Key community and social mobilization principles (see Chapter Six) can also be considered major influences in the practice of constituency relations.

In public health, several organizations and institutions increasingly recognize the role of constituency relations. For example, in 1999 the U.S. National Institute of Mental Health launched the Constituency Outreach and Education Program, a nationwide initiative to "focus the energy of advocacy groups on merging science with service" and provide them with tools and information to develop health communication programs that will increase access to appropriate medical interventions by patients who suffer from mental illnesses (Cave, n.d.). The program, now called the Outreach Partnership Program, has enlisted over the years "national and state organizations in partnerships to help bridge the gap between research and clinical practice by disseminating the latest scientific findings; informing the public about mental disorders, alcoholism, and drug addiction; and reducing the stigma and discrimination associated with these illnesses. The program also provides the National Institute of Mental Health with the opportunity to engage community groups across the United States in developing a national research agenda grounded in public health need" (National Institute of Mental Health, 2006).

Constituency relations can help advance several disease-specific or social objectives within a health communication program. Some of the key areas or issues on which constituency relations can help are discussed later in this chapter.

RECOGNIZING THE LEGITIMACY OF ALL CONSTITUENCY GROUPS

Positive relationships with organizations, opinion leaders, and individuals who have a stake in a specific health issue often lead to creating a favorable and receptive environment for the key messages and activities of a health communication program. However, relationships should extend beyond groups or individuals who share common ideas and goals. Recognizing the legitimacy of all constituents, including groups that may have an opposite point of view, is an integral component of the practice of constituency relations (Burson-Marsteller, 2006).

Understanding opposing opinions as well as the key facts that may lead to them is one step toward anticipating and managing criticisms as well as gaining the respect of those who advocate opposite causes or solutions for the same health issue. In some cases, it may help find common ground, minimize differences, or propose solutions that may be acceptable to all parties.

Although it is not always possible to bridge different opinions, it is important to convey the impression of being for or against an issue and not against someone personally. At a minimum, contacts with opponents or information about their activities can guide communication efforts and tactics.

A relevant example is the ongoing debate on animal rights versus animal research that has been taking place for decades in Europe and the United States. Some of the animal rights organizations in the United States have long recognized that "an uncompromising, vegetarian-only, anti-medical-progress philosophy has a limited appeal" (Center for Consumer Freedom, 2006) with key constituencies, including the general public and policymakers. In some European countries, animal welfare organizations had to react to increasing support as well as petitions in favor of animal research by scientists, doctors, and reputable opinion leaders from the medical community. As a result, some of them have somewhat changed the focus or the tactics used in their efforts (Constance, 2005).

In recognizing the legitimacy of all constituencies, many of the skills and theoretical bases of interpersonal communications and other health communication areas come into play in managing criticisms as well as looking for common ground whenever possible. In fact, constituency relations use many of the tools and tactics of these communication areas (for example, public advocacy, one-on-one meetings, issues management) to address criticisms as well as develop alliances with key constituency groups that share similar values and goals.

At the same time, constituency relations is an integral component of all the other areas of health communication. For example, public advocacy (see Chapter Five) is often used to attract new constituents to a health issue. At the same time, establishing and maintaining relationships with key representatives of the mass media is fundamental to media advocacy efforts and uses many of the principles of constituency relations.

CONSTITUENCY RELATIONS: AN EFFECTIVE AND STRUCTURED APPROACH

As with other areas of health communication, constituency relations is both an art and a science. Health organizations that approach this field for the first time may require changes at the individual, team, and organizational levels in order to succeed in their constituency relations efforts. Still, as experience has shown, constituency relations and building are critical elements in the process for addressing existing and new public health recommendations and challenges (Kimbrell, 2000).

Health organizations and communication teams may want to consider building internal capabilities to establish and maintain relationships with key constituencies and, ideally, develop strategic partnerships and coalitions. This transformation usually starts with key management (for example, executive directors, board members, and communication directors) and extends to all levels of the organization. Encouraging a constituency relations and partnership-oriented mind-set among staff and consultants has these key components:

- Identifying constituency relations and outreach champions and, when resources allow, establishing professional positions or departments dedicated to this area. For example, the U.S. National Institute of Mental Health has an Office of Constituency Relations and Public Liaison. Also, the Campaign for Tobacco-Free Kids, "one of the United States largest nongovernmental initiatives ever launched to protect children from tobacco addiction and exposure to second-hand smoke" (Campaign for Tobacco Free Kids, 2006), has several staff members dedicated to constituency relations as well as a vice president of constituency relations.

- Emphasizing the importance of teamwork, listening, and negotiation skills, as well as balancing different needs and sharing credit for success with other organizations.
- Training staff members.
- Sharing results with other organizational departments.

In addition, organizations and health communication teams need to develop a long-term vision about key constituency groups as well as their key issues and priorities. They also need to establish and cultivate long-term relationships with all of these groups. Table 8.1 gives examples of the dos and don'ts of establishing and preserving relationships with key constituents.

DEVELOPING ALLIANCES TO ADDRESS HEALTH OR SOCIAL ISSUES AND TO EXPAND PROGRAM REACH

One of the common outcomes of constituency relations is the development of partnerships, coalitions, or other kinds of collaborations. Coalitions often grow out of partnerships and require a more formal structure, including written memoranda of communication agreements, by-laws, a dedicated management team, and common tools, as well as a long-term commitment to the coalition's cause. A relevant example is the Coalition for Health Communication (2006), "an inter-organizational task force whose mission is to strengthen the identity and advance the field of health communication." The coalition, which includes several groups, associations, and U.S. federal agencies, has a common Web site, a management team, and common activities and tools.

Regardless of their format, partnerships, coalitions, and other forms of collaborations can help advance health and social goals by strengthening the credibility and relevance of a specific issue; giving a structured voice to constituencies that can influence policymakers, the press, and other key stakeholders; expanding the program's reach; or combining different resources and expertise. Box 8.1 features an interview with key staff members from Physicians for Human Rights, an international nonprofit organization, and provides a practical perspective on the importance of constituency relations.

TABLE 8.1. GUIDELINES FOR ESTABLISHING AND
PRESERVING LONG-TERM RELATIONSHIPS

Do	Don't
Understand the mission, strategic priorities, and focus of key constituency groups.	Look down at constituency groups if they are smaller in size or in favor of a different approach to a health issue.
Reach out to these groups at the program's onset.	Assume they will support every aspect of your health cause or communication program.
Keep an open mind in exchanging relevant information.	
Consider their worries and concerns.	Give the impression they are not accountable for their responsibilities if a partnership is established or do their share of the work.
Recognize and respect cultural, ethnic, or other kinds of differences.	
Look for shared goals and priorities.	Try to control or micromanage them.
Act to establish long-term relationships based on trust and mutual respect.	
When of interest, address barriers to potential partnerships.	
If a partnership is established, honor deadlines, financial commitments, and mutually agreed-on procedures and roles.	
Encourage and maximize participation by all partners in program design, implementation, and evaluation.	

Box 8.1

How Constituency Relations Can Help Advance an Organization's Mission: A Practice-Based Perspective

The following perspective on constituency relations reflects a telephone interview and personal communications in 2006 with Gina Cummings, deputy director of operations, and Nancy Marks, director of outreach, for Physicians for Human Rights.

Physicians for Human Rights (PHR), founded in 1986, mobilizes health professionals to advance the health and dignity of all people through actions that promote respect for, protection of, and fulfillment of human rights. In 1997 PHR shared the Nobel Prize for Peace as a founding member of the Steering Committee of the International Campaign to Ban Landmines. PHR is a membership organization of physicians, nurses, public health experts, forensic scientists, human rights experts, and others dedicated to advancing health and human rights. Health care professionals are a reputable voice in society and have the power and credibility to advocate for human rights protection.

Over the past twenty years, the organization has evolved in its mission and has made many changes to engage health care providers (including physicians, nurses, and medical, nursing, and public health students) from the United States and many other parts of the world in studying the impact of human right abuses on the health status of populations as well as advocating for change with policymakers and other relevant parties. PHR built a U.S.-based professional constituency that provides expertise and document abuse and advocates for new policies and practices. It is currently beginning to cultivate a similar constituency in Africa to work on issues related to the prevention of HIV/AIDS and treatment and care of HIV/AIDS patients.

Medical, nursing, and public health students are key constituencies in the organization. PHR believes that students represent the future of public health and human rights. Student volunteers raise awareness of health care disparities, persuade policymakers about the importance of viewing HIV/AIDS as a global crisis with an impact on health care and health care systems, and work to end the genocide in Darfur, Sudan.

PHR work has been focusing not only on building and supporting new constituencies but also on maintaining and cultivating relationships with existing constituency groups and other stakeholders,
including U.S. policymakers, ministries of health in developing countries, the World Health Organization, and other human rights organizations, including Amnesty International. PHR is often a resource
for policymakers and other key constituencies; for example, it provides
scientific content about human rights and health issues and proposes
strategic solutions. PHR also acts as a convener of stakeholders in
meetings, workshops, and summits that aim to establish consensus
on potential solutions of health and human rights issues, as well as a
clear path to achieve them.

For example, in recognizing that most health centers in rural
Africa are attended by nurse practitioners, PHR partnered with the
U.S. Association of Nurses in AIDS Care to organize an HIV summit
that included the participation of twenty-five to thirty nurses working
with AIDS in Africa. These nurses not only had an opportunity to exchange information on best clinical practices in HIV/AIDS treatment
and prevention but were also able to meet with U.S. policymakers to
address issues related to the funding of HIV prevention, care, and
treatment in Africa. The summit also addressed the issue of the increasing shortage of health care professionals in developing countries
due to deteriorating socioeconomic conditions. PHR gave to the project its expertise in human rights, while the nurses' association was instrumental for technical competence and wealth of knowledge in the
HIV/AIDS field.

Building a constituency is often the result of speaking with organizations or people who understand the specific health or human
rights problem and its potential solutions. It also requires a clear understanding of roles and responsibilities of different constituencies,
expected outcomes of potential partnerships, the time frame of all
joint efforts and collaborations, and the decision-making process that
will be used for joint efforts.

Most people understand the nuances of the work required in constituency relations only after many years of practice. This is the kind
of professional competence that one learns on the job. Nevertheless,
it is important to become familiar with the values and key principles
of this important area as part of formal education and training.

KEY STEPS IN DEVELOPING STRATEGIC PARTNERSHIPS

Building strategic partnerships requires hard work in both the exploratory and the maintenance phases. It is important to identify potential partners early in the process as well as to be aware of organizational restrictions and administrative requirements of one's organization that may prevent or regulate partnerships.

The decision about developing partnerships should be made early in program development. In doing so, health organizations and communication teams should be aware of the potential drawbacks of partnerships and be prepared to address them efficiently (National Cancer Institute and National Institutes of Health, 2002).

In general, most drawbacks can be successfully addressed if all partners have established and agreed on well-defined objectives for the specific partnership, standard procedures, shared workload, and common goals. All of these elements are usually addressed as part of the partnership plan component of a health communication program (see Chapter Twelve).

Nevertheless, partnerships take time and commitment. Being aware of some of the potential drawbacks is a step forward in overcoming barriers and preserving long-term relationships. Table 8.2 lists potential drawbacks. Some of them may be minimized by choosing the right partners.

TABLE 8.2. POTENTIAL DRAWBACKS OF PARTNERSHIPS

Feelings of loss of control over program development

Time-consuming process

Partners who may go "off strategy"

Lack of partners' participation or real commitment to the project

Too many administrative roadblocks

The cost (economic or human resources) of maintaining and managing the partnership

---

Sources: National Cancer Institute and National Institutes of Health (2002); Weinreich (1999).

CHOOSING THE RIGHT PARTNERS

Since the list of potential partners is often quite long, the following criteria may help identify partners and organizations that are best suited to support and contribute to the health communication program or the mission of a specific health organization:

- Mutual mission and goals, which often starts with a common vision but sometimes can be the result of an engaging communication process in which common interests and solutions are identified, negotiated, and selected to the satisfaction of all potential partners.
- Background and experience in relation to the specific health issue or audience the program is seeking to address. It also includes relevant experiences in different fields that may function as a model for new health communication interventions.
- Access to intended audiences through existing communication vehicles or because of the reputation of potential partners with key audiences, the mass media, or other key stakeholders.
- Preexisting relationships with one's organization.
- Enthusiasm about overall program goal and content.
- Access to additional resources and skills.
- Ease of process in terms of the review process for materials and messages, as well as lack of excessive standard protocols that are not flexible to accommodate partners' working styles and routine procedures.
- Costs (economic, time, and resources) that need to be dedicated to establishing and managing a specific partnership.

In short, it is always better to identify partners that have organizational, professional, or audience-related objectives that in the long term can contribute to the achievement of the health communication program's goals and objectives. If and when partnerships with commercial companies are considered, most nonprofit organizations have written or informal criteria and policies that guide such partnerships. These criteria are set to preserve the nonprofit organization's credibility and independence, as well as the overall reputation of the partnership. Usually they are also welcomed and endorsed by most commercial entities.

Box 8.2 provides the U.S. National Cancer Institute guidelines for the evaluation of commercial partners that may participate in health communication interventions or other institute efforts. Specific criteria and steps also apply to other special kinds of partnerships such as coalitions, *public-private partnerships* (such as any collaboration between public authorities such as local or central governments, and private companies or organizations; National Council for Public-Private Partnerships, 2006), and *collaborative agreements* (such as those that involve universities, health care professionals, and organizations). Appendix A includes a select list of resources in relation to special kinds of partnerships.

Box 8.2

National Cancer Institute Guidelines for Considering Commercial Partners

Policies

- The National Cancer Institute will not consider any collaboration that endorses a specific commercial product, service, or enterprise.
- The National Cancer Institute name and logo may be used only in conjunction with approved projects and only with the written permission of NCI. NCI retains the right to review all copy (e.g., advertising, publicity, or for any other intended use) prior to approval of the use of the NCI name and logo.
- The National Cancer Institute will formally review each proposal for partnership.
- No company will have an exclusive right to use the NCI name and logo, messages, or materials.
- Confidentiality cannot be guaranteed for any collaboration with a federal program.

Criteria for Reviewing Corporations
Prior to Partnership Negotiations

- Company is not directly owned by a tobacco company and is not involved in producing, marketing, or promoting tobacco products.

- Company does not have any products, services, or promotional messages that conflict with NCI policies or programs (e.g., the company does not market known carcinogens or market some other product that NCI would not consider medically or scientifically acceptable).
- Company is not currently in negotiation for a grant or contract with NCI.
- Company does not have any unresolved conflicts or disputes with NCI or NIH [National Institutes of Health].
- Establishing a partnership with this company will not create tensions/conflicts with another NCI partner or federal program.
- Company or institution satisfactorily conforms with standards of health or medical care.
- There is evidence that the company would be interested in becoming a partner with NCI.

Source: U.S. National Cancer Institute and National Institutes of Health. *Making Health Communication Programs Work.* National Institutes of Health, Publication No. 02-5145, 2002, p. 37.

In conclusion, the practice of constituency relations, as well as the potential for partnerships or other kinds of collaborations that derive from this practice, is a valuable asset in all health communication areas. For example, when planning the professional medical communications component of a health communication program, it is critical to understand and involve health organizations and groups that can influence physician behavioral change. At the same time, constituency relations rely on many of the theoretical assumptions and tools of other areas of communication (for example, interpersonal communications) and can be considered a strategic communication area of its own. Often new communication programs and approaches as well as the decision to focus on a specific health issue start with an informal meeting or telephone call in which constituency groups are involved. From this starting point, the road to effective interactions, collaborations, and partnerships is as complex and gradual as described in this chapter.

KEY CONCEPTS

- Constituency relations is a key area of health communication as well as a critical component of all other action areas of communication.
- In health communication, constituency relations can be defined as the process of convening, exchanging information, establishing, and maintaining strategic relationships with key stakeholders and organizations with the intent of identifying common goals that can contribute to the outcomes of a specific communication program or health-related mission.
- Constituency relations is commonly used in the public health, nonprofit, and commercial sectors as a fundamental area of communication.
- One of the fundamental premises of constituency relations is the importance of recognizing the legitimacy of all constituency groups, including those that may have opposite opinions on or approaches to a health issue.
- Establishing and maintaining positive relationships with groups that share common values and goals depends on a number of factors.
- Building a constituency around a health issue or developing strategic partnerships and collaborations requires hard work and several fundamental steps. These steps are usually summarized in the partnership plan component of a health communication program (see Chapter Twelve).

FOR DISCUSSION AND PRACTICE

1. Discuss examples of partnerships or coalitions of which you are aware, and highlight their role in advancing public health or organizational goals.
2. Review Table 8.1, and describe a professional or personal experience in which any of the dos or don'ts in the table have influenced the process of establishing and preserving long-term relationships. Rank the dos and don'ts in the table in order of importance, and provide a rationale for your ranking order.
3. How do constituency relations fit in health communication? Provide examples to illustrate key concepts explored in this chapter.

PART THREE

PLANNING, IMPLEMENTING, AND EVALUATING A HEALTH COMMUNICATION PROGRAM

CHAPTER NINE

OVERVIEW OF THE HEALTH COMMUNICATION PLANNING PROCESS

IN THIS CHAPTER

- Why Planning Is Important
- Approaches to Health Communication Planning
- The Health Communication Cycle and Strategic Planning Process
- Key Steps of Health Communication Planning
- Elements of an Effective Health Communication Program
- Establishing the Overall Program Goal: A Practical Perspective
- Outcome Objectives: Behavioral, Social, and Organizational
- Key Concepts
- For Discussion and Practice

Most health organizations have or expect to have a communication plan at some point in their life cycle. However, many of them have difficulties converting plans into actions that have an impact on their constituencies, their mission, or the visibility of their organization. Most of the problems rest in a lack of understanding of the fundamental steps of a health communication plan and how to design communication interventions that fit the organization's mission, as well as the needs of its key constituencies and stakeholders. In other words, there is often lack of clarity about what the plan should do for the organization and its key audiences (Adams, 2005).

A practical example is the use of mandated cigarette warnings as part of the U.S. public policy strategy "to educate consumers about the risks of smoking" (Krugman, Fox, and Fischer, 1999, p. 95). Cigarette warnings have been used for many years but have proven to be ineffective communication tools. Part of the problem is that they were designed as the result of negotiations between the U.S. federal government and the tobacco industry and "neither developed nor implemented with specific communications goals in mind" (p. 95).

It is important that policymakers clearly understand and establish at the onset of the warning program what they expect warnings to accomplish. Should warnings be designed to communicate the risks associated with smoking or attempt to prevent smoking initiation? Did the current design and message length take into account how much time consumers would spend reading the warning? Did warnings aim to reach primarily adolescents or also other age groups? What about the graphic appeal of the warnings in contrast with the flashy images of tobacco industry ads? Understanding all of these factors and many others that are not listed here may increase the efficacy of cigarette warnings if they become part of a comprehensive health communication program (Krugman, Fox, and Fischer, 1999).

This example reinforces several of the fundamental premises of this book: know your audience; be clear about what you want them to do or believe; use a multifaceted and participatory approach to affect their core beliefs and behavior; and help them own the change process. In health communication, planning is a rigorous research-based process. Health communication terminology is important in guiding the different planning and implementation steps.

This chapter, the first in Part Three, which provides a step-by-step guide to health communication planning, implementation, and evaluation, discusses why planning is important and highlights the key steps of the health communication process. It provides an overview of this process, which will be discussed in further detail in the remaining chapters and, using practical examples, defines the meaning of "overall program goal" and provides practical guidance in establishing these goals at the onset of the program together with behavioral, social, and organizational change objectives.

WHY PLANNING IS IMPORTANT

Too often health organizations operate on emergency mode and use communication primarily as a tool to respond to emerging needs or sudden crises. This frequently leads to difficulties in securing adequate funding or response to what appear to be last-minute needs. The truth is that most needs can be anticipated and many crises averted if communication planning is one of the standard protocols and activities of the organization.

Communication planning is a research-driven process. An in-depth understanding of the health communication environment as well as the needs, preferences, and expectations of key audiences and stakeholders on a health issue may result in multifaceted and well-orchestrated interventions that are far more effective than single and sporadic approaches to communication. Even when the health communication intervention is part of a larger public health or corporate effort, which happens in most cases, "a plan specific to the health communication component is necessary" (National Cancer Institute and National Institutes of Health, 2002, p. 16).

A health communication plan can help clarify how an organization can:

- Advance its mission
- Involve others in a health issue and its solutions
- Expand the reach and implementation of its ideas, recommended behaviors, and practices
- Ultimately support health behavior change

Moreover, planning can help in other ways too:

- Provide further knowledge on the health issue being addressed and key factors influencing its potential solutions.
- Develop a clear understanding of key audiences' characteristics, culture, preferences, needs, lifestyle, and behavior.
- Engage key audiences and stakeholders in the design and implementation of the health communication intervention.
- Become clear about what the program is asking key audiences to do and whether the proposed change is feasible.

- Evaluate the strengths, weaknesses, and cost-effectiveness of different approaches that can be used to support change.
- Set communication priorities.
- Select potential partners.
- Evaluate the organization's internal capability and resources to address the health issue.
- Develop culturally appropriate tools and activities.
- Define program time lines, roles, and responsibilities, as well as budget parameters.
- Establish evaluation parameters designed to facilitate program assessment.

An example illustrates one of the benefits of planning: gaining knowledge on the health issue. Imagine an organization that initially thought about launching a communication program to reduce sodium consumption among young women, with the ultimate goal of reducing the incidence and morbidity of hypertension in this age group. Before focusing exclusively on sodium consumption, the organization should explore the importance of sodium in the pathology of hypertension versus other contributing factors, as well as lessons learned from previous experiences that focused on only one element of a multifactorial condition. These are just a few of the many areas that should be addressed in order to gain understanding of the health issue and its potential solutions. Research will help the organization validate its original idea or, depending on key findings, may prove the need for a much broader approach.

APPROACHES TO HEALTH COMMUNICATION PLANNING

While there may be variations in the number of phases different authors use to describe communication planning, the fundamental steps and principles of the overall planning process are always the same and are described in the next section of this chapter. However, from a theoretical perspective, there are many differences between the traditional approaches to planning and a more participatory approach (National Planning Council, Colombia,

2003). Most of them are related not only to the actual process of planning but also to the potential outcomes of the health communication program.

In general, *traditional planning* is "centralized," "vertical (from the top to the bottom)," "technical (done by experts)" and "recognizes a certain population as an object that will benefit from the plan." In contrast, *participatory planning* is "decentralized," "horizontal and agreed upon (from the bottom to the top)," "dialogue-based," "democratic," and "recognizes social actors as active subjects in their own development" (National Planning Council, Colombia, 2003).

However, in looking at the characteristics of traditional planning versus participatory planning, it is important to remember that the word *participation* may have different meanings to different people, groups, or cultures. Ideally, key audiences should be involved as much as possible in the research, planning, implementation, and evaluation of a health communication program. Behavioral and social changes are always more likely to occur if people are part of the process. "Social efficacy is a key concept in the field of health communication. For it to be achieved, groups' and persons' social skills must be made use of and influence program design" (Ader and others, 2001, p. 190).

Still, critics of the participatory approach, especially in Asia, have highlighted that often "participatory models were premised on Western-styled ideas of democracy and participation that do not fit political cultures somewhere else." In other words, participation may not always be welcomed by all communities and cultural groups, at least not to the extent and with the same implications with which it is conceived in the Western world. It is important to acknowledge that in some cases the community may not be interested in investing time in a democratic decision-making process and may have other priorities. In certain contexts, "recommendations for participation could be also seen as foreign and manipulative by local communities" (Waisbord, 2001, p. 22).

Moreover, there are situations in which one of the two approaches may be better suited to address a specific health issue or avert a crisis and limit its negative consequences. For example, "in some cases such as in epidemics and other public health crises,

quick and top-down solutions could achieve positive results" (Waisbord, 2001, p. 21). Instead, a participatory approach to planning
is better positioned to achieve long-term and sustainable behavioral and social outcomes. In other circumstances, characteristics
of a specific planning process are mixed and matched from the
two approaches.

Finally, some of the traits mentioned above are attributed to
participatory and traditional planning and may vary from situation
to situation and country to country. Therefore, they should be interpreted only as general tendencies of these two approaches,
which may diverge from the above elements or should be customized to meet the needs of specific audiences, cultures, and situations. This is not very different from other aspects of health
communication. In fact, theories, models, and approaches should
always be considered part of a tool box with multiple options.

THE HEALTH COMMUNICATION CYCLE
AND STRATEGIC PLANNING PROCESS

Different authors and models may describe the phases of communication planning or the general health communication cycle in
divergent ways. However, the general premises and steps of the
health communication cycle tend to stay the same:

- Understand how health communication can contribute to the
  resolution of a health problem or advance the mission of a
  health organization.
- Research the health communication environment and the key
  characteristics and needs of intended audiences.
- Establish a multidisciplinary team, which should include representatives of key program audiences.
- Determine the best approach and channels to reach intended
  audiences, and involve them in the communication and behavioral and social change process.
- Develop communication messages, materials, activities, and
  tools, and seek feedback from intended audiences.
- Implement the health communication program.
- Evaluate program effectiveness in relation to behavioral,
  social, organizational, or other key outcomes and parameters

that were set in advance and agreed to by all team members and partners.
- Refine or validate program elements in agreement with lessons learned and evaluation analysis.

Figure 9.1 describes the phases of health communication planning and shows how strategic planning is directly connected to the other two stages of the health communication cycle (program implementation and monitoring, and evaluation, feedback, and refinement). In fact, effective strategic planning influences the success of the implementation experience, as well as the overall evaluation process and potential outcomes. In turn, planning is influenced by observations and lessons learned during the implementation and evaluation phases, which may validate or call for changes in all or some of the elements of the initial communication plan. Finally, all steps of the planning phase are interdependent. Failure to complete all steps may limit the program's ability to meet the expectations and needs of intended audiences as well as effectively address any given health issue.

FIGURE 9.1. HEALTH COMMUNICATION CYCLE

Planning
- Research- and audience-based
- Structured approach
- Strategic process

Implementation and Monitoring
- Hard work to ensure spotless execution
- Monitor progress, results, and audience feedback

Evaluation, Feedback, and Refinement
- Starts during planning
- A continuing part of the communication process

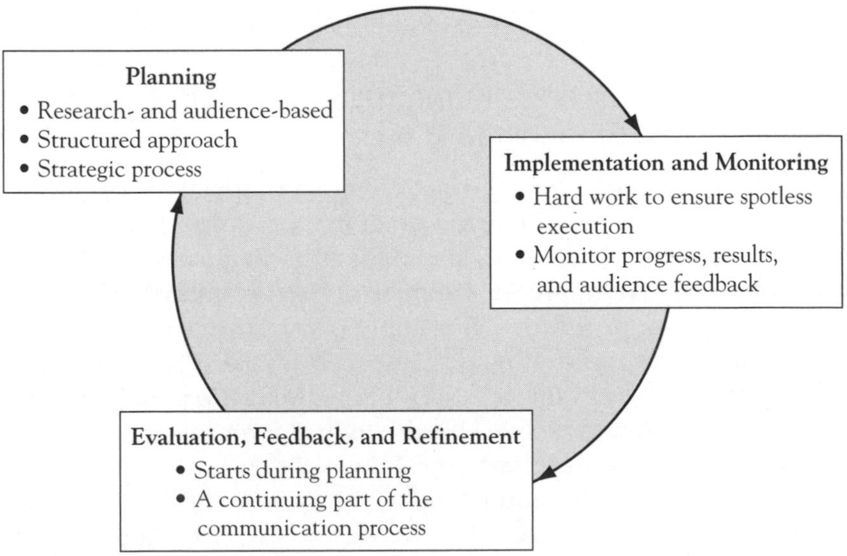

KEY STEPS OF HEALTH COMMUNICATION PLANNING

The steps listed in this section are key to effective strategic planning and reflect actual communication practice. All of them are described in further detail in the following chapters as well as in Appendix A, which includes worksheets and other practical information to develop a health communication plan. Since health communication planning is a step-by-step process in which all phases are interdependent and each informs and guides the next one, following this sequence is important. Figure 9.2 shows the key steps of health communication planning, which are further described below.

OVERALL PROGRAM GOAL

The goal is a brief description of the "overall health improvement" (National Cancer Institute and National Institutes of Health, 2002, p. 22) that the health communication program is planning to achieve—for example, "contribute to the elimination of health disparities among African Americans," "reduce the morbidity and mortality associated with asthma among children under age ten," or "help reduce the number of deaths associated with vaccine-preventable childhood diseases." This goal should inspire and guide the design of the health communication intervention.

OUTCOME OBJECTIVES: BEHAVIORAL, SOCIAL, OR ORGANIZATIONAL OBJECTIVES

This is the statement of a specific behavioral, social, or organizational result that is sought by the program and supports the overall program's goal. Behavioral, social, or organizational objectives (**outcome objectives**) are the ultimate desired results of the health communication program. They complement the program's goal and should be validated by the research phase. They explicitly highlight what key audiences should do (**behavioral objectives**), what policy or new practice should be implemented and institutionalized (**social objectives**), and how an organization should be perceived or act in relation to the health issue or be supported in its mission (**organizational objectives**). Ideally, behavioral objectives (World Health Organization, 2003) and other kinds of out-

Figure 9.2. Key Steps of Health Communication Planning

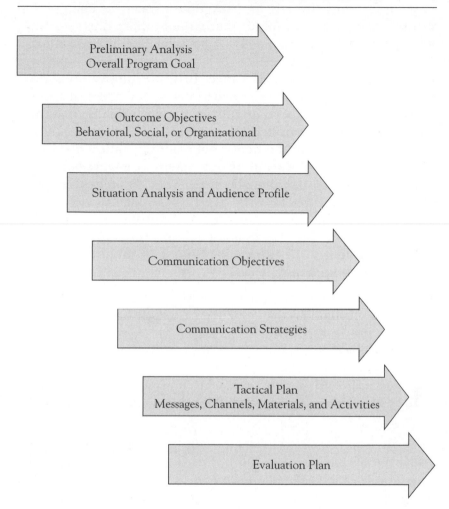

Preliminary Analysis
Overall Program Goal

Outcome Objectives
Behavioral, Social, or Organizational

Situation Analysis and Audience Profile

Communication Objectives

Communication Strategies

Tactical Plan
Messages, Channels, Materials, and Activities

Evaluation Plan

come objectives should be time bound and measurable since they are often used as key indicators for program evaluation. Social and organizational objectives are usually achieved as a result of the attainment of a series of behavioral objectives. Therefore, behavioral change is a key milestone of any kind of change. Examples are, "Prompt U.S. mothers of children under age two to immunize their children against flu [behavioral objective—to be quantified with actual percentages of intended population and dates, whenever possible]"; "Promote adoption, by the year 2003, of a U.S. health policy recommending pediatric flu immunization [social change objective]"; and "Initiate and sustain a process of change that would make pediatric immunization the number one priority of KIDS TODAY [fictional name] by the year 2009 [organizational objective]."

Some authors (National Cancer Institute and National Institutes of Health, 2002) consider behavioral, social, or organizational objectives as one type of communication objectives. Other authors and communication models (World Health Organization, 2003; Donovan, 1995) separate them from communication objectives, which are considered the intermediate steps to achieve behavioral and other kinds of outcome objectives. This chapter as well as all other chapters in Part Three are based on the latter models. Therefore, outcome objectives are distinguished from communication objectives. In practice, after establishing the overall program goals, there are some key questions that resonate or should resonate in communication planning meetings:

- What do we want our audience to do? What are some of the key actions that may lead to a decrease in disease incidence, morbidity, or mortality?
- What kind of policy, social structure, or norm would support the overall program goal?
- What kind of change do we need to make in our organization to be able to implement a program that would serve the goal we have just established?

Establishing outcome objectives early in program planning helps guide the development of key audience and marketing research questions for the initial planning steps, as well as inform all other program elements. This is also instrumental to reaching consensus among team members on what the program wants to achieve.

SITUATION ANALYSIS AND AUDIENCE PROFILE

This step is a detailed and research-based description of all factors that influence a specific health issue and its potential solutions, as well as the adoption of new behaviors, clinical practices, and policies. It includes an in-depth analysis of the health communication environment as described in Chapter One (see Figure 1.1) in relation to the specific health issue and all related factors. The situation analysis is integrated by a comprehensive and research-based audience profile for intended audiences as well as individuals and groups whose opinions or actions are most important to the success of the health communication intervention.

COMMUNICATION OBJECTIVES

These objectives describe the intermediate steps that must be taken to achieve the program's goals (UNICEF, 2001). They may coincide with behavioral, social, or organizational objectives when the audience's readiness, the specific situation, or the overall lack of complexity of the health issue allows for simplified programs that expect to produce an immediate behavioral, social, or organizational change.

Typically communication objectives describe changes in knowledge, attitudes, and skills that, in support of the overall program's goal, can lead to behavioral, social, or organizational change. In these circumstances, they are the intermediate evaluation parameters of the potential effectiveness of a communication effort. Whenever possible, they should be measurable. Examples are, "Increase the awareness of HIV preventive measures and services among 10 percent of young women in the United States by the year 2010," "Fifteen percent of adolescents in the target group will report by the year 2009 to know about the risk associated with using recreational drugs," and "Increase clinician recognition of the importance of early diagnosis and treatment of primary nocturnal enuresis among 70 percent of health care providers in urology clinics in the United Kingdom."

COMMUNICATION STRATEGIES

This step results in a broad statement on how the program will reach its outcome and communication objectives. Strategies are not tactical. In other words, they do not mention in detail flyers, brochures, media campaigns, workshops, or other tactical elements. They are conceptual descriptions of the communication actions that need to be undertaken to reach specific objectives. Strategies are audience specific—for example, "Promote among women aged eighteen to nineteen short-term family planning methods as well as their safety and efficacy via health care providers counseling" (O'Sullivan, Yonkler, Morgan, and Merritt, 2003),

"Leverage natural opportunities (for example, annual conferences) to highlight pertussis severity and cycle of transmission among physicians and other professional audiences," and "Create a social and professional network to support high-risk groups in their intention to seek screening for prostate cancer."

TACTICAL PLAN

The tactical plan provides a detailed description of all communication messages, materials, activities, and channels, as well as the methods that will be used to pretest them with key audiences. It is audience specific and usually consists of a strategic blend of different areas of health communication (for example, interpersonal communications and public relations) as described in this book. The tactical plan also includes a detailed time line for the program implementation, an itemized budget for each communication activity or material, and a partnership plan with roles and responsibilities that have been agreed on by all team members. (How to develop a tactical plan is addressed in detail in Chapters Twelve and Thirteen.)

EVALUATION PLAN

The plan includes a detailed description of the behavioral, social, or organizational indicators, as well as other evaluation parameters, to be used to assess program outcomes. Expected outcomes and other evaluation parameters need to be mutually agreed on by all team members and program partners. The plan should also describe methods for data collection, analysis, and reporting, as well as related costs. (See Chapters Twelve and Thirteen for a comprehensive discussion on how to develop and implement an evaluation plan as well as current theories, models, and topics on the assessment of health communication programs.)

ELEMENTS OF AN EFFECTIVE HEALTH COMMUNICATION PROGRAM

Only well-planned and well-executed health communication campaigns have the potential to achieve long-term and sustainable results. Key elements of effective health communication interventions are listed in Table 9.1 and briefly discussed here.

TABLE 9.1. KEY ELEMENTS OF AN EFFECTIVE HEALTH COMMUNICATION PROGRAM

Careful analysis of the situation, opportunities, and communication needs

Understanding of constituency and audience needs

Early agreement on expected outcomes and evaluation parameters

Well-defined communication objectives

Strategies designed to meet the objectives

Multiple and audience-specific vehicles

Adequate funding and human resources

CAREFUL ANALYSIS OF THE SITUATION, OPPORTUNITIES, AND COMMUNICATION NEEDS

Health communication is a research-based discipline. Only a true understanding of the political, social, and market-related environments can lead to the design of optimal interventions. This analysis should rely on a variety of approaches and research methods described in Chapter Ten.

UNDERSTANDING OF CONSTITUENCY AND AUDIENCE NEEDS

Since the audience is at the center of the health communication approach, its evolving needs should be understood and considered in communication planning and execution. Communicators should be open to redefine interventions on the basis of their understanding of the needs, preferences, and cultural values of key audiences and constituency groups (see Chapter Eight). This process, which starts with the development of an audience profile as part of communication research and planning, should continue throughout the communication process and rely on the input of representatives of interested audiences.

EARLY AGREEMENT ON EXPECTED OUTCOMES AND EVALUATION PARAMETERS

A question that is too often asked in the evaluation phase of communication interventions is, "Why were our donors [or clients or partners] not satisfied with the results of our program even if we achieved the program's objectives?" A common answer to this kind of question is that partners, donors, constituencies, or clients were not involved in defining expected outcomes of the communication program.

Establishing mutually agreed-on outcome objectives and evaluation parameters with key stakeholders is the latest wisdom in evaluating health communication programs, at least in the private and commercial sectors. This allows the extended communication team to share early on their vision about expected outcomes as well as minimizes the potential for disappointment that may result in changes in program funding or a decrease in the level of commitment and participation by the program's partners. Moreover, early agreement on evaluation indicators and parameters informs and shapes the development of all other elements of health communication planning.

Ideally, planning frameworks and evaluation models should stay consistent at least until the preliminary steps of the evaluation phase of a program are completed. This allows communicators to take advantage of lessons learned and redefine theoretical constructs and communication objectives by comparing program outcomes with those that were anticipated in the planning phase.

WELL-DEFINED COMMUNICATION OBJECTIVES

Communication objectives need to respond to the audience's needs. For example, if the audience is not aware of being at high risk for oral cancer, communication efforts should address the need to raise awareness of that risk. If instead the audience is aware of the high risk for oral cancer but does not know how to prevent it, communication efforts should focus, for example, on key risk factors and how to make lifestyle changes or how to discuss with dentists and other primary health care providers the importance of regular oral cancer screening. Sometimes several communication objectives can be defined and achieved in the same time frame. At other times, communicators need a more gradual, step-by-step approach in which different objectives are achieved at different times. These kinds of decisions need to be based on an in-depth analysis of the audience's needs and levels of receptivity to the communication effort (see Chapter Ten).

As for outcome objectives and evaluation parameters, communication objectives also need to be discussed and mutually agreed on with representatives of intended audiences, key constituencies, and partners. In this way, all members of the extended communication team will have in mind similar program outcomes and can work toward achieving them (see Chapter Eleven for a more comprehensive discussion).

STRATEGIES DESIGNED TO MEET THE OBJECTIVES

There may be many good ideas in health communication, but just a few of them may actually support communication objectives. Since communication strategies represent how communication objectives are met, they should always support objectives and represent a creative and cost-effective solution to reach them.

MULTIPLE AND AUDIENCE-SPECIFIC VEHICLES

Creating and identifying multiple and audience-specific vehicles and messages are among the keys to the success of well-planned health communication programs. Messages and vehicles need to respond to audience needs, preferences, and literacy levels. Consumer-targeted messages and channels need to be different from messages on the same topic that are intended for key opinion leaders, policymakers, or health care providers. For example, in many countries in the developing world, theater and puppet shows that travel from village to village to spread AIDS prevention or immunization-related messages have been effective vehicles to reach the general public in areas where low literacy levels and the absence of more sophisticated communication outlets may jeopardize the use of alternative channels. At the same time, communication efforts targeted to health care providers have been taking place using more traditional venues and vehicles, such as professional meetings and peer-reviewed journals.

ADEQUATE FUNDING AND HUMAN RESOURCES

Too often well-designed communication programs fail to achieve projected outcomes because of insufficient funds or human resources. An adequate budget and human resources estimate is an important component of effective planning. Budget estimates should also include contingency funds for potential crises or changes in plans that may become necessary to meet audience needs or other specific circumstances. Failure in estimating adequate funds or human resources may affect the program's quality as well as the perception of the overall effectiveness of health communication interventions in the eyes of partners, clients, or funding agencies.

This leads to the next point related to this topic: the role of health communication professionals in advocating for adequate funding of communication interventions by proving their added value in the health care field. In fact, "despite the proven success of communication programs, communication activities often do not receive adequate funding. They are often considered optional and, therefore, vulnerable to being cut in budget shortages" (Waisbord and Larson, 2005, p. 2).

Unfortunately, this happens also in clinical areas, such as childhood immunization, where several studies have shown "a positive association between communication campaigns and behavior" (p. 2). In the United States, the recent emphasis on health communication by federal agencies and reputable organizations and sources such as *Healthy People 2010* may contribute to improve funding resources for health communication interventions in the nonprofit and public health sectors. Still, program planning is one of the most important opportunities to argue for the value of communication interventions by showing their strategic connection with health outcomes.

ESTABLISHING THE OVERALL PROGRAM GOAL: A PRACTICAL PERSPECTIVE

In establishing health communication among its priorities, *Healthy People 2010* sets the goal to "use communication strategically to improve health" (U.S. Department of Health and Human Services, 2005, p. 11-3). Improving health is also one of the strategic goals of health communication and is reflected in the definition of the overall program's goal in communication planning. In fact, program goals are developed to reflect and meet a specific need. They express the reason that a program is considered, initiated, and developed. They should be viewed as the rationale for seeking funds or asking a health organization to invest in communication.

As for the other elements of health communication planning, the program goal is evidence based. At the time program goals are developed, the communication team should already have conducted some preliminary research (for example, a literature review or one-on-one conversations with key stakeholders, representatives of key audiences, potential partners or clients, or organizational departments) or received a briefing on the health issue that allows them to state the need to address a specific health problem. In this phase, the situation analysis and audience profile may still need to be completed. Still, the goal can be established by keeping in mind the preliminary research findings or briefing. As previously stated, the program goal highlights the health improvement or "the overall change in the health or social problem" (Weinreich, 1999, p. 67) the program is seeking to attain. At this stage, the program goal is preliminarily defined and will need to be validated and clearly stated once a comprehensive situation analysis and audience profile (see Chapter Ten) is finalized. Among the practical examples of program goals are these:

- Contribute to decrease HIV incidence rates among Hispanic men.
- Help limit the impact of women's depression on family and work-related settings.
- Decrease the incidence of mild traumatic brain injury among young people in the United States.

Health communication interventions are almost always part of larger public health or corporate initiatives. Therefore, using words such as *contribute* or *help* may serve to acknowledge that change is always the result of comprehensive efforts, of which communication is an important element but nevertheless just one element. It may also help the communication team and its audiences focus on what communication can and cannot do (see Chapter One for a discussion of this topic), so that program design is based on realistic expectations, and seek achievable results.

At this stage, the health communication team in research settings may have already selected the theoretical framework or model that will guide their key assumptions and logical thinking throughout program planning or at least for some of its phases (for example, applying the steps of a behavior change theory to the development of the audience profile). Although this approach may not be rigorously applied in other contexts (for example, in the nonprofit or commercial sectors), it is still important to use consistent models and assumptions throughout program planning and evaluation.

OUTCOME OBJECTIVES: BEHAVIORAL, SOCIAL, AND ORGANIZATIONAL

Outcome objectives (behavioral, social, and organizational) complement the program goal and should be initially established after the preliminary research or briefing on the health issue. As for the program goal, these objectives would need to be refined and validated by the key findings of the situation analysis and audience profile (see Chapter Ten). Still, stating the behavior, social, or organizational change objectives at the onset of the planning process helps focus all research efforts (for example, literature review, one-on-one interviews, and focus groups) that lead to the situation analysis and audience profile, and ultimately, the development of adequate communication objectives. The communication objectives should support the program goal and help achieve the behavioral, social, or organizational change that is sought by the program. In fact, "the early stages of any communication planning model should explicitly link the overall program's broad goals, specific outcome objectives, and individual behavior change objectives to the communication component of the program" (Donovan, 1995, p. 215). Such objectives should be established by outside experts or the intended community depending on the nature of the health communication intervention.

Behavioral objectives refer to what key audiences should do in relation to a specific health issue or situation, social change objectives highlight the policy or social change that the program is seeking to achieve, and organizational objectives refer to the change that should occur within an organization in terms of its focus, priorities, or structure in relation to the specific health issue. Key program outcomes will be measured against these outcome objectives as well as other intermediate parameters that may correspond to the communication objectives or be specifically identified and agreed on by the health communication team. Still, this assumes that all these objectives support the attainment of the overall program goal and are critical to it.

Outcome objectives should be measurable and realistic. Setting the right expectations is critical in defining the percentage of the population or group in which any change is expected. Human behavior is difficult to change, so expecting 30, 40, or 50 percent of the intended audience to make a change is quite unrealistic. Sound objectives may look at a 3 to 5 percent change in a realistic time frame that may extend for several years (E. Rogers, cited in Atkin and Schiller, 2002; Health Communication Unit, 2003a; National Cancer Institute and National Institutes of Health, 2002). This time frame as well as the percentage of people being affected by a health communication intervention may vary according to the health issue or program. Many of the methods and considerations that go into developing communication objectives (see Chapter Eleven) also apply to the definition of outcome objectives.

Most important, behavioral, organizational, or social change in health communication should be considered instrumental to a reduction of the burden of disease. Therefore, behavior, social, and organizational objectives should refer to changes that make possible the attainment of the overall program goal.

Additional examples of behavioral, social, or organizational change objectives are included in Exhibit 9.1 and refer to the prevention of asthma severity and mortality in inner cities in the United States. Asthma is a leading cause of death "among children ages 3 to 12 years old" (Dumke, 2006, p. 304). It is a condition that can be aggravated by several indoor triggers, for example, dust or mold (Ad Council, 2006a, 2006b; Centers for Disease Control, 2006f). In addition, lack of medical insurance or inadequate knowledge may jeopardize the prevention and management of asthma attacks (Lara, Allen, and Lange, 1999).

KEY CONCEPTS

- Health communication planning is a research-based and strategic process that is necessary for effective health communication interventions.

EXHIBIT 9.1. EXAMPLES OF OUTCOME OBJECTIVES
FOR A PROGRAM ON PEDIATRIC ASTHMA

Overall Program Goal

Reduce the severity and mortality of asthma among children less than
twelve years of age who live in inner cities in the United States

Behavioral Objectives	*Social Objectives*	*Organizational Objectives*
Within 3 years from program launch, prompt XX% of parents or caretakers of asthmatic children in target neighborhoods to: • Recognize early signs of an asthma attack • Go immediately to the emergency room By the year 2010, persuade XX% of parents or caretakers in the intended group to: • Get rid of triggers (for example, mold, dust mites, cats and dogs) of child asthma attacks in their homes • Keep their health care providers abreast of progress Within the next year, prompt XX medical practices in target neighborhoods to discuss pediatric asthma with children and their families: • At routine visits • Using bilingual materials and interpreters, when needed	By the year 2010, reduce by XX% disparities in health outcomes among children who suffer from asthma Remove by the year 2020 existing health insurance barriers to adequate access to services and medications for asthmatic children in inner cities	By the year 2010, become recognized as a leading medical professional organization in pediatric asthma management by XX percent of health care providers, donors, and other key stakeholders in the field (for example, in the case of a professional organization that has a new vision; believes in its potential to contribute to the overall program goal; wants to develop and disseminate new solutions or guidelines; and understands that its reputation in the field is instrumental to its cause)

Note: The goals and objectives in this exhibit are an example. The definition of actual goals and objectives for a program on pediatric asthma in inner cities should be based on an in-depth situation analysis and audience profile.

- Planning is a fundamental stage of the communication cycle, which also includes implementation and monitoring; and evaluation, feedback, and refinement.
- Strategic planning helps clarify what health communication programs should do for an organization and its audiences.
- There are variations in some of the stages and categories that different authors or organizations use to describe the health communication cycle as well as the planning process. Still, the overall general premises tend to stay the same and describe the overall function of each step or stage in the process.
- The key elements of a health communication plan are:
  - Overall program goal
  - Behavioral, social, and organizational objectives (outcome objectives)
  - Situation analysis and audience profile
  - Communication objectives
  - Communication strategies
  - Tactical plan (including communication messages, channels, activities, and materials)
  - Evaluation plan
- The key elements are research based and interdependent. Each affects decisions in relation to the others.
- Health communication planning terms serve to increase clarity about the different steps of communication planning.
- The overall program goal is evidence based and describes the overall "health improvement" (National Cancer Institute and National Institutes of Health, 2002, p. 22) or "overall change in a health or social problem" (Weinrich, 1999, p. 67) that the program is seeking to achieve.
- Behavior, social, and organizational change objectives (outcome objectives) complement the overall program goal and should be defined early in program planning. They help focus the research phase, which leads to the next steps of the planning process as well as to the development of adequate communication objectives.
- Program outcomes should be measured against outcome objectives as well as other intermediate evaluation parameters, which are refined and finalized on the basis of the key findings of the situation analysis and audience profile (see Chapter Ten).

FOR DISCUSSION AND PRACTICE

1. In your opinion, why is planning important? List and discuss what you see as the top three reasons for a structured and rigorous approach to planning in health communication.

2. Luciana is a nineteen-year-old Italian woman who loves spending time at the beach and is unaware of the risk for skin cancer associated with prolonged sun exposure. (For additional detail on Luciana's beliefs, behavior, and social context, see Box 2.1 in Chapter Two.) Apply the core definitions in this chapter to:

   • Establish the preliminary overall program goal of a health communication program targeted to Luciana and her peer group.

   • Develop measurable outcome objectives (behavioral, social, and/or organizational) for this program. For organizational objectives, think of professional or consumer organizations that may have an interest in participating in a program on skin cancer prevention.

3. Imagine you are a health communication consultant who has been hired to develop a health communication plan. Identify the steps in your planning process using (a) a traditional, expert-led approach to planning and (b) a more participatory approach involving intended audiences and key stakeholders. Discuss the pros and cons of the two approaches and the steps you have envisioned.

CHAPTER TEN

SITUATION ANALYSIS AND AUDIENCE PROFILE

IN THIS CHAPTER

- How to Develop a Comprehensive Situation Analysis and Audience Profile
- Organizing and Reporting on Research Findings
- Common Research Methodologies
- Key Concepts
- For Discussion and Practice

Health communication planning can be compared to a tower with many building blocks. Think about the potential verbal or written briefing that health communicators may receive from an organization, agency, or team that seeks to address HIV/AIDS prevention among young women in the United States. This briefing can be regarded as the first building block that allows communicators to establish, share, and discuss the preliminary program goals, as well as the potential behavioral, social, or organizational objectives with team members and other key program stakeholders. Most likely the briefing has been complemented by some preliminary research, including a few conversations with key opinion leaders in the HIV field and an initial literature review.

Still, the foundation of the health communication tower is not yet solid. The team members will have many gaps in their knowledge that they will have to close in order to implement the health communication program. These gaps may include the team's actual understanding of the extent and severity of HIV/AIDS among young women, as well as all factors contributing to potentially higher incidence rates and limited use of preventive measures. The tower's foundation will be built only by using a comprehensive situation analysis, including an audience profile for all interested groups and communities the program intends to reach. Ideally this analysis should enlist the participation of intended audiences in defining the health issue and its potential solutions.

The situation analysis is a fundamental building block in the communication tower. A well-executed situation analysis informs and guides all the other steps of health communication planning. It also makes sure that all the building blocks in the tower are not at risk of falling for lack of the research- and audience-based glue that holds them together.

This chapter focuses on how to build a solid foundation for health communication programs by developing an in-depth situation analysis and audience profile. In doing so, it provides a step-by-step guide on how to research and analyze all key factors contributing to a health problem, as well as to select and prioritize the information that is instrumental to the development of health communication objectives and strategies. The information in this chapter is complemented by a detailed worksheet included in Appendix A (see "Situation Analysis and Audience Profile Worksheet: Sample Questions and Topics").

HOW TO DEVELOP A COMPREHENSIVE SITUATION ANALYSIS AND AUDIENCE PROFILE

The term *situation analysis* has different meanings in different contexts. In this book, it is used as a planning term and describes the analysis of all individual, community, social, political, and behavior-related factors that can affect attitudes, behaviors, social norms, and policies about a health issue and its potential solutions. This analysis is integral to the development of communication objectives and strategies.

The situation analysis is not just a compilation of data and statistics. It is an analytical and selective report on the health communication environment (see Figure 1.1 in Chapter One) and all audience-related factors. It helps communicators gain an in-depth understanding of how these factors influence the health issue and how health communication can affect the environment. All topics in the situation analysis are selected, prioritized, and covered only to the extent that they are relevant to a specific health issue and its audiences.

Ultimately the situation analysis helps identify what may work and what has not worked. For example, in Nigeria, a situation analysis report on the government's efforts to prevent sexually transmitted infections (STIs) showed that "past actions have lacked coordination, failed to establish linkages between projects and actions, and suffered from insufficient financial allocations" (Soul Beat Africa, 2006). The report also identified the lack of involvement of many key sectors of society in previous initiatives as well as the absence of critical information on key audiences (Soul Beat Africa, 2006).

Some authors distinguish the situation analysis from the audience profile and consider them as two separate steps. In this book, the audience profile is described as one of the key sections of the situation analysis. This also reflects actual health communication practice.

The audience profile focuses only on the audience's characteristics, demographics, needs, values, attitudes, lifestyle, and behavior. These descriptive factors are also used to segment key audiences. However, practical experience has shown that often many of the issues pertaining to an audience are also related to the health communication environment described within the situation analysis. For example, the social stigma that in many countries is attached to certain health conditions such as HIV/AIDS should be analyzed not only as part of the social environment of a community or group but also as part of the audience profile. Fear, poor knowledge of HIV transmission modalities, and a lack of empathy for a disease that may appear to be self-inflicted (International Center for Research on Women, 2003) may feed social conventions and at the same time be reinforced by them. Social norms, policies, and audience beliefs, attitudes, and behaviors are all mutually influenced. When the audience profile is part of the situation analysis, this connection and mutual interdependence may become easier to understand. For this reason, the audience profile, which refers to a detailed description of the key program's audiences as well as groups that influence them, is included in this book as part of the situation analysis.

These practical tips may help in developing a situation analysis:

- Never feel as though you have spoken with too many people about a health issue or condition. Gathering multiple perspectives is essential to the planning process.
- Use a team approach in collecting data and relevant information. Brainstorm in advance about research needs and methods, as well as potential difficulties and strategies to overcome them.
- Involve representatives of key audiences across the various research and analysis phases.
- Do not get discouraged if it is difficult to find a specific piece of information (O'Sullivan, Yonkler, Morgan, and Merritt, 2003). Be persistent.
- Share and solicit feedback on research findings, as well as the final situation analysis, from key audiences and as many people as possible in your organization or team.
- Use data strategically to develop sound communication objectives and strategies, but do not jump ahead. Do not include communication objectives and strategies as part of the situation analysis. Program planners should be able to develop adequate communication objectives and strategies only after reviewing, discussing, and analyzing key findings (see Chapter Eleven).
- Look for signs suggesting there is sufficient information in support of a basic framework of understanding of the specific health issue and its audiences. Examples are the emergence of recurring trends or multiple data from different sources that point to similar conclusions.

All of these points provide practical guidance in completing the steps of a situation analysis as illustrated in Figure 10.1.

DEFINE AND UNDERSTAND THE HEALTH PROBLEM

The first step in developing a situation analysis is to gain an in-depth understanding of the health issue: its medical and situational causes, risk factors, severity, and statistical significance among different au-

FIGURE 10.1. KEY STEPS OF SITUATION ANALYSIS

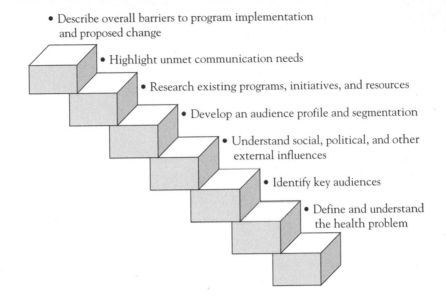

- Describe overall barriers to program implementation and proposed change
- Highlight unmet communication needs
- Research existing programs, initiatives, and resources
- Develop an audience profile and segmentation
- Understand social, political, and other external influences
- Identify key audiences
- Define and understand the health problem

diences and groups. This step leads to identifying the audiences or audience segments the program would prioritize reaching.

For example, decisions about the design and key audiences of a program on sudden infant death syndrome (SIDS), a condition that has been associated with many risk factors, including improper infant sleeping position (National Institutes of Health, 2003; Centers for Disease Control, 2002), may be influenced by the higher mortality rates among African American children than among other U.S. children (National SIDS/Infant Death Resource Center, 2006; National Institute of Child Health and Human Development, 2005). If economic and human resources limit the program's ability to reach multiple audiences or the general public, it may make sense to focus all resources on reaching out to African Americans, where the risk for SIDS deaths is higher. Of course, these decisions are influenced by many factors, including the organizational competence to address a specific group or population.

Other important information to include in this first step of the situation analysis are data and opinions on current treatment and prevention strategies, recent scientific progress, anticipated preventive or therapeutic options, best clinical practices, and existing guidelines. If a new health product or practice is involved, information about its major advantages and disadvantages, as well as how they compare with existing products or services, should be obtained at this stage. Such data can be obtained by a literature review as well as telephone or in-person interviews with key opinion leaders and professional organizations. Understanding current clinical practices and available tools helps shed light on the behavior or practice change that needs to be addressed at a patient, health care provider, or policymaker level, to name a few potential audiences.

Finally, information about the health issue or condition needs to be evidence based. Whenever possible, use statistically significant parameters to define the problem:

- Incidence—the number of new cases of a health condition that are occurring or are expected to occur in a given population within a specific time frame—for example, "HIV/AIDS cases in Africa are expected to increase by X percent in the next five years."
- Prevalence—the total number of cases of disease in a given population at a specific time, often expressed as a percentage of the population—for example, "X percent of U.S. children age six and over have suffered from primary nocturnal enuresis at any time during the past five years."
- Mortality—the total number of people who died of a health condition during a specific time frame—for example, "In 2002, there were X deaths due to pertussis in the United States."
- Morbidity—the number of people who present with severe symptoms of a disease and are either temporarily or permanently disabled as a result—for example, "In 2003, X percent of U.S. adults forty to fifty years old who were severely obese were hospitalized for longer than one week."
- Cost of the health condition to individuals, health organizations, communities, groups, or the society as a whole—for example, "In 2005, depression accounted for X number of lost workdays, which resulted in X dollars in lost earnings among people suffering from depression."
- Morbidity or mortality of other conditions associated with the primary health condition or issue—for example, "Serious

head injuries as a result of falls among Alzheimer's patients is a common disease complication and occurs in X percent of patients."

- Percentage of people who received or had access to adequate preventive or treatment options—for example, "In 2006, X percent of Canadian children received all the immunizations in the recommended childhood immunization schedule."

Ideally, all of these parameters should be explored and defined by age, gender, and ethnic and cultural group or other relevant variations at the population level. Peer-reviewed publications, organizational Web sites, and other relevant literature can be used to gather specific information related to this step.

Identify Key Audiences

This step entails identifying the primary and secondary audiences of the health communication intervention. The *primary audiences* of a health communication program are the people the program seeks to influence: the people who are at risk for a certain medical condition or are suffering from it; parents or caregivers who are responsible for pediatric care decisions for their children; and other audiences (for example, health care providers and policymakers) in cases where programs are small and target only a specific group or constituency (for example, through professional communications or government relations). *Secondary audiences* are all individuals, groups, communities, and organizations that have an influence on the decisions and behaviors of the primary audiences. In other words, secondary audiences include those people who can help reach the primary audience. Primary and secondary audiences can change or switch over time when, for example, some of the program objectives are achieved and the program focus is redefined.

Take the example of the human papilloma virus (HPV), which is a sexually transmitted infection and can present with almost no symptoms (Weinstock, Berman, and Cates, 2004). Persistent HPV infection with specific types of the virus has been described as one of the leading causes of cervical cancer (Sellors and others, 2003). In 2006, the U.S. Food and Drug Administration (FDA) approved the first vaccine against HPV (U.S. Food and Drug Administration,

2006). The vaccine is approved for use in women "9 to 26 years of age" (U.S. Food and Drug Administration, 2006). Primary audiences of a health communication program aiming at reducing HPV incidence by getting people vaccinated might include adolescents and young adults, as well as parents of children nine to twelve years old who can influence their preteens' decision to be immunized. The decision on selecting one of these two groups (or both of them) as the primary audience of a health communication intervention should be based on a number of factors, including audience risk for HPV, organizational competence to address an audience's needs, current policies and medical practices, and the chance for success in convincing people to comply with immunization.

Secondary audiences should be selected by using a similar process and include all groups (for example, family members, health care providers, peers, student associations) that may have an influence on the primary audiences. In the case of HPV, one obvious secondary audience is health care providers, including pediatricians (when the primary audience consists of parents of children ten to twelve years old), as well as family practitioners, gynecologists, nurses, and family planning counselors. In fact, health care providers are a credible source of information on HPV and can support the decision to be immunized.

While identifying potential audiences, both primary and secondary, it is important to start grouping them by age, professional associations, cultural or ethnic factors, religious beliefs, gender, current attitudes, practices, and behaviors, as well as other distinguishing characteristics that contribute to the makeup of a specific group or community. This information will be used and analyzed to complete the audience profile and segmentation.

UNDERSTAND SOCIAL, POLITICAL, AND OTHER EXTERNAL INFLUENCES

Once the health problem has been defined and potential audiences identified, the next step is to understand the external factors that influence the current situation or may represent a challenge or opportunity for change. This phase takes into account the social nature of human interactions and decision making. Individual decisions often are influenced by peers, institutions, social norms, and policies. Medical practices and government policies are often shaped by the communities to which legislators or health care providers belong, as well as their constituencies and the public at large.

Consider the fictional example of Adriana, a forty-five-year-old Italian woman who takes care of her brother, Mario, who has suffered from schizophrenia since age twenty. He is now thirty-five years old and lives with his seventy-year-old mother. Adriana is married with four children but spends her time between her own home and her mother's home.

Like her brother, she lives in a small town where family values are strong and dictate people's involvement in the care of less fortunate family members. Still, the community is also dominated by a lack of understanding of mental illness and feelings of fear about anyone who suffers from it. Adriana's work colleagues and many friends have isolated her and her family and seem to expect that she may also become "crazy" at any moment. In a way, the community values are contradictory: on the one hand, Adriana is supposed to take care of her family, while on the other hand, almost no one is able to offer the emotional and social support she and her brother need.

Over time Adriana and her mother have been influenced by social prejudice against mental illness. They kept Mario's illness a secret for a long time, and Mario avoided treatment and counseling at the local mental health clinic for fear of being seen there by his neighbors and friends. He accepted professional help only at a late stage of his illness. Overall, the lack of social support and high level of family stress this created affect Mario's ability to comply with treatment and have had a negative impact on his health. This also prevents him from holding a steady job or performing other regular daily activities.

Unfortunately, most countries and communities are still overridden with social prejudice against mental illness. People tend to believe that mentally ill patients are dangerous (Corrigan, 2004). However, many of them are in a middle group: "struggling with mental illness [yet] living on their own with a full-time job" (Medscape, 2004).

Prejudice may be reinforced by or, in some cases, lead to specific local policies and practices. For example, some U.S. states have laws "that undermine a person's [with mental illness] ability to have a family, to vote, and things like that" (Medscape, 2004). Discrimination may also apply to the quality of health care mentally ill patients receive. For example, people with mental illness appear to be less likely to receive cardiac care (Medscape, 2004; Druss and others, 2000). Finally, additional disadvantages in health insurance policies "also reflect the stigmatization of people with mental illness" (Gaebel, Baumann, and Phil, 2003, p. 657).

In the case of schizophrenia, "delayed intervention leads to greater secondary morbidity" (Hustig and Norrie, 1998, p. 58). A social, medical, and policy environment that does not encourage early intervention and instead contributes to family and patient stress may have a negative impact on patient outcomes.

The mental illness example shows why social and medical practices, as well as existing policies and regulations, need to be analyzed and included as part of the situation analysis of a health communication program. Stigma is only one of many elements that are influenced by multiple factors that are all interdependent. Others include:

- People's beliefs, attitudes, and behaviors
- Cultural, ethnic, gender, religious, and age influences
- Social norms, policies, and regulations
- Health insurance policies or other practices related to the health care system
- Overall ideas of health and illness within a specific population or subgroup
- Market- or environment-related considerations, such as the way a disease is portrayed by the media
- Disease-related stereotypes

This step of the situation analysis focuses primarily on analyzing all relevant external factors related to the social, scientific, market, and policy environment, including these aspects that may be specific to a given health issue or region of the world. In completing this step, it is important to take into account how people are influenced by these factors, as well as what they can do to shape the environment in which they live.

DEVELOP AN AUDIENCE PROFILE AND SEGMENTATION

Developing the audience profile and segmentation in groups with similar characteristics and behavioral stages is one of the most significant steps of the situation analysis. "Know your audience" is probably the most important mantra of health communication. In fact, no one can attempt to influence people without making an effort to know them first.

Only health communication interventions that are based on a true understanding of the audiences have any chance of succeeding and meeting expected program outcomes. Depending on the type of health communication intervention, either representatives of intended audiences or large segments of the community should be involved and complement expert efforts to profile and analyze key findings about the needs, characteristics, beliefs, attitudes, and behaviors of intended audiences.

In most cases, profiling an audience also includes segmenting it into groups with similar characteristics and needs. This helps make sense of the audience's complexity and guides the allocation of resources as well as the development of adequate communication objectives and strategies for each segment. Audience segmentation may lead to several different combinations of attributes for each segment. However, there are cases in which segmentation is not necessary because the audience presents with similar characteristics and behavioral stages.

A number of obvious categories should be used in profiling, grouping, and segmenting an audience:

- Demographic characteristics, including age, gender, race, ethnic background, language, marital status, number of children, and literacy level
- Common beliefs, attitudes, and behavior in relation to the health issue, including perceived or existing barriers to the adoption of new behaviors or the use of new health services and products
- Geographical factors, such as location, rural versus urban environment, size of city or county, climate, and means of transportation

- Socioeconomic factors, such as income level, education, and professional status
- Lifestyle and cultural characteristics, such as preferred pastimes, risk behaviors, work versus family balance, cultural values, ideas about health and illness, religious beliefs, media habits, and preferred media channels
- Physical or medical factors, such as health status, medical history, comorbidities, and group and individual risk factors
- Other factors that may be issue or audience specific

Sometimes all of these categories apply to the health issue being analyzed. At other times, only a few of them are significant. For example, an analysis of the transportation system of a specific region may be relevant in northeast Brazil, where there are large distances and very few well-equipped health centers (Stock-Iwamoto and Korte, 1993; Tannebaum, 2006). In contrast, transportation issues and related audience preferences will not be relevant to interventions intended to promote screening for breast cancer among U.S. women under age fifty who live in metropolitan areas, where public transportation and access to health care facilities are generally diverse and widespread.

The most important parameter for audience segmentation is the stage of the audience's beliefs, attitudes, and behaviors in relation to the health issue being addressed. How far are policymakers from passing legislation that would increase the number of available public health clinics? Are they convinced about the importance of this issue? Do they feel it is important to their constituencies? Do they care? Are they normally empathetic about the rights of underserved and underprivileged people?

Some authors (Weinreich, 1999) suggest using the stages of behavior change model (see Chapter Two) to segment key audiences on the basis of their attitudes and behavior. The five steps of this theory (precontemplation, contemplation, preparation, action, and maintenance) are described in Chapter Two.

In general, if we think about human behavior and the reason that people may decide to immunize their child, use condoms on a regular basis, or protect their skin from the risk for cancer, the main reasons for adopting or not adopting a recommended behavior can be summarized in the following categories of people:

"Don't know; know, but see too many obstacles; know, don't see obstacles, but don't see benefits; know, don't see too many obstacles, see benefits, but don't care" (Southwest Center for the Application of Prevention Technology, 2001), and know, don't see too many obstacles, see benefits, care but don't have the time, resources, tools, or support to implement the change.

Interventions targeted to each of these segments may be quite different and will need to take into account the other characteristics of each segment (for example, socioeconomic factors, age, lifestyle). Sometimes because of the diversity of the approaches that are required to reach different segments or subgroups of a population, health communicators may decide to focus on only one group or include other groups gradually. Exhibit 10.1 shows a practical example of audience segmentation that uses the categories set out here.

Once the segments have been defined, there are some general criteria and questions that can help prioritize audience segments and allocate appropriate resources:

- Is the segment at greatest risk for the health condition (Weinreich, 1999)?
- Can it be influenced given the current level of competence of the health organization to address the audience's needs and the specific health situation?
- Does change in a particular segment need to happen before focusing on other audience segments because of the group's ability to lead the process of change?
- Is the segment ready to make a behavior change (Weinreich, 1999; Hornik, 2003), or would this require economic and human resources that go beyond the current program estimate?
- What is the segment size (Hornik, 2003)? Is it worth a large investment, or should resources be proportional to its size?

Secondary audiences should be profiled using a similar process and the same categories described earlier in this section. In addition, there are a few specific criteria that apply to the process of profiling and segmenting secondary audiences: the level of influence exerted on the primary audience, potential benefits (for example, visibility, mission fulfillment) that secondary audiences may derive

Exhibit 10.1. Audience Segmentation Example

Audience: U.S. women over age fifty-five who suffer from Type 2 diabetes and are severely overweight or obese

---

Stage of Knowledge, Attitude, or Behavior	*Examples of Potential Segments*
Don't know	Women who are not aware of the association between obesity and Type 2 diabetes. They may attribute diabetes to other causes or consider it a normal part of aging.
Know, but see too many obstacles	Women who know about the association between obesity and Type 2 diabetes. However, they feel they will never succeed in losing weight because of one or all of the following obstacles: • Peer and family pressure to eat fast food or other kinds of unhealthy food • Lack of time to cook or implement lifestyle changes • Insufficient health club or gym presence in their neighborhood or cost of membership • Overall feelings of being unable to make a change • Others
Know, don't see many obstacles, but don't see benefits	Women who know about the association between obesity and Type 2 diabetes, don't see many obstacles or are confident they can overcome them. Still, they don't believe that at this point losing weight would make any difference in regard to their diabetes or any other comorbidities of obesity. For example, they

EXHIBIT 10.1. AUDIENCE SEGMENTATION EXAMPLE, CONT'D.

Stage of Knowledge, Attitude, or Behavior	*Examples of Potential Segments*
	may regard diabetes as a lifetime condition on which nothing can have an impact.
Know, don't see many obstacles, see benefits but don't care	Women who know about the obesity-diabetes association, don't see many obstacles to change, see benefits but don't care for any of the following potential reasons:
	• They currently are able to control diabetes with medications, so, what's the big deal? • They have a fatalistic view of health and illness and feel they cannot do anything about it (whatever it is, it is). • They have many other conflicting priorities in their life and feel this is not one of them. • Others.
Know, don't see many obstacles, see benefits, care, but don't have the time, resources, tools, or support to implement change	Women who know about the obesity-diabetes link don't see obstacles to change and see benefits and care. They consider losing weight one of their top priorities but are overwhelmed about the process and may need help or tools to
	• Learn how to integrate exercise into their busy lifestyle or find cost-effective options for physical activity

EXHIBIT 10.1. AUDIENCE SEGMENTATION EXAMPLE, CONT'D.

Stage of Knowledge, Attitude, or Behavior	Examples of Potential Segments
	• Engage peers and family in their lifestyle change
	• Ask the right questions of their health care providers about weight loss
	• Become aware of quick recipes for healthy meals they can prepare after work
	• Find the right weight loss program
	• Others

Source: With the exception of the last stage in this exhibit, the stages of knowledge, attitude, or behavior are from Southwest Center for the Application of Prevention Technologies (2001).

from their involvement in the program, and barriers to their involvement (Weinreich, 1999). Other criteria should include the level of difficulty in working with them, the audience commitment to the health issue, and existing opportunities (for example, ongoing communication channels, annual venues) that have been developed by secondary audiences and may expand program reach.

Box 10.1 is an example of audience profiling and segmentation. This example refers to the Centers for Disease Control (2006h) campaign "Got a Minute? Give It to Your Kids!" which is targeted to less involved parents and uses social marketing as a planning framework and theoretical model.

Box 10.1

Audience Profile: Got a Minute? Give It to Your Kids!

The Audience

The intended audience for this campaign is parents who are less involved with their 9- to 12-year-old children—that is, those who are less likely to eat dinner with those children, know where those children are during the day, help those children with homework, or otherwise be involved in those children's lives. These are parents who need to become more involved if they are to help their children reject the lure of tobacco.

Why Are We Addressing Only Less-Involved Parents?

Segmenting or identifying a group of people who have enough in common that you can reach them or motivate them in the same way is an essential component of a successful social marketing campaign. The more precisely we can describe a group, the stronger our campaign can become. After all, the goal is to influence behavior among the largest number possible with the available resources.

We identified less-involved parents as our target audience after looking at extensive research: in 1998, CDC hosted 60 parenting experts at a meeting to determine how parents should be characterized. After that we looked at consumer data from sources like HealthStyles and Prizm and conducted focus groups with parents. Our analysis showed us a distinction between three main clusters of parenting attitudes and behaviors:

- On-target parents—those doing all the right things according to the research.
- Non-enforcers—those who were involved with their children and set clear rules but then failed to enforce those rules.
- Less-involved parents—the group targeted with the *Got a Minute?* campaign.

Who Are Less-Involved Parents?

It is not hard to empathize with less-involved parents. Parenting preteens is not easy. As they age through this period, children who were once running to their parents for help are suddenly running away, seeking independence. Parents can feel they have lost control. For our target audience, this is especially true. Less-involved parents want to be involved with their children, but they don't know how, when, or what to do. And as their children enter adolescence, the distance between parent and child often grows, placing these preteens at greater risk for tobacco, drug, and alcohol use.

Compared with the other groups, less-involved parents are overwhelmed. Time that may have been set aside for their children is quickly absorbed in household chores, work, or just trying to find a moment to relax. Although they work similar hours to other parents, our target audience can't find enough time to get organized and plan activities with their preteens or even with other adults. In short, for less-involved parents, efficiently managing their time is one of the largest barriers to participating in activities with their children.

The lack of time and general organization for less-involved parents is not due to involvement in activities without their children. This group seldom visits friends. They are typically not members of social clubs, churches, or volunteer organizations. In fact, nearly half would call themselves "couch potatoes" and most (62%) consider television their primary form of entertainment.

A powerless feeling is a defining characteristic of less-involved parents. They reported the lowest self-efficacy on a wide range of behaviors. They are often aware of a need to change unhealthy habits and daily patterns, but they don't believe they can.

Regarding parenting, our intended audience knows they should spend time with their children but believe they are unable to change current behavior patterns. They are less confident about protecting their children from behavioral risks than other groups of parents and are less likely to create, develop, and enforce rules with their children.

Snapshot of Less-Involved Parents

- 69% indicated consistently feeling a great deal of pressure.
- 43% see their home as chaotic.
- 90% feel they work very hard.
- 39% do not have their children do chores on a regular basis.
- 43% reported household incomes over $50,000.

What Do Less-Involved Parents Look Like?

Our intended audience can be found anywhere. They cross lines of ethnicity, education level, socioeconomic status, and marital status. Less-involved parents can be blue- or white-collar workers. They are more likely than the other groups to be part of a parenting dyad (nearly one-quarter of less-involved parents are likely to be separated, divorced, or never married). Most also fall within the low-middle to upper-middle household income levels. Not unlike the other groups, they want to be perceived as ambitious (75%), hardworking (98%), and courageous (88%), and they want their children to exceed their current socioeconomic status.

What Are Their Current Parenting Behaviors?

Although our intended audience wants to spend time with their children, they are not able to identify possible activities or actions they can take to increase or improve their time together. For example, a majority (54%) of less-involved parents do not usually eat dinner together as a family. They think food preparation should take as little time as possible and are less likely to feel guilty about serving convenience food.

Concerning rule enforcement and monitoring of children's activities, many parents in our intended audience are not requiring that their children do chores on a regular basis, and their children are usually not checking in with them regarding their after-school or weekend activities.

Overall, less-involved parents are not satisfied with how their lives are currently going (52%)—including their relationships with their children. They feel overwhelmed with obligations, have low self-confidence, and feel like they are never going to get a grasp on their parenting obligations.

How Do We Reach Them?

Our intended audience is open to ideas on how to improve their parenting behaviors. They are willing to listen to various communications channels and are not that selective about the messenger. If it seems like a good idea, they will try it. However, they are likely to resent messages that do not provide a choice or that criticize their current behaviors. One subtle distinction goes to the heart of this: they want ideas, not advice.

Thus, the *Got a Minute?* campaign is designed to offer help, not issue orders or encourage guilt. At its core, the campaign simply provides ideas about how to connect with their children—just what less-involved parents are seeking.

Source: Centers for Disease Control and Prevention. "Got a Minute? Give It to Your Kid: Audience Profile." http://www.cdc.gov/tobacco/parenting/audience.htm. Retrieved Feb. 2006. Used by permission.

Key Stakeholders and Constituency Groups

Stakeholders are all individuals and groups who have an interest or share responsibilities in a given health issue. They may represent the primary audience (for example, AIDS activist groups or breast cancer survivors' groups) or influence them. As part of the audience profile and segmentation, key stakeholders need to be identified, cultivated, and engaged in the early phases of program planning to secure their potential commitment and endorsement of communication objectives and strategies.

For example, in designing a program that aims to reduce flu transmission from health workers to patients by promoting immunization of nurse practitioners and other health workers, it makes sense to speak with the organization that represents nurse practitioners. In doing so, communicators can solicit their feedback on key research findings about current beliefs, attitudes, and behaviors, as well as potential communication objectives and strategies. Moreover, brainstorming with them about communication activities and their involvement in the program provides invaluable insight into the design of the communication intervention and increases the likelihood that the program will effectively reach nurse practitioners.

Stakeholders are either individuals, such as physician opinion leaders in a field, or constituency groups, such as the nurse association described above, that represent and influence specific communities, groups, or people who share common interests and goals. Securing the endorsement of program elements by key constituency groups as well as managing criticisms and different viewpoints by key influential groups is an important component of the health communication process and should be a key priority in the planning process.

Key resources to identify stakeholders and constituency groups include the Web, existing literature, articles or broadcast clips from mass media outlets, interviews, and other personal encounters with representatives of key audiences, colleagues, and disease experts.

Preferred Communication Channels,
Vehicles, and Venues

Health communication is audience specific. Understanding the media habits and preferences for different kinds of communication channels of each primary and secondary audience is an integral part of the audience profile section of the situation analysis. Special consideration should also be given to audience-specific venues, such as annual conferences or existing community or chapter meetings.

In this book, the term *communication channel* refers to both the means and the path selected to reach the intended audience with health communication messages and materials. Communication channels can be divided into three broad categories:

- **Mass media channels**: print and broadcast media, the Internet, and other new media
- **Interpersonal channels**, such as counseling, one-on-one meetings, provider-patient encounters, peer education, stakeholder-led meetings, or other interactive channels
- Other **community-specific channels** and venues, such as local or traditional media, poetry, traditional folk media, theater, existing community meetings, churches, local markets, or annual conferences

The U.S. Agency for International Development (1999) analyzes benefits and challenges of diverse communication channels on the basis of three key parameters: ease of message control, interactivity, and ease of boundary control. In this model, radio and television are the less interactive channels, and peer education and counseling are considered the most interactive. Interactivity is considered more likely to influence a group to take action.

In general, the most appropriate channels for a given health communication program are audience specific, reflect the audience's preferences, and depend on several criteria that should inform research objectives on this topic as well as the analysis of relevant findings:

- *Message content and complexity.* Complex messages cannot rely on only the use of the mass media; they also need to be delivered using interpersonal channels and other community-specific media to reinforce mass media messages. Consider, for example, the mother of a twelve-year-old boy who may have read in a national newspaper about the recent increase in U.S. pertussis incidence (Centers for Disease Control, 2005). She may be aware of the need to immunize adolescents to protect them from contracting the disease and transmitting it to more vulnerable segments of the population such as infants and young children (Centers for Disease Control, 2006i). However, the decision to immunize her child would need to be supported by her physician as well as her peer group. This would be particularly important in the absence of school mandates and other specific regulation in her community. Health communication programs in this field should also include the use of interpersonal channels and tools to facilitate peer-to-peer interactions as well as provider-parent communications. Ideally, interpersonal channels such as one-on-one meetings or community-specific channels such as local government newsletters and meetings could also be used to support the introduction of school-based mandates at local government level.

• *Audience reach.* A common criterion in selecting communication channels is the number of people a channel can reach. In the case of print and broadcast media, this number is expressed in terms of audience circulation (see Chapter Five). In other cases, it may be the number of people in the intended audiences that a workshop or community meeting is estimated to attract. These numbers are important to define the most suitable and effective channels to reach the largest number of members of key audiences. Audience reach is one of the key parameters to consider in designing cost-effective interventions.

• *Cultural and issue appropriateness.* Even within the variety of channels that are specific to a given audience, a distinction needs to be made in selecting those that are culturally appropriate for discussing or breaking news about a specific health issue. For example, Bernhardt and others (2002) reported that African American and European American men who participated in a study on Internet-based health communication on human genetics were interested in the great potential for Internet communication but "voiced concerns about the credibility and accuracy of on-line information, lack of trust in many websites, and fear of safeguarding privacy" (p. 325). Conversely, people coping with HIV infection appear to regard the Internet as a source of empowerment that "augments social support and facilitates helping others" (Reeves, 2000, p. 47).

• *Cost-effectiveness.* Since cost-effectiveness is one of the key elements of health communication (see Chapter One), possible channels need to be assessed on the basis of budget parameters and priorities. Cost-effectiveness assessments should be based on a cost comparison of options that will lead to comparable results. This analysis should also include an evaluation of existing programs and resources as potential channels for the delivery and distribution of health messages and materials. Cost-effectiveness assessment naturally leads to the next step of the situation analysis (existing programs, initiatives, and resources) and is one of the many reasons for researching past and ongoing programs.

Even within the same kind of communication channel (for example, interpersonal channels), it is important to consider the impact on behavior that different speakers or messengers may have on intended audiences. For example, a study by Holtzman and Rubinson (1995) showed differences in the behavioral outcomes of parent communications versus peer communications on HIV/AIDS among high school students. In fact, "young women were influenced more by HIV discussions with parents, while young men were influenced more by discussions with peers" (Holtzman and Rubinson, 1995, p. 235). Peer discussions were more likely to lead to multiple partners and unprotected sexual intercourse.

Once the key stakeholder analysis has been completed, further consideration should be given to the stakeholder access, level of comfort, and effectiveness with different communication channels. This analysis intersects with the assessment of key communication channels and may influence resource allocation for the development of tools, materials, or activities specific to a given channel.

The analysis of communication channels is one of the last steps of the audience profile section of the situation analysis. Of course, other audience- or issue-specific factors may not be included in this book's description.

Once channels have been researched and analyzed, it is important to understand overall audience preferences and reactions to different communication vehicles. In health communication, the term *communication vehicles* refers to the specific means or tools that are used to deliver a message using communication channels (Health Communication Unit, 2003b). It includes communication activities, events, and materials. For example, if the communication channel is print media, such as a consumer magazine, potential vehicles include feature articles and advertorials. Communication vehicles are audience and channel specific. All criteria that apply to the analysis of which communication channels to select also apply to communication vehicles. In health communication practice, the terms *vehicles* and *channels* are sometimes used interchangeably, which may lead to confusion. In order to avoid confusion, the term *tactics* in this book is primarily used to indicate the same category (for example, activities, materials, and events). However, *tactics* also has a strategic connotation because of the connection of the communication vehicles being used with the other elements of the tactical plan (see the Glossary and Chapter Twelve).

RESEARCH EXISTING PROGRAMS, INITIATIVES, AND RESOURCES

There are several reasons to research and analyze past and existing programs, initiatives, and resources:

- Lessons learned and key success factors of past and ongoing programs.
- Opportunities for partnerships, material distribution, message delivery, and overall enhanced access to key audiences.
- Existing tools and communication channels that may complement the new program's messages and materials or be used with them. Capitalizing on existing tools and channels may reduce the new program's costs for material development and audience outreach.
- Knowledge of programs or approaches that may be in opposition to the health communication program goal and objectives. For example, if the program being developed is in support of animal research, it may be helpful to understand the rationale and tools used as the basis of health communication programs that advocate against animal research.

These should all be considered key components of this analysis. Key resources to collect information on past or existing programs and initiatives include the Web, communication or public affairs directors of health organizations in the field, health communication listservs or chatrooms, mass media articles, peer-reviewed literature, and field experts.

HIGHLIGHT UNMET COMMUNICATION NEEDS

This step complements and expands on the analysis of existing programs. In fact, the previous step may help identify unmet communication needs that have not been addressed by past or current programs or may help distinguish a program and attract the attention of key audiences. However, this analysis is often integrated by information collected through interviews with key stakeholders and representatives of intended audiences, focus groups, literature review, or other research methods, which should contribute to highlighting specific communication needs and priorities for each audience.

DESCRIBE OVERALL BARRIERS TO PROGRAM IMPLEMENTATION AND PROPOSED CHANGE

Health communication programs that are poised to address potential barriers to behavioral or social change or program implementation are more likely to achieve expected outcomes (Grimshaw, Eccles, Walker, and Thomas, 2002). Therefore, a description of barriers should be included in the situation analysis along with an initial vision for how to address and overcome them. This vision should be defined using the input of representatives of key audiences, stakeholders, and constituency groups or, depending on the program characteristics and planning needs, the community at large.

Among the potential barriers are these:

- Cost, which is the actual financial cost of the product the program asks people to use, or the human cost or sacrifices in terms of time, lifestyle, or supportive relationships needed to adopt a new behavior, policy, or practice
- Lack of adequate tools and resources to facilitate the integration of the proposed behavior into people's lifestyle
- Lack of capacity or technical competence that, for example, may help people become independent in adopting a new behavior (for example, lack of knowledge on how to perform a breast cancer self-exam) or advocating for a new policy
- Poor or inadequate local infrastructure that limits access to the recommended health behavior—for example, lack of

health services in a region that is asked to become more pro-active in using family planning methods or lack of hospitals that perform HIV screening within a certain geographical distance
- Lack of clear guidelines or clinical standards
- Time constraints
- Inadequate policies
- Individual or group factors such as social norms, lack of communication training, existing prejudices, or language barriers
- Lack of organizational commitment to health communication and its funding
- Inadequate economic or human resources

All potential barriers should be analyzed by reviewing key findings of the situation analysis and listing all the factors and data that may point to potential difficulties in program execution or the achievement of expected results. There are circumstances in which existing barriers require a significant economic or human resource commitment for their removal. In these cases, it may be advisable to prioritize health communication efforts and initial resource allocations on minimizing or removing such obstacles. This will still require a behavioral- and social-oriented mind-set. In fact, the focus of this initial barrier-conscious intervention would be, for instance, convincing local health authorities to improve access to health services or products; or changing existing social norms and removing prejudice within a community; or attracting additional funds and resources to the program's mission and overall goal.

ORGANIZING AND REPORTING ON RESEARCH FINDINGS

Once the research phase of the situation analysis has been completed, the next step is to prioritize, present, and discuss findings with team members, representatives of key audiences, clients, health organizations, organizational departments, and, depending on the nature of the program, everyone who has a stake in the health communication intervention. Since not all of the data being collected are likely to be relevant to the program, the first step is to select and expand on the information that will lead to the development of communication objectives and strategies. This tends to be all information that has been confirmed as relevant by multiple sources and appears to meet current audience needs and preferences in relation to the behavioral, social, or organizational outcomes that are sought by the program. This also represents the core briefing for the development of communication objectives and strategies.

In organizing and presenting key findings and related conclusions, it may be helpful to divide the situation analysis in the same categories described in this book for its different steps (see "Situation Analysis and Audience Profile Worksheet: Sample Questions and Topics" in Appendix A). Other logical categories can be added if they improve the overall organization and clarity of the analysis. Another practical tip is to think in terms of key issues—in other words, the facts, data, or information that are critical to the health issue and its audiences as well as to the achievement of outcome objectives.

A common practice in the private and commercial sector is the use of a SWOT (strengths, weaknesses, opportunities, and threats) analysis to organize the information about a particular product, behavior, social, or organizational change. Other authors have already suggested a much broader use of this tool in health communication planning (O'Sullivan, Yonkler, Morgan, and Merritt, 2003). SWOT analyses help in gaining a clear understanding of the situation and present with an easy-to-digest format to share the information with partners and team members. Exhibit 10.2 includes a practical example of a SWOT analysis.

The situation analysis leads to communication objectives and strategies. Still, it would be premature to develop communication objectives without first validating the initial program's goal as well as key behavioral, social, and organizational objectives.

Consider the example of the program goal of an asthma program that was originally established on the basis of preliminary data pointing to a higher disease incidence in a specific group. The overall program goal was to reduce the incidence and morbidity of asthma in that group. Yet more conclusive evidence has shown that asthma incidence in the target group is actually comparable to rates for the general population. The key health issue is not asthma incidence but the disease severity and mortality because of

EXHIBIT 10.2. SWOT ANALYSIS FOR THE CARIBBEAN CERVICAL
CANCER PREVENTION AND CONTROL PROJECT

Strengths

1. Communication system that allows wide reach
2. Previous initiatives to build and improve on
3. Dedicated workers
4. Enabling environment for use of media
5. Established culture of health communication
6. Media houses with space and time dedicated for health
7. Access to performing arts for health communication

Weaknesses

1. Gaps in information
2. Limited resources
3. Limited reach and understanding of the message and material
4. Deficiencies in academic curriculum for health workers
5. Lack of control over media placement (when message will be aired)
6. Conflicting message at all levels and in all sectors
7. Inadequate monitoring and evaluation
8. Lack of a sustainable communication program
9. Limitations of access to services promoted
10. Inadequate social-marketing expertise

Opportunities

1. Destigmatization of cancer
2. Ability to link with other programs
3. A fertile environment for the cervical cancer program
4. Several potential partners in health CBOs, NGOs, private sector, opinion leaders, and so on
5. Greater access to creative skills
6. Capacity for networking among countries, agencies, and programs

Threats

1. Myths in the society
2. Gender roles and patterns
3. Differences in interpretation or presentation
4. Multichannel media making reach more difficult and costly
5. Loss of human resources from public to private sector and overseas (brain drain)
6. Limited buy-in from health professionals

Source: Adapted from Caribbean Epidemiology Center. "Report of Communication Advisory Committee Meeting, Sub-Committee of the Technical Advisory Group." Caribbean Cervical Cancer Prevention and Control Project (CCCPC), 2003, p. 2. http://www.carec.org/documents/cccpcp/communication_advisory_report.doc. Used by permission.

the lack of knowledge and communication tools to help prevent and manage severe asthma attacks in that community. Therefore, the final program goal should reflect the conclusions of the situation analysis and be restated as following: Reduce the severity and mortality rates of asthma in a given group. Outcome objectives should be established to meet such goal.

COMMON RESEARCH METHODOLOGIES

Health communication practitioners and students need to be aware of key research strategies and methods in order to complete the research phase of the situation analysis and audience profile, as well as some other steps of the health communication process. This is equally important for cases in which more formal research is needed; as a consequence, the health communication team may need to interview, hire, and supervise the work of a marketing and communication research firm.

Before moving to the definition of core methodologies, it is important to make a distinction between *market research* and *marketing research*. Although these terms are often used interchangeably, *market research* defines the process of gathering information about a market and its dynamics, and *marketing research* is a systematic approach to research that includes more than a description of market factors and dynamics and applies to much broader research needs, including audience profile and segmentation (QuickMBA, 2006). As discussed in Chapter Two, this systematic, rigorous, and analytical approach to research is one of the most important contributions marketing has made to the health communication field and heavily influences communication research.

Another important distinction is between qualitative and quantitative research. **Qualitative research** refers to techniques and research approaches that are used to collect data in relatively small groups. Qualitative data are not statistically significant and focus on opinions, trends, and insights (Andreasen, 1995). Qualitative research is often used in the preliminary research phase to establish initial program goals and behavioral objectives and tends to provide in-depth details on motivations, attitudes, and behaviors. It is also frequently used to assess the format and needs for quantitative data. Qualitative research sometimes can include approximate numbers (for example, percentages) of a trend, opinion, or behavior.

Quantitative research refers to research methods and data that are statistically significant and are usually collected from large samples. Regardless of its focus (for example, health behaviors, media habits of intended audiences, frequency of physician-patient encounters on a health issue, or level of awareness about a medical condition), the aim of quantitative research is to provide the health communication team with exact numbers about different kinds of audience- or environment-related factors.

Many health communication programs rely solely on well-planned and well-executed qualitative research, but there are cases in which it is necessary to collect statistically significant data (for example, when statistically significant data are needed to convince key stakeholders of the relevance of a specific health issue and the significance of the health communication intervention). Table 10.1 lists some of the key characteristics of qualitative versus quantitative research.

This section provides a brief overview of key communication research methodologies for qualitative and quantitative research, as well as practical advice on how to select and use them. It also examines key principles in identifying and selecting a suitable marketing and communication research firm to provide technical assistance with the research process in case this is needed.

TABLE 10.1. QUALITATIVE VERSUS QUANTITATIVE RESEARCH METHODS

Qualitative	Quantitative
Provides depth of understanding	Measures level of occurrence
Asks "Why?"	Asks "How many?" and "How often?"
Studies motivations	Studies actions
Is subjective; probes individual reactions to discover underlying motivations	Is objective; asks questions without revealing a point of view
Enables discovery	Provides proof
Is exploratory	Is definitive
Allows insights into behavior and trends	Measures levels of actions and trends
Interprets	Describes

Source: From *Methodological Review: A Handbook for Excellence in Focus Group Research* by M. Debus. Copyright 1988 by The Academy for Educational Development, Washington, D.C. Reprinted with permission.

All methodologies described here apply at least to a certain extent to all research phases of the health communication process (Freimuth, Cole, and Kirby, 2000):

- Formative research, which consists of all research efforts that precede program design and implementation: the research conducted for the situation analysis and audience profile in order to assess the health communication environment and the key needs and characteristics of all intended audiences and the **pretesting** of messages, materials, and activities with intended audiences (discussed in further detail in Chapter Twelve). A pretest is an analysis of an audience's reactions that takes place prior to the dissemination and implementation of messages, materials, and activities.
- Process-related research, which aims at assessing and monitoring the implementation phase of a health communication program. This process often relies on marketing research methodologies and means of contacts, such as stakeholder interviews and surveys, to secure feedback by key audiences on program elements and their execution.
- Summative research, which refers to the research conducted as part of the evaluation phase of the program to assess the effectiveness of the program's strategies, the overall program reach, and its impact on the program's goals and key objectives.

Depending on the nature of the health communication program, all research phases may be completed by the health communication team and other experts or by the community itself with the guidance and technical assistance of outside experts and facilitators. The latter option is at the core of participatory research, which involves and gives authority to intended audiences for the design, implementation, and analysis of research efforts. Although the degree of participation of key audiences in research design and implementation may vary depending on the project and audience characteristics, this book advocates for the inclusion of at least key stakeholders and representatives of intended audiences in the process of sharing information, as well as providing feedback and analyzing research findings.

SECONDARY DATA

Secondary data are all information that has been collected, published, or reported by others in different formats (for example, unpublished reports, existing presentations, posters, Web sites, mass media articles, public health reports, guidelines, peer-reviewed articles) and in relation to different programs. The individuals or groups who analyze and use the data were not involved with the initial design and implementation of the research.

Potential examples of secondary data that may be relevant to a specific health communication program include information about key audiences' demographics and cultural or religious beliefs, other countries or programs' experiences in relation to the same health issue, and data from surveys or focus groups related to similar topics and audiences.

Several authors (Saunders, Lewis, and Thornhill, 2003; Andreasen, 1995) have already highlighted many of the limitations that apply to the use of secondary data. However, all of them also agree on the value of secondary data at least in the initial research phase. Among the limitations are these:

- Secondary data were gathered for different projects and purposes and may be incomplete in exploring topics critical to the health communication program.
- The credibility of secondary data varies and should be carefully assessed (for example, in relation to specific Web sites and Internet resources).
- Secondary data may be difficult to interpret in the absence of the original research design or protocol.
- Secondary data can be outdated.

Nevertheless, secondary data are important in the exploratory research phase to help gather critical background knowledge on the health issue and its audiences. Sometimes this knowledge is current and relevant to a given health communication program. Other times, it needs to be supplemented by new research. In most cases, it is advisable to gather additional information at least through one-on-one interviews with key stakeholders and representatives of intended audiences. In these cases, secondary data will provide a valuable framework to develop key questions and engage key stakeholders during the interview and in relation to the overall health communication process on a given health issue.

The following sections look briefly at several sources and methods to research secondary data.

Literature Review

A review of existing literature can include peer-reviewed journals, press clips, broadcast segments, trade journals, unpublished reports, PowerPoint presentations, annual reports, and other types of publications by local and international health organizations, among others. University and public libraries are good places to start a search. They also provide access to databases and online journals that may save time and facilitate the research process. However, most health organizations now have the internal capability to conduct these searches from their offices.

Database and Internet Search

In Western countries, where computer and Internet use are widespread, most searches for existing literature or other secondary data can take place over the Internet. In most parts of the world, the number of online publications and virtual libraries is rapidly increasing and includes several thousand peer-reviewed journals, magazines, newspapers, newsletters, and other kinds of publications.

The Internet also eases access to PowerPoint presentations, health organizations' annual reports, program descriptions, meetings proceedings, clinical guidelines, and a wealth of additional information. There are a huge number of available databases and search engines.

Search engines catalogue information from the public, private, news media, and academic sectors. Most people try more than one search engine or database while researching for a specific kind of information. In the United States, Google and Yahoo! have been the two search engines most used in the past few years (Sullivan, 2006).

Relevant databases for health communication research include Medline, the online database of the U.S. National Library of Medicine (NLM); LexisNexis, a searchable archive of U.S. and international magazines, newspapers, business, and legal documents;

and several commercial databases to which users can subscribe or access using a public library system.

Users who are searching the Internet for data compilation and analysis must use objective criteria to evaluate information credibility. The information source (the author or organization, for example) is one of the key parameters to assess credibility (Montecino, 1998; Jitaru, Moisil, and Jitaru, 1999). Is the author well published (Montecino, 1998)? In other words, is the author published in reputable journals and outlets, or does he or she have a substantial number of publications? Does he or she have practical experience on the subject? Is the author affiliated with a reputable organization? Do other organizations or stakeholders recognize the credibility and authority of the organization that endorsed or publicized specific health data or information? Did the author or organization have any personal or group interest to support a given viewpoint? These are only some of the key questions that should be asked about the information source.

Other key criteria for the evaluation of online information include the editorial review process (Does the editorial board include recognized experts in the field?) and currency (Does the information reflect current data and trends? How often does the information appear to be updated?) (Jitaru, Moisil, and Jitaru, 1999). Finally, Web sites that clearly disclose the author's or organization's intent or mission as well as contact information and potential grants or conflicts of interest are likely to be more credible.

Web Sites of Existing Organizations

Web sites of professional organizations, patient groups, government offices, universities, and other groups may be valuable sources for information on existing health communications programs or other initiatives, case studies, potential partners, and best clinical practices, to name a few topics. They may also be helpful in identifying key stakeholders in a specific health field, who usually tend to be part of advisory boards or mentioned frequently on reputable Web sites.

The same criteria that apply to assessing the credibility of other online information are also relevant to Web sites and should be used to evaluate them. Table 10.2 includes additional criteria that apply more strictly to health-related Web sites and are concerned

TABLE 10.2. FREQUENCY OF EXPLICIT CRITERIA FOR EVALUATION
OF HEALTH-RELATED WEB SITES BY CRITERIA GROUPS

Criteria groups	Frequency (%) (n-165)
Content of site (includes quality, reliability, accuracy, scope, depth)	30 (18)
Design and aesthetics (includes layout, interactivity, presentation, appeal, graphics, use of media)	22 (13)
Disclosure of authors, sponsors, developers (includes identification of purpose, nature of organizations, sources of support, authorship, origin)	20 (12)
Currency of information (includes frequency of update, freshness, maintenance of site)	14 (8)
Authority of source (includes reputations of source, credibility, trustworthiness)	11 (7)
Ease of use (includes usability, navigability, functionality)	9 (5)
Accessibility and availability (includes ease of access, fee for access, stability)	9 (5)
Links (includes quality of links, links to other sources)	5 (3)
Attribution and documentation (includes presentation of clear references, balanced evidence)	5 (3)
Intended audience (includes nature of intended users, appropriateness for intended users)	3 (2)
Contact addresses or feedback mechanism (includes availability of contact information, contact address)	2 (1)
User support (includes availability of support, documentation for users)	2 (1)
Miscellaneous (includes criteria that lacked specificity or were unique)	33 (20)

Note: Of five authors who assigned weights or priorities to their proposed criteria, four cited content and one cited peer review (categorized as miscellaneous) as the most important criterion. The percentage total does not equal 100 because of rounding off.

Source: Kim, P., Eng, T., Deering, M. J., and Maxfield, A. "Published Criteria for Evaluating Health Related Web Sites: Review." *British Medical Journal,* 1999, *318,* p. 648. Used by permission.

not only with the credibility of the information but also with the overall quality of the site, which may be another credibility indicator. These criteria (165 in total) were compiled from twenty-nine published rating tools and journal articles and were assessed on the basis of their frequency (Kim, Eng, Deering, and Maxfield, 1999).

One-on-One Contacts and Interviews

In regions where the Internet is less accessible (for example, in some developing countries), gathering secondary data may be challenging. A good way to start is by contacting university researchers, local public health departments, nonprofit organizations, government officers, corporations, and all other stakeholders who can point to the existence of previous reports, documents, and data and perhaps share them together with their own professional experience. While this approach is extremely valuable in situations where Internet research is not an easy option, contact with those in the field should be sought in all cases to confirm the validity of secondary research findings, supplement other data and professional experiences, and make sure that potential or actual stakeholders can have an opportunity to contribute to analyzing them.

PRIMARY DATA

Primary data include all information gathered specifically to address the research needs of a given health communication program. Such data are collected directly by program planners or marketing research firms by direct observation of specific facts and behaviors or using systematic research approaches. Program planners and other researchers involved in the project are directly responsible for the design, implementation, and analysis of primary research efforts. Primary research can be quantitative or qualitative or both.

Since they are collected specifically for the purpose of informing and shaping program decisions, primary data are the most valuable resource in program planning. In the case of participatory research, members of key audiences or the community at large are also involved in most steps of research design, implementation, and analysis.

OVERVIEW OF QUALITATIVE VERSUS QUANTITATIVE RESEARCH METHODS

Primary research relies on direct communication methodologies, which include all means of contact researchers use to gather data by communicating directly with research subjects "either in person, through others, or through a document such as a questionnaire" (Joppe, 2006).

The following techniques are common in qualitative research:

- *One-on-one in-depth interviews.* These can be telephone or in-person interviews with internal and external stakeholders, members of key audiences, representatives of relevant health organizations. Whenever possible, it is preferable to conduct in-depth interviews in person.
- *Focus groups.* One of the most common research methodologies, this consists of small group discussion. Participants are usually representatives of key program audiences (for example, mother of children under two years of age; African American men who are over forty-five years old; emergency room physicians who work in metropolitan areas).
- *Case study analysis.* This method yields a detailed description and analysis of experiences and programs that are related to a given health communication program. It relies on a combination of in-depth interviews with representatives of the organization where the experience, or "case," took place, with an analysis of secondary data, such as existing literature and press reports.

Quantitative research relies primarily on surveys of large segments of key audiences, which can be conducted by telephone or distributed over the Internet, by mail, or at meetings or other venues and tend to be self-administered by respondents. Following is a closer look at key considerations and parameters in using qualitative and quantitative research methods.

One-on-One In-Depth Interviews

Stakeholder interviews, the most common form of in-depth interview, as well as other kinds of one-on-one encounters, require specific skills, advance preparation, and the ability to create rapport with the individuals being interviewed. It is always a good idea to precede the interview with a preliminary conversation, e-mail, or other form of communication that addresses the overall focus and purpose of the interview. Advance preparation should also include a tentative list of key questions and a review of some background information on the organization that the interviewee may represent. In today's competitive and busy work environment, wasting anyone's time for lack of preparation is not a good way to encourage their interest in helping with a specific health issue.

Often one-on-one interviews may become the forum to discuss the potential for partnerships or other topics that may digress from the initial focus but are still relevant to the specific health communication program. In general, in-person interviews are preferable to telephone interviews. However, the telephone interviews are increasingly common and help break down barriers related to lack of time or geographical distance. The average interview lasts 30 to 120 minutes.

Some general criteria apply to the process of interviewing and may help establish a rapport with the person being interviewed. Although these criteria are particularly important in the case of one-on-one interviews, they generally apply to other research methods, such as focus groups and telephone surveys.

For example, it is important to ask general and nonintrusive questions first. Breaking the ice by making a joke or telling something about oneself helps create feelings of comfort among people being interviewed. Confrontational questions (for example, about an article the interviewer read that supports opposite views about the work of the interviewee) should always be asked toward the end of the interview. By then, the interviewee trusts the interviewer and may feel more comfortable addressing controversial topics. Also, whenever possible, it is a good idea to repeat and summarize some of the key points that the interviewee raised. This may help correct potential misunderstandings as well as organize the information once the interview has been completed. Other practical tips help the interview proceed smoothly:

- List the questions in a logical order.
- Use simple language, and avoid technical words.
- Divide a complex question into multiple questions.
- Avoid leading questions, such as yes or no questions.

All interviewers, regardless of whether they are involved in one-on-one interviews, focus groups, or telephone surveys, should be trained and become familiar with all questions and potential follow-up inquiries in advance of the actual research implementation.

Focus Groups

Focus groups are facilitated group discussions. Many of the general principles discussed for one-on-one interviews also apply to these groups. However, in the case of focus groups, the facilitator and interviewer, who is usually called a moderator, needs to be aware of group dynamics in order to make sure that all participants feel comfortable and encouraged to contribute to the discussion.

Focus groups are one of the most common means of contact in communication research. They are used to gather data for the situation analysis and audience profile; test the words and questions of a survey's questionnaire; secure the audience's feedback on the message and graphic concepts of communication materials and activities; and understand the audience's reaction to a specific health product or service or behavior, to name a few applications. They may reveal unexpected details about audience preferences and beliefs. For example, a focus group study on the use of insecticide-treated nets for malaria protection in Angola revealed that users would prefer nets to be in bright colors (yellow, orange, and pink) instead of white because of concerns with white nets, which can become visibly dirty shortly after installation (Schiavo, 1998, 2000).

As with other research methods, focus groups are regulated by several codes of ethics (Office for Human Research Protections, 2006; National Institutes of Health, 2006) to protect participants in the research and make sure that they are fully informed about the research methodology and objectives. Although focus group participants usually receive and sign a consent form, which should include a description of the research's purpose and methodology, the group should begin by reviewing this information. The focus group moderator should:

- Facilitate introductions and provide the rules for interactions within the group.
- Avoid asking leading or yes or no questions. Most questions should be open-ended.

- Monitor topics to make sure the discussion stays focused on the research topic.
- Have a clear understanding of the research goals and the kind of information that needs to be collected.
- Show respect for all participants and their opinions.
- Make sure everyone understands there is no right or wrong answer (National Cancer Institute and National Institutes of Health, 2002).
- Shield shy participants from more verbal or aggressive panelists (Hester, 1996).
- Make sure everyone has an opportunity to express his or her opinion.

In participatory research, a community member may decide to act as the moderator of the focus group. He or she may be a representative of a local organization, a member of the intended audience, or a local government officer, for example. In this case, a health communication and research expert will likely be present at the focus group and provide technical assistance. The expert should also train the community member for the moderator role well in advance to the focus group. A troubleshooting session to identify potential pitfalls and difficult situations that may arise during the focus group, as well as how to address them, should be included in the training.

Surveys

Surveys are a common technique used in collecting quantitative data. There are two primary types of surveys: telephone and self-administered. Among self-administered surveys, Internet-based surveys are gaining prominence in Western countries (Solomon, 2001). Some authors (Joppe, 2006; National Cancer Institute and National Institutes of Health, 2002) also mention in-person surveys, but these are rarely used because of their high cost.

If the survey is well designed and implemented, it can be an excellent and accurate method to acquire information about a given population. Also, surveys rely on standard questionnaires that in some cases can be applied to different subgroups of the same population. This allows researchers to compare attitudes, behaviors, beliefs, and other information from one group to another.

Moreover, using standard questionnaires ensures higher reliability and accuracy of the information being collected because the findings are not influenced by differences in interviewers' styles or other subjective parameters that can influence qualitative research findings.

The survey sample needs to be clearly defined early in the survey design phase. This needs to be representative (in terms of percentage) of the target population and include a relative homogeneous group of people (for example, parents of six- to eleven-year-old children; women under thirty-five years of age). If different racial and ethnic groups are included, as they should be, it may be worth defining in advance the percentage of the total sample each group would represent. In the case of a health issue that is quite widespread in the general population (for example, the recent epidemic of childhood obesity in the United States; Kaur, Hyder, and Poston, 2003) but is more prevalent among some at-risk groups, it makes sense to oversample these specific groups or run a specific survey targeted to them.

Self-administered surveys require respondents to complete the questionnaire by themselves and in their own time. Self-administered questionnaires are usually distributed at professional meetings, by direct mail, or posted online on relevant Web sites. In general, the response rate of self-administered surveys tends to be lower than that of telephone surveys (Wiggins and Deeb-Sossa, 2000). For example, even with telephone reminder calls, mail surveys have a lower response rate than telephone surveys (Ngo-Metzger and others, 2004). Although some of these facts are rapidly changing with the rise of caller ID and cellular phones, telephone surveys are still one of the best methods for quantitative research.

Other elements contribute to response rates for both self-administered and telephone surveys. These include the clarity and length of the survey, the relevance of the topic it addresses, and other audience-related factors. For example, if the survey targets working parents of children younger than ten years of age, the time at which a telephone survey is administered may affect the response rate (Dillman, Sinclair, and Clark, 1993; Bogen, 2006). Weekends may be the best time to reach these parents since in the morning they are at work and in the evenings are probably busy with the children, dinner, and household chores.

Telephone surveys tend to be commonly used and offer the advantage of quick methods for sample randomization. Random sampling facilitates "the extrapolation of characteristics from the sample to the population as a whole" (Joppe, 2006). One of the most common randomization methods is random digit dialing: all numbers are selected randomly on the basis of the last four digits or first three numbers of a telephone prefix, which are chosen by the interviewers.

Finally, survey questionnaires need to be developed by keeping in mind the limited time the audience may have to reply to all questions, as well as literacy levels and the importance of language clarity and simplicity. In addition to initial demographic questions (to confirm the respondent's age, sex, and other key sample information), the survey questionnaire can include different types of questions such as yes and no questions, scale questions (for example, "On a scale from 1 to 5, how do you rate this specific health service?"), and multiple-choice questions.

WORKING WITH MARKETING RESEARCH PROFESSIONALS

In some cases, the health communication team does not have the expertise, time, or human resources to conduct formal marketing research. In this situation, selecting a marketing and communication research firm or consultant may be the best option.

The selection process should start by giving a detailed briefing to several marketing research firms or consultants who are invited to respond with recommendations and an estimated budget on the basis of this key information. This briefing can be delivered in person at an initial meeting or in writing. Written briefings may be better to ensure that all firms that participate in the selection process have access to the same information and to limit potential misunderstandings. Regardless of its format, the briefing should ideally include these components:

- A brief description of the health issue
- Overall program goals
- Key research and information needs
- The research sample being envisioned
- Preferred research methods

- Total available budget
- All other program- or audience-related information that may be relevant to research efforts
- What is expected from the research consultant or firm

The last point is extremely important in establishing the right relationship from the start. A marketing research firm or consultant can be hired for different purposes, which may include helping with the research design, the actual research implementation and fieldwork, data analysis and reporting, or technical assistance throughout the process. For example, in the case of community-led participatory research, chances are that the research firm or consultant would help facilitate the overall process and provide technical assistance. Other times, they will conduct the entire research study or participate only in data analysis.

Finally, key parameters in selecting a firm or consultant are reputation (it is important to ask for references); previous experience on health communication (which should be an ideal prerequisite) or the specific health issue; the consultant's compliance with current codes of ethics and research parameters; affordability; dedicated staff; professionalism; and others that vary from case to case. Regardless of the firm or consultant selected, program planners should stay close to the overall research process, actively participating in all or most of its phases and supervising it. This is an opportunity for program planners to learn about their audiences.

KEY CONCEPTS

- The situation analysis is a fundamental step in program planning and should be the foundation of health communication programs. In fact, health communication is a research-based field.
- In this book, *situation analysis* is used as a planning term. It describes the research and analysis of all individual, community, social, and behavior-related factors that can affect attitudes, behaviors, social norms, and policies about a health issue and its potential solutions.
- The situation analysis has a number of steps, which include an audience profile for all primary and secondary audiences.

Including the audience profile as part of the situation analysis may facilitate a full understanding of the mutual interdependence between audience and environment-related factors.

- Audience segmentation in groups with similar characteristics and behavioral stages is required for most programs.
- Once segments have been defined, ranking them can help guide resource allocation as well as the overall focus of the health communication intervention.
- There are several criteria that apply to audience segmentation and ranking and serve as a framework to guide the completion of these steps.
- There are several communication and marketing research methodologies. This chapter highlights the difference between market research and marketing research, qualitative versus quantitative research, secondary and primary data as well as frequently used research methods (one-on-one in-depth interviews, focus groups, and surveys). Practical suggestions on how to use common research methodologies or to select a marketing and communication research firm or consultant conclude the chapter.

FOR DISCUSSION AND PRACTICE

1. Using again the fictional example of Luciana, the nineteen-year-old Italian woman who spends a lot of time at the beach and is unaware of the risk for skin cancer (see Box 2.1 as well as the previous chapter), list and discuss questions that need to be addressed as part of the situation analysis and audience profile of a program targeted to her and her peer group. The worksheet in Appendix A (see "Situation Analysis and Audience Profile Worksheet: Sample Questions and Topics") provides additional guidance.
2. Provide situations in which you would use qualitative research methods versus quantitative methods. List all factors that may influence your decision to use a specific research method.
3. Review key concepts in this chapter, and discuss what in your opinion links the situation analysis to the other steps of health communication planning.

CHAPTER ELEVEN

IDENTIFYING PROGRAM OBJECTIVES AND STRATEGIES

IN THIS CHAPTER

- How to Develop and Validate Communication Objectives
- Outlining a Communication Strategy
- Key Concepts
- For Discussion and Practice

The communication objective of a health communication program by Radio Salankoloto, a local radio station in Burkina Faso, Africa, is to tackle HIV/AIDS by increasing knowledge and understanding of HIV/AIDS preventive measures (Fisher, 2003). In the United States, one of the key objectives of the communication component of *Healthy People 2010*, the U.S. public health agenda, is "to improve the health literacy of persons with inadequate or marginal literacy skills" (U.S. Department of Health and Human Services, 2005, pp. 11–15).

In both cases, the objectives support the overall goal of the health communication program or public health intervention as well as the behavioral and social objectives the two programs try to achieve. In the case of HIV/AIDS in Burkina Faso, the overall goal of the health communication intervention is to help reduce the increasing incidence of HIV/AIDS in that country (Fisher, 2003) by prompting people to use preventive measures (behavioral objective). In the case of *Healthy People 2010*, improving health literacy is considered instrumental to "longer life, improved quality of life, and reduction of chronic diseases and health disparities"

(National Institutes of Health, 2005), key goals of the U.S. public health agenda. In order to achieve these goals, people need to understand and act on health information (behavioral objective).

Several strategies have been developed or suggested by Radio Salankoloto and *Healthy People 2010* in support of communication objectives and have highlighted not only the focus of the intervention but also the strategic use of communication tools and approaches to reach such objectives. In Burkina Faso, Radio Salankoloto uses popular forms of expression (radio drama) to reach its program's objectives and help people identify with the story. *Healthy People 2010* identified two strategic areas to improve health literacy: "the development of appropriate written materials and improvement in skills of those people with limited literacy" (U.S. Department of Health and Human Services, 2005, pp. 11–15).

This chapter focuses on defining communication objectives and strategies while highlighting the connection of these two important steps to other phases of the planning process that precede or follow them. By providing a practical guide on the dos and don'ts of establishing communication objectives and strategies, this chapter helps build knowledge of the technical skills that are needed to complete this step of health communication planning.

How to Develop and Validate Communication Objectives

Communication objectives are the intermediate steps (National Cancer Institute and National Institutes of Health, 2002) that need to be attained in order to meet the overall program goals as complemented by specific behavioral, social, and organizational objectives. Often communication objectives are expressed as follows:

"To raise awareness"

"To increase knowledge"

"To break the cycle of misinformation"

"To change attitudes"

"To facilitate interactions"

"To help build expertise or skills"

The outcomes highlighted by communication objectives all refer to the different components of the mental process of change that communication can affect. In fact, often communication objectives are about changes in knowledge, attitudes, beliefs, motivation, and human interactions (Colle and Roman, 2003), which are all intermediate and critical steps in the achievement of behavioral, social, or organizational objectives and, ultimately, the overall program's goal. Such changes can take place at the individual, group, organizational, or societal level as the result of communication interventions with well-defined objectives. Sometimes communication objectives coincide with behavioral objectives, but in most cases they address intermediate steps that lead to behavioral outcomes. For example, in the case of breast cancer prevention, some communication objectives could be "to raise awareness among Latino women over age forty of the need for annual mammograms" or "to facilitate provider-patient interactions on breast cancer–related questions." Both objectives support the behavioral (outcome) objective that aims at prompting women to have annual mammograms.

Sometimes communication objectives are written to emphasize the role of the audience in making the change. For example, the first of the two objectives on breast cancer screening can be stated as follows: "Latino women over forty years of age will report to be aware of the need for annual mammograms."

Whenever possible, communication objectives should include specific measurable parameters that can be used in the program evaluation phase to assess the success (or lack of) of the communication strategy in support of such objectives. Many authors agree that communication objectives should describe: "WHO will do or change WHAT by WHEN and by HOW MUCH" (Weinreich, 1999, p. 68). This rule also applies to outcome objectives such as behavioral, social, and organizational objectives.

Under this rule the possible objectives of breast cancer screening can be restated:

- To raise awareness by the year 2010 of the need for annual mammograms among X percent of Latino women over forty years of age who live in target neighborhoods (or, for broader programs, in the United States)

- To facilitate by the year 2012 provider-patient communications
  on breast cancer as reported by X percent of health care
  providers in fifteen selected medical practices in the target
  neighborhood

In practice, especially in the private sector, including both
commercial and nonprofit organizations, communication objectives rarely specify quantitative measurements (for example, by
"how much" and "when"). Sometimes they may include an approximate estimate of how long it may take to achieve them. This
overall tendency is motivated by perceived difficulties and limitations of measurement, which also require the allocation of adequate funds.

In many corporations and nonprofit organizations, communication departments simply do not get funded to do measurement.
The culture of too many health organizations supports the idea of
measurement but often does not justify or provide a means of pay-
ing for it. Other parameters, primarily process oriented, activity
specific, or financial, are used to assess the success of a program.
When changes in knowledge, beliefs, attitudes, or behavior are
measured, it is usually on a qualitative basis, by stakeholder interviews that are conducted before and after the intervention. In academic settings, in contrast, measurement of the quantitative
parameters used to define outcome and communication objectives
tends to be a standard practice for research-based efforts and other
kinds of interventions in health communication.

While it is true that all quantitative measurements of outcome
and communication objectives require in-depth pre- and postintervention analyses in concentrated geographical areas and time
periods (see Chapters Twelve and Thirteen), setting measurable
objectives is still an excellent practice for health communication.
Measurable objectives are important for program evaluation (after
all, communication objectives are the intermediate milestones of
the program); creating agreement among team members, partners, and other key stakeholders on success factors and parameters; and helping focus program planners on what communication
can do and by when. However, health communicators, partners,
donors, and key stakeholders should always take into account that
measurement in health communication faces several limitations,

which are discussed in detail in Chapters Twelve and Thirteen and relate to many of the points introduced in this section.

In general, a model that can be used in developing communication objectives as well as outcome objectives such as behavioral, social, and organizational objectives is SMART. Under SMART, objectives should be (O'Sullivan, Yonkler, Morgan, and Merritt, 2003, p. 79; Piotrow, Kincaid, Rimon, and Rinehart, 1997):

Specific	They describe who should do what.
Measurable	They are defined by quantitative parameters.
Appropriate	They reflect audience needs and preferences.
Realistic	They can be reasonably achieved.
Time bound	They can be achieved within a specific time frame.

SMART has been endorsed by several organizations and planning guides (UNICEF, 2006; O'Sullivan, Yonkler, Morgan, and Merritt, 2003; Health Communication Unit, 1999).

Exhibit 11.1 shows the sample communication objectives that relate to a specific program goal as well as to a specific behavioral objective. Of notice, changes in individual or social behavior are more difficult to achieve than changes in knowledge, attitudes, or skills. Therefore, it is always more likely that in a given time frame outcome objectives will be attained in a smaller percentage of intended audiences when compared to changes in knowledge, attitudes, or skills that are defined by communication objectives.

SETTING COMMUNICATION OBJECTIVES

The first step in setting communication objectives is to consider all data that have been gathered for the situation analysis and audience profile. It is important to prioritize the findings that point to a specific communication or audience need or preference. Research findings should also be carefully analyzed in reference to the behavioral stages of the primary audiences as well as secondary audiences (individuals, groups, or stakeholders who may exert an influence on primary audiences). Communication objectives need to reflect and be consistent with the information gathered on these topics.

Before establishing communication objectives, it is important to validate the overall program goals, as well as the behavioral, social, and organizational objectives that were determined on the basis of

Exhibit 11.1. Sample Communication Objectives: Understanding
the Connection with Other Program Elements

Overall Program Goal

Reduce the incidence and mortality of adult melanoma cases
associated with early and excessive sun exposure during
childhood (by the year 2020)

Behavioral Objective: By the year 2012, 5 percent of U.S. parents who live
in Florida will use sunscreen, sun hats, and other preventive measures
to protect their children from the damaging effects of prolonged and
excessive sun exposure.

Communication Objectives (if all relevant to the specific stages of audience
beliefs, attitude, skills, and behavior, they should be implemented in
different program phases because they are in excess of the recommended
limit of two to three objectives per audience): By the year 2008, 10
percent of U.S. parents who live in Florida

- Will be aware of the association between excessive sun exposure
  during childhood and the risk for adult melanoma
- Will be able to define "excessive sun exposure"
- Will report having conversations with their health care provider
  about preventive measures
- Will know how to protect their children from excessive sun exposure
  and feel capable of doing so
- Will have instructed all of their children's caretakers to adopt the
  same protection measures
- Will advocate within their community for the widespread use of sun-
  protection measures

---

the preliminary briefing or literature review. The framework for
this validation should be provided by data from the situation analysis and audience profile, which by now should have been finalized.
This will ensure that communication objectives are set to meet realistic and accurate program goals and outcome objectives.

Once this preliminary step has been completed, the health communication team can start brainstorming to set and prioritize
communication objectives. The following sections discuss practical tips and examples on how to develop adequate communication
objectives.

Make Sure Communication Objectives Are Audience Specific

Consider again the case of a program that aims to reduce the incidence of pertussis, a vaccine-preventable childhood disease that in its severe forms is characterized by a prolonged cough with a typical whoop. As for other vaccine-preventable childhood diseases, it is possible that young health care providers in the United States may have never seen a case of pertussis and may feel it is no longer a priority in their practice. Still, the disease is on the rise (Centers for Disease Control, 2005), and there have been a number of deaths among infants and young children from this disease. If interviews with key opinion leaders in this medical area show that there is low physician awareness of pertussis and its potential life-threatening consequences as well as on how infants and young children can contract it (Cherry and others, 2005; Tan, 2005; Greenberg, von Konig, and Heininger, 2005), one of the communication objectives should address the need for increasing knowledge of pertussis, its cycle of transmission, and key characteristics among health care providers in the pediatric and primary care settings. The communication objectives that may be set for parents may be completely different and address other kinds of needs that can be highlighted by research findings.

Do Not Include Tactical Elements

A good practice in developing communication objectives is to leave out information related to tactical elements, such as communication activities, materials, and channels. At this point, program planners should focus on what communication should accomplish and not worry whether the mass media, online events, interpersonal channels, or other kinds of activities would be used by the program (Health Communication Unit, 1999). All of these elements will be defined as part of the tactical plan and guided by the communication strategy.

Limit the Number of Communication Objectives

Too many communication objectives often result in too many messages. Since behavioral and social change is a gradual process, having too many objectives (and related strategies and messages) may be confusing for target audiences. When research findings point to multiple communication needs, it is critical to prioritize communication objectives that are more likely to lead to the achievement of the program's goal. Another possibility is to distribute them over time in a logical sequence that addresses the most important communication needs first. Therefore, even if it is appropriate to start brainstorming about multiple objectives, the final communication objectives should not include more than two or three objectives per audience.

Identify and Prioritize Objectives

Consider existing levels of knowledge as well as attitudes and common beliefs. Look at existing policies and social norms, as well as past and ongoing programs that address individual behavior and community needs. Think about what kinds of attitudes, beliefs, skills, policies, or norms need to be in existence to attain the behavioral, social, or organizational objectives that have been established and validated in support of the program goal. Think about the existing situation and how communication can help.

These steps should lead to identifying the most important communication objectives, which normally correspond to the key steps of the mental, behavioral, and social process of change. An audience segment might be teenagers who are unaware of the health risks associated with smoking and have just started smoking. If audience awareness of these risks is low among teenagers, the decision to focus on increasing knowledge about smoking cessation methods and programs may leave out a large percentage of teenagers. In fact, communicating about how to quit smoking is a lower priority in the absence of a high level of audience awareness on the health damages caused by smoking. Although there are cases in which both objectives could be met at the same time (it is always a good idea to provide solutions while alerting people of specific health risks), focusing on smoking cessation methods without raising awareness of the health consequences of smoking is unlikely to lead to results in this audience segment.

Selecting and applying one of the behavioral or social theories described in Chapter Two can help identify and prioritize communication objectives. In fact, these theories can provide a logical framework to organize one's thoughts and prioritize communication objectives by taking into account the key steps of behavioral or social change.

Analyze Barriers and Success Factors

After prioritizing and selecting communication objectives, program planners should analyze potential barriers that may delay or jeopardize the attainment of these objectives. It is possible that additional communication objectives would need to be established and focus on removing such barriers. In a case in which smoking cessation may be perceived as a very low priority because the community or the country's cultural and policy context supports it, potential communication objectives are (1) to persuade policymakers about the relevance of a smoke-free environment for some of their key constituencies or (2) to inform them about the risks associated with smoking and their responsibility to protect the communities they govern. This may help remove some of the barriers to change. For example, in January 2005, "the Italian government banned smoking in all indoor public places" (Gallus and others, 2006, p. 346). Until then, the only smoke-free areas had been selected public spaces such as airports and libraries, but not necessarily restaurants, bars, or offices. Preliminary analyses on the impact of the ban on smoking habits showed that the new policy is associated with a decrease of 8 percent in tobacco consumption (Gallus and others, 2006).

In other cases, other issues need to be addressed to promote people's compliance with smoking bans. In fact, smoking bans and regulations are not always enforced (Godfrey, 2005; European Network for Smoking Prevention, 2005; Borg, 2004).

Of course, if social objectives had been established at the onset of program planning, policy changes should be part of the overall plan. Still, it is worth taking an additional look at all barriers in the context of the development of communication objectives. This will help establish the time sequence and priority by which changes need to happen and set realistic expectations about the overall behavioral, social, or organizational change process.

Success factors in achieving communication objectives should also be analyzed. However, the analysis of these factors is relevant primarily to the development of communication strategies and tactical plans (see the next section as well as Chapter Twelve). In fact, an analysis of estimated success factors may point to the key strategic approaches or activities that may lead to achieving the communication objectives.

Define Time Frames

This step is related to establishing the time frame within which a communication objective can be achieved. Many factors can affect this time frame. In addition to external factors (for example, existing behaviors, policies, specific circumstances, clinical practices, or potential barriers), which are usually highlighted by the situation analysis and audience profile, there are several program- or health organization–related factors that can influence the overall time frame for the attainment of communication objectives:

- Available funds, which determine the program reach as well as the speed with which materials and activities can be implemented.
- Human resources, which need to be adequate in all phases of program implementation, monitoring, and evaluation.
- Organizational competence and experience in a specific health field or in reaching its key audiences. Health organizations with limited experience or reputation in a health field may need longer to achieve communication objectives because of the need to establish themselves with target audiences or in the specific disease area.
- A clear understanding of team members' roles and responsibilities, as well as core contributions by program's partners.
- A specific time line that is shared with and endorsed by all team members and partners.
- Overall program span, which may condition the interval between activities as well as the timing of specific communication objectives. For example, in health emergency situations, communication objectives need to be achieved much more rapidly than in the case of interventions that attempt to tackle chronic situations or diseases.

MOVING TO THE NEXT STEP

Since all elements of health communication planning and the health communication process itself are interconnected and dependent on each other, communication objectives set the stage for the development of communication strategies. Well-designed communication objectives influence and guide the rationale used in the next steps of communication planning, as well as in the allocation of resources.

OUTLINING A COMMUNICATION STRATEGY

A *communication strategy* is a statement describing the overall approach used to accomplish the communication objectives. It highlights how people can become aware of a disease risk, gain knowledge about prevention methods, or improve patient-provider communications on sensitive health issues, among others.

Communication strategies shape the tactical elements of a health communication program; they are directly connected to and serve the overall program goal and the behavioral, social, and organizational objectives and communication objectives. In fact, communication strategies are often highlighted as part of a strategy plan that includes all of these other elements. This approach showcases the evidence and logical sequence that has led to specific communication strategies.

As for the objectives, communication strategies are audience specific and research based. Consider again the example of teenagers who are not aware of the health risks associated with smoking and have just started smoking. In this case, a potential communication objective is, "To raise awareness of the health risks associated with smoking among 5 percent of teenagers from thirteen to nineteen years of age who live in the United States." This communication objective has been established to support the overall program goal of reducing the incidence of smoking-related morbidity among U.S. teenagers. The communication objective also supports the behavioral objective of prompting teenagers to quit smoking.

A number of potential strategies can support this objective—for example:

- *Use teenage role models* to highlight the risks of smoking.
- *Create a peer support network* to facilitate discussion of smoking risks.
- *Engage high schools* in establishing smoking risk awareness programs.

- *Use natural opportunities* (for example, teen meetings, publications, concerts) to raise awareness of the health risks of smoking.
- *Provide tools to parents* to speak with teenagers about health risks associated with smoking.
- *Develop core communication tools and activities* on smoking health risks that can be easily distributed and customized by primary and secondary audiences.
- *Establish partnerships with local youth organizations* to include discussion of smoking risks in their agenda and enhance program reach.
- *Promote smoking risk awareness* through one-on-one counseling at routine medical visits.
- *Focus on the limitations* that smoking poses to physical performance and excellence in sports.

None of these examples of potential strategies mentions any tactical elements such as flyers, brochures, press releases, and workshops. In fact, a communication strategy is an overall concept and describes in general terms how to achieve objectives. It is the guiding framework under which messages and tactics will be established. Communication strategies identify and describe in broad terms the right combination of channels, messengers, and settings and guide message development.

Key Principles of Strategy Development

As described so far in this chapter, once health communicators have analyzed all findings from the situation analysis and audience profile and established sound outcome and communication objectives, they usually move to consider several strategic approaches that may resonate with intended audiences. The process of identifying, rating, prioritizing, and selecting communication strategies relies on many steps, which are described next.

Review Research Evidence

The first step in strategy development is a careful review of the situation analysis and audience profile. This step is common to all phases of planning that follow the initial research steps. In the case of strategy development, research findings should be analyzed to identify the most suitable audience- or situation-specific approaches that would help meet the communication objectives. Audience preferences for specific communication channels and messengers should be considered and analyzed as part of this additional data review.

Make Sure All Communication Strategies Are Audience Specific

Similar to objectives, communication strategies are audience specific. Usually different strategies are needed for different audiences. Also, multiple strategies are often needed to attain the communication objectives for a specific audience.

Evidence-based strategies always include a rationale for their development that is likely to be used to present the program to partners, perspective donors, and intended audiences (O'Sullivan, Yonkler, Morgan, and Merritt, 2003). It is therefore important that the rationale for the development of a specific strategy is clear to all members of the extended communication team, including partners and key stakeholders.

A logical approach in developing a communication strategy is to have an audience-centered mind-set, so the strategy will be established in response to the audience's needs, preferences, pastimes, and influencing factors. Sound strategies should also consider strengths, weaknesses, opportunities, and threats (SWOT) as identified as part of the situation analysis. For instance, the examples of strategies provided in this chapter support awareness of the health risks associated with smoking among teenagers in these ways:

- Relying on the audience's needs or preferences (create a peer support network; use teenager role models)
- Tapping into the work, credibility, and networks of existing organizations (establish partnerships with local youth organizations)
- Exploiting natural opportunities (for example, teen meetings, publications, concerts)
- Identifying potential communication angles that may be relevant to teenagers (focus on the limitations that smoking poses to physical performance and excellence in sports)

- Identifying secondary audiences or settings that can exert an influence on teenagers (provide parents with tools; engage high schools)

Other categories can be chosen in relation to specific health issues, products or services, and related audiences. Among them, the category that focuses on identifying potential communication angles that may be relevant to key audiences is particularly important in message development. In fact, this category helps define all attributes of a specific behavior, health service, or product that should be incorporated in communication messages in order to make them appealing to intended audiences. Obviously this should be complemented by awareness-, risk-, or action-oriented messages. This strategic category, as well as the specific message development process that this influences, is part of *positioning*, a core concept in marketing and social marketing. Positioning identifies the fit between what target audiences are seeking and what the product could actually deliver or represent for them (Kotler and Roberto, 1989). It has to do with the long-term identity of a behavior, health service, or product that would make it desirable to intended audiences and facilitate the change process related to its acceptance and adoption (O'Sullivan, Yonkler, Morgan, and Merritt, 2003).

In health communication, the concept of identifying and focusing on communication angles and topics that are relevant and resonate with intended audiences goes beyond the idea of selling a health behavior, product, or service. In fact, it is often an organizing principle for individuals, groups, communities, and key stakeholders to get together about a health problem. For example, in the case of smoking cessation, many parents and teenagers agree about the benefits and rewards of a physically active life (Centers for Disease Control, 2001, 2006g). Sports and athletic competitions have been used as a motivating factor for keeping children away from smoking, drugs, and risky behaviors by many kinds of programs and interventions (Castrucci, Gerlach, Kaufman, and Orleans, 2004). The sense of pride that goes with practicing a sport or seeing a loved one excel in its performance motivates communities around the world to create athletic clubs, programs, and facilities where children can play and be together. Since the long-term effects of smoking include a reduction in physical fitness (American Heart Association, 2006b), focusing on this health consequence may become an organizing principle for communities and interested groups.

In summary, the rationale of a communication strategy should always state the reason that the strategy has been established and selected over other approaches (O'Sullivan, Yonkler, Morgan, and Merritt, 2003).

Rate, Prioritize, and Select Strategic Approaches

Different strategies have the potential of supporting a communication objective; however, some of them may be best suited to achieve communication objectives in an efficient, time-saving, cost-effective, or audience-friendly manner. In evaluating communication strategies, serious consideration should be given to the strategy's sustainability, credibility with intended audiences and key stakeholders, and implementation costs and barriers. Other factors may be issue or audience specific and include whether the strategy can accommodate an adequate and integrated blend of tools and activities; is innovative and suited to secure people's attention, especially in relation to issues for which many programs may exist; and is best suited to meet audience's needs.

In the end, this kind of analysis aims at selecting strategies that are best positioned to meet the program's goals and objectives. It should be conducted for each of the strategies under consideration.

The process of ranking and selecting adequate communication strategies can be organized to address the following issues:

- Key benefits: for example, the strategy can accommodate an integrated use of tools and activities or the messenger has credibility with the intended audiences.
- Disadvantages: for example, the implementation time needed is lengthy.
- Potential barriers to implementation: examples are a lack of existing policies that support the strategy or a social stigma that would prevent patient survivors to be involved in the program.
- Ability to secure community or key stakeholder endorsement.
- Available resources, which should be adequate to strategy implementation.
- Organizational capability and competence in executing the strategy.

Appendix A includes a worksheet, "Ranking and Selecting Communication Strategies," that incorporates all of these categories and can be used as a model to rank and select communication strategies.

BRINGING THE STEPS TOGETHER

All elements of health communication planning are interconnected. In fact, in the early phases of health communication planning, most of the efforts are concentrated on linking the overall program goal with outcome objectives (behavioral, social, or organizational) and, in turn, with communication objectives and strategies. Preliminary and formative research informs and guides all of these steps.

Prior to the development of the tactical and evaluation plans, it is helpful to take a look at the progress in establishing these important foundations of the health communication program, as well as to appreciate the link and interdependence of all of these elements. Finally, the potential success of effective communication objectives and strategies is dependent on the quality and execution of the tactical plan that will be developed to execute them. This reinforces the concept of a health communication cycle in which key steps are interdependent.

KEY CONCEPTS

- Communication objectives and strategies are interdependent and connected with all other components of the health communication program.
- Communication objectives are the intermediate steps or changes that are needed to achieve behavioral, social, and organizational objectives, as well as the overall program goal.
- Sometimes communication objectives coincide with behavioral objectives. More frequently, given the complexity of human behavior, which calls for many intermediate steps in order to achieve behavioral or social change, communication objectives focus on addressing these intermediate steps.
- Communication strategies are designed to serve the communication objectives of the program, as well as its outcome objectives (behavioral, social, and organizational).

- Communication strategies describe the approach used to meet the objectives. In other words, they focus on how the changes sought by the communication objectives will be attained.
- Neither communication objectives nor strategies focus on or describe tactical elements. Communication strategies inform and guide the development of the tactical plan (including communication messages, channels, materials, and activities).

FOR DISCUSSION AND PRACTICE

1. Discuss the difference between outcome objectives (behavioral, social, and organizational) and communication objectives. Use practical examples.
2. Using again the fictional example of Luciana in relation to skin cancer prevention among her peer group (see Box 2.1. as well as the discussion sections of previous chapters in Part Three), think of suitable communication objectives and strategies, and state them according to the methods and concepts included in this chapter.
3. Rank in order of importance and suitability all strategies you have developed for the previous question (for additional guidance on ranking key strategies, see the "Ranking and Selecting Communication Strategies" worksheet in Appendix A).

CHAPTER TWELVE

DEVELOPING TACTICAL AND EVALUATION PLANS

IN THIS CHAPTER

- Overall Definitions of Tactical and Evaluation Plans
- Key Elements of a Tactical Plan
- The Evaluation Plan: An Overview of Models and Trends
- Key Concepts
- For Discussion and Practice

The tactical plan is the step of health communication planning that many in the health communication profession consider enjoyable. Creativity comes into play in this phase of planning, which relates to selecting a strategic blend of messages, channels, activities, and materials in support of the program strategies and objectives. All elements of the tactical plan are related to the different communication areas as defined in this book. For example, the tactical plan of a program by the U.S. Centers for Disease Control and Prevention (CDC) that aims at reducing colorectal cancer deaths by encouraging prevention and early detection includes public service announcements (PSAs), online informational materials, community-based events for low-income people, and many other communication tools (Centers for Disease Control, 2004/2005, 2006c). The tactics in this program are related to different communication areas (for example, public relations, professional communications) and support communication objectives and strategies.

The selection of communication areas and tools should be inspired by more than creativity and what may work. The word *strate-*

gic is critical to understanding how to develop an effective tactical plan that will serve the program's strategies and objectives. This chapter focuses on some of the key attributes of strategic tactical plans, as well as the key steps in developing them. The chapter also establishes the need for developing a detailed evaluation plan prior to program implementation. It provides an overview of trends and models in program evaluation as well as practical guidance in developing evaluation plans that reflect key program assumptions, goals, and objectives.

OVERALL DEFINITIONS OF TACTICAL AND EVALUATION PLANS

The title of this chapter is directly linked to the origins and literal meaning of the two key words of these two steps of communication planning: *tactics* and *evaluate*. It also reflects the connection of these key steps to each other as well as the other phases of the health communication cycle.

TACTICAL PLANS

Tactics are defined as a "procedure or set of maneuvers engaged in to achieve an end, an aim, or a goal" (*American Heritage Dictionary of the English Language*, 2004). Although the term may evoke military procedures, it refers to a plan of action that includes communication messages, activities, materials, and channels and is developed to serve the program's strategies and objectives. Other authors and models (World Health Organization, 2003) use the term *action plan* to define this program component.

The term *tactical plan* is widely accepted in health communication practice and refers to a detailed description of the program components:

- Audience-specific messages, actions, materials, and related channels that are developed and implemented as part of the health communication program (including program launch activities and materials)
- A detailed pretesting plan that should describe key research methods (for example, focus groups, in-depth interviews) and

questions that will be used to secure audience feedback on **communication concepts** ("ways of presenting information to intended audiences"; National Cancer Institute and National Institutes of Health, 2002, p. 55, and the overall kind of appeal that will be used in reaching them) as well as draft messages, materials, and activities
- A partnership plan that will list all program partners, their roles and responsibilities, and key contact people
- A program time line for each activity
- A budget estimate for each activity, including evaluation activities, and all materials

Further consideration should be given here to the term *strategic* in the context of tactical plans. In fact, the tactical plan is nothing more than a detailed extension of the broad outline for action established by communication strategies. It describes how to accomplish key objectives on a level of tactical details that strategies do not address. However, the tactical plan is still supportive of the same objectives that have been established for the program and the development of key strategies. In other words, the health communication cycle never ends.

Consider the example of a communication program that aims at reducing the impact of depression on work performance and family interactions among women over forty-five years of age. The behavioral objectives of the program are to prompt women to (1) seek help when they feel depression is affecting their work and family lives and (2) comply with best practices in the treatment and management of depression. If depression is still stigmatized in a specific population or country, as it is in Australia (Barney, Griffiths, Jorm, and Christensen, 2006) and among African Americans (Das, Olfson, McCurtis, and Weissman, 2006), a social objective may be to foster a change in social attitudes toward depression, so that this condition can be accepted and discussed in social and professional contexts by the year 2020. The program has set the following communication objectives and strategies:

Communication Objectives

- Raise awareness of strategies and methods to cope with depression among women over forty-five years of age who suffer from depression or are at high risk for this condition (quantitative parameters to be included).

- Dispel common myths and correct misinformation about depression among the general public in the United States (include quantitative parameters).

Communication Strategies

- Create a social and peer support network that will rely on women who successfully manage to minimize the impact of depression on work performance and family interactions.
- Use women role models to personalize depression and show the human face of this condition.

There are many ways to execute each of these strategies—for example:

- Establish peer-to-peer communications meetings at local health clinics, major hospitals, and other venues.
- Train women spokespeople, and create a media speaker bureau to react to and offer perspectives on recent news on depression as well as encourage media coverage of strategies and messages to cope with depression.
- Conduct outreach through women's magazines.
- Develop radio and TV PSAs pointing to a toll-free number or Web site for professional help and peer support meetings.
- Organize Internet chats on top women's Web sites.

Since tactics are audience and strategy specific, some of these activities may be better suited to support and execute one of the two strategies. Others may support both of them or perhaps should be discarded if they are not as effective as other options in serving the communication strategies. For example, the first of the tactics, "establish peer-to-peer communication meetings," may be suited to execute the first strategy, while the others may be used to support both strategies but may have unequal effectiveness. The selection of specific messages, activities, materials, and channels is related to research findings and audience preferences, as well as many criteria that are specific to the health issue and its environment.

EVALUATION PLANS

While most authors, organizations, and experiences support the importance of developing evaluation parameters and plans prior to program implementation and early in the planning process (National Cancer Institute and National Institutes of Health, 2002; World Health Organization, 2003; O'Sullivan, Yonkler, Morgan, and Merritt, 2003), too often measurement is considered only toward the end of a health communication program. This frequently leads to confusion and disagreement about the measures of success. For example, if activity-related outcomes are being evaluated for an online discussion, potential measurement parameters can include the number of participants, the quality and significance of the questions and opinions they expressed, or the overall contribution of the discussion to audience or marketing research for future programs or changes in knowledge, attitudes, and behavior among intended audiences. All of these may be valuable evaluation parameters, but different team members and partners may have different ideas about what can be called a successful online discussion.

Including an evaluation plan early in program planning helps health communicators, team members, and partners to focus on the program's ultimate goals and objectives, agree on expected outcomes, and combine their efforts to achieve them. This is only one of the many important benefits of early evaluation plans.

Sound evaluation plans should include a comprehensive description of key measurement parameters and expected outcomes to consider when evaluating the program, as well as the methods that will be used to collect and analyze data in relation to these parameters. This format applies to the different phases of evaluation (formative, process, and summative) as defined and described in this chapter, as well as to related research methods (see Chapter Ten).

Finally, further insights into the importance of evaluation and early definition of key parameters and methods is provided by the literal meaning of the word *evaluate,* which is defined as "to ascertain or fix the value or worth of [something]" (*The American Heritage Dictionary of the English Language,* 2004). People tend to ascertain the value of things they intend to buy or to which they are considering committing significant personal or professional time well in advance of moving ahead with their final decisions. For example, it is likely that house buyers will conduct some research on current prices for comparable houses in the same neighborhood. This information helps them determine what they are willing to pay for the house they are considering and whether it is worth their investment. Why should it be different for health communication planning? The worth of financial, human resources, and time investments should be evaluated prior to the use of these resources.

One of the fundamental premises of this book is that health communication is an intrinsic part of everyone's life (Du Pré, 2000). As in other aspects of life, health communication interventions should establish early in the process the worth of each investment in relation to specific outcomes and measurement parameters. This practice is also critical in establishing the overall value of the health communication field in the public health and private sectors by avoiding, or at least minimizing, potential disappointments among key stakeholders, partners, donors, supervisors, and clients about the return of their investment. However, it is important to recognize the limitations and costs associated with the evaluation of health communication programs, another of the key topics of this chapter.

Key Elements of a Tactical Plan

The success of a tactical plan is highly dependent on several key elements that should guide its development. This section examines the most important features of well-designed tactical plans.

Integrated Approach

In designing a tactical plan that supports core communication strategies and objectives, multiple approaches and channels from different areas of health communication are likely needed to address a given health issue. The concept of an integrated approach, in which all tactical elements support and are complementary to each other, is commonly used in commercial marketing. In the private sector, integrated marketing communications (IMC) is one approach to organize and manage communications tools and activities, so that information takes into account the beliefs, attitudes, preferences, and perceptions of the consumers (Nowak and others, 1998; Renganathan and others, 2005).

The concept of an integrated approach to communication is well established in health communication practice and incorporated at different levels in communication models for behavior and social change. In fact, IMC is one of the many influencing disciplines and factors of the WHO Communication for Behavioral Impact (COMBI) model (see Chapter Two) for strategic behavior communications (Renganathan and others, 2005). Similarly, the communication for the social change model (see Chapter Two) is defined as "an integrated model for measuring the process and its outcomes" (Figueroa, Kincaid, Rani, and Lewis, 2002) that relies on multiple approaches and tools. In addition, the health communication chapter of *Healthy People 2010* often refers to the integration of different communication areas (for example, "mass media with community-based programs") in existing or past communication campaigns (Department of Health and Human Services, p. 11-4).

Similar to other characteristics of health communication and its planning process, the concept of integrated communications draws on everyday life. Communication, and more specifically health communication, is a common part of social exchanges and contexts, from personal and professional encounters to the mass media and traditional forms of expression such as theater and poetry, as well as informal conversations in barber shops, churches, restaurants, markets, and other public places (Exchange, 2006). Tactical plans should reflect this diversity of communication approaches and channels to match how communication actually takes place. "What works in communicating about health depends on the context, and the way different communication processes and approaches are linked together or remain separate" (Exchange, 2006). Depending on how communication is used, different approaches can help "build momentum around some issues, but also isolate some social groups and conversations" (Exchange, 2006). A well-designed, well-integrated, and multifaceted tactical plan can help bridge gaps between current beliefs, attitudes, and behaviors and what is needed to achieve desired behavioral and social outcomes.

CREATIVITY IN SUPPORT OF STRATEGY

This book supports the ability and role of health communication practitioners to redefine the theory and practice of health communication by incorporating lessons learned and great ideas that worked well in related programs. But health communication needs to be strategic. This means that great ideas are acceptable as long as they support communication strategies and objectives and are connected to the other elements of the planning cycle.

Many health communicators can recall colleagues who were in favor of a specific communication approach, channel, or tactic and used it in all programs. And communication consultants or vendors that specialize in a specific communication channel or tool (for example, PSAs and videos) may have a partial view of the infinite possibilities for strategic tactics. Making videos for the sake of making videos does not help advance the communication goals and objectives the program is seeking to achieve, no matter how innovative and well designed the video may be. It is better to discard all great ideas that do not support communication strategies.

COST-EFFECTIVENESS

Cost-effectiveness should be one of the parameters to guide the comparison of different tactical approaches. Ultimately this kind of analysis should still aim for selecting the best approach, but in the case of multiple options, it may provide an objective criterion to prioritize and rank different tactics with similar effectiveness. This type of analysis needs to address a number of questions—for example:

- How do different approaches compare in serving core communication strategies? If they all serve the strategy with similar effectiveness, is there any difference in their cost, including economic cost and the investment of time and human resources?
- Are there any existing programs that could be used as a communication vehicle in support of communication strategies?
- Is there any potential for partnerships or collaborations with other organizational departments or external players that may

save costs or time for the implementation of a specific communication activity?

Saving costs and using human resources strategically are important not only in the case of limited funds or resources. Even
when resources or costs do not appear to be an issue, which is almost never the case in health communication, there is no reason
to waste them. The careful allocation of resources is one of the key
elements of strategic health communication and related tactical
plans.

IMAGINATION

In developing a tactical plan, it is important to envision how communication messages, channels, and activities can have an impact
on program strategies. Careful consideration should also be given
to potential barriers and pitfalls in implementing all tactics, so that
these can be prevented or minimized. As in all other steps of communication planning (see Chapter Nine), communication models, theories, case studies, and past experiences, if adequately
understood and selected, can help develop this vision. In the case
of the tactical plan, case studies and past experience are fundamental to foresee potential pitfalls, barriers to implementation, estimated impact on program goals and objectives, time, and human
resource investment, among others. Still, there is also an intuitive
quality to imagining and visualizing future activities and potential
pitfalls that can be developed over time as a result of experience.

CULTURALLY COMPETENT COMMUNICATION MESSAGES, CHANNELS, AND VEHICLES

Many observations throughout this book establish the influence of
cultural, ethnic, geographical, socioeconomic, age, and gender-
related factors on people's lifestyle, preferences, concepts of health
and illness, reaction to illness, and overall health outcomes (see
Chapter Three). The information gathered as part of the situation
analysis and audience profile should guide the selection of messages, channels, and vehicles that reflect the cultural characteristics and preferences of the intended audiences. Selecting culturally

competent communication tools is critical to the potential success of a health communication program.

For example, focus groups conducted in two geographical regions of Angola in sub-Saharan Africa with members of the local communities showed that interpersonal channels such as home visits and school- or church-based meetings were strongly favored by study participants. In one of the regions, strong preference was given to television versus radio when mass media were considered among potential channels. Finally, printed materials such as posters and brochures were excluded because of the high level of illiteracy among intended audiences. Focus group findings suggested that if printed materials were considered at all, they should rely more on graphics than words (Schiavo, 2000).

It is almost never possible to use any kind of one-size-fits-all communication strategy and related tactics anywhere in the world. For example, communication materials or messages that have been translated from English to Spanish can be confusing to Spanish speakers and audiences. And the literal meaning of expressions adapted from English may be perceived as offensive. Therefore, communication messages and materials intended for Hispanic audiences should be developed directly in Spanish and tested with members of these audiences.

Similarly, in developing the graphic content of printed, online, or broadcast materials that address health issues of large public interest, it is important for different ethnic groups to be represented among the models featured in all images so that people are able to recognize themselves and feel included in the message. In selecting adequate photos, health communicators should be aware that many stock photos (collections of photography and other kinds of images that can be purchased, used, and reused for design purposes by publishers, graphic designers, and health communication teams) tend to reinforce common stereotypes and misconceptions and need to be analyzed in detail. The contribution of members of health organizations who serve or represent intended audiences in the selection of adequate imaging and photos may help avoid or minimize the possibility of offending the people for whom communication materials are meant.

The first step in developing communication concepts, messages, materials, and activities is to keep an open mind and not assume that a specific message, workshop, or brochure may work for all. Formative research should guide the development of the tactical plan, which should be validated by pretesting with representatives of key audiences.

Concept Development

In health communication, *concepts* are preliminary to message and material development. They describe "ways of presenting the information to intended audiences" (National Cancer Institute and National Institutes of Health, 2002, p. 55) as well as the overall kind of appeal (for example, fear, hope, action, progress) that will be used in reaching them.

Communication concepts apply to actual messages as well as the content and graphic format of key materials and activities. For example, the logo of a health communication program that aims at prompting health workers to get immunized against flu can evoke fear (for example, a stop sign that crosses out the word *flu*) or wellness (a smiley face with a "feeling well" message around it). A communication campaign aimed at reaching drug abusers and convincing them to embrace the path to recovery can focus on eliciting fear for the life-threatening consequences of drug abuse or appeal to the sense of responsibility drug users may have for their children or other loved ones. Of course, both examples highlight only partial aspects of complex problems that need to be addressed by multiple interventions and messages.

A number of categories of communication concepts are commonly used in message development—for example (Weinreich, 1999; National Cancer Institute and National Institutes of Health, 2002; R. W. Rogers, 1975, 1983; Witte and Allen, 2000):

- *Fear appeal:* Concepts developed to evoke fear and refer to an emotional response
- *Action step:* Specific recommended actions
- *Rewards or benefits,* highlighting key advantages associated with recommended change
- *Perceived threat:* The audience's perception about its own risk levels for a specific health condition; refers to an audience response that is information based
- *Perceived efficacy:* The audience's perception about its own

ability to perform recommended actions and behavior, as well as the impact of such actions on the actual threat
- *Hope:* Conveys that following the recommended behavior will lead people to unexpected milestones or changes

Table 12.1 lists examples of concepts for a health communication program on childhood immunization that is directed to parents. As with all other kinds of concepts, these are raw messages. Final messages should be selected to reflect key issues and informational needs that have been highlighted by formative research, cultural values, audience preferences, and reactions to each of these possibilities. Notably, Table 12.1 includes a concept category of barriers, which refers to presenting information in a way that shows that perceived or existing barriers to behavioral or social change can be addressed and eliminated.

Prior experiences and research studies should also guide the selection process and provide information on the overall effectiveness of specific concepts. For example, fear appeal has been studied and applied over the years. Although many health communication practitioners and researchers believe that "fear appeals backfire," further analyses of communication interventions have suggested that "strong fear appeals produce high levels of perceived severity and susceptibility, and are more persuasive than low or weak fear appeal messages" (Witte and Allen, 2000, p. 591).

TABLE 12.1. EXAMPLES OF COMMUNICATION CONCEPTS
FOR A PROGRAM ON CHILDHOOD IMMUNIZATION

Benefits:	Immunization protects children from severe childhood diseases.
Barriers:	Childhood vaccines are safe and effective. The benefits of immunization are by far larger than the risk for side effects.
Consequences:	Vaccine-preventable childhood diseases can have long-term effects on a child's physical and mental development.
Action Steps:	Immunize your child. Talk to your health care provider about vaccines.

Moreover, fear appeal encourages behavior change, especially when coupled with high-efficacy messages.

In practice, the use of fear appeal in a strong or moderate way, or not at all, depends on the audience's characteristics and reactions, as well as the nature of the health issue being addressed. Raising fears or awareness of existing threats should always be coupled with messages and tools that build people's skills and make them feel confident that they can succeed on their own. There is nothing worse than informing people about potential risks or health conditions without giving them a way to prevent or manage them.

Recall the example of the parents of a nine-year-old boy who still wets the bed at night as the result of primary nocturnal enuresis, a common medical condition. Once the parents become aware that this is actually a medical condition and not a character flaw or behavioral problem (Cendron, 1999), they are likely to want to do something about it. They have already gone through many months of stress and shame and may feel relieved that help may be on the way. Suggesting they talk to a health care provider or go to a specialized health center is an important element of effective communication.

Similarly, think about the case of Maristela, the mother of five children who lives in a small village in northeast Brazil. She recently heard about the death of a child who used to play with her children. Apparently the child had visceral leishmaniasis, which is also known as kalazar, a parasitic disease spread by the bite of infected sand flies and is found in Central and South America, Africa, and some Asian countries. Kalazar presents with vague symptoms such as fever, weight loss, fatigue, and an enlarged spleen and liver (Centers for Disease Control, 2006j), also known as a pot belly. Rapid diagnosis, which starts with the initial suspicion of the disease in the presence of a pot belly, is critical to saving lives and is normally part of emergency control plans (Arias, Monteiro, and Zicker, 1996).

Maristela is scared of kalazar, does not understand it, and feels powerless about the possibility that her children might contract it. A health communication program intended for Maristela and other parents in her village is likely to be more successful if, in addition to raising awareness of the disease and its early symptoms, incorporates action steps and self-efficacy concepts and messages.

Among others, these could encourage disease suspicion (when a child has a pot belly) and prompt early intervention (such as rushing to the closest health care facility) and inquiry to health care providers about the possibility the child may have kalazar.

All of the examples in this section establish that communication concepts and messages are research based and should address the intended audience's specific needs and characteristics. Whenever possible, they should also be designed to show the path to behavioral or social change by highlighting a series of steps or actions leading to that. Most important, they should be validated by intended audiences through pretesting methods and analysis.

Box 12.1 presents a case study by the U.S. National Cancer Institute (NCI) that shows how communication messages were developed from a variety of initial communication concepts and on the basis of audience feedback. Practical tips on message development and an overview of pretesting methods and principles are addressed in the following sections.

Box 12.1

NCI's Cancer Research Awareness Initiative: From Message Concepts to Final Message

In 1996, the NCI's Office of Communications (OC), then the Office of Cancer Communications, launched the Cancer Research Awareness Initiative to increase the public's understanding of the process of medical discoveries and the relevance of discoveries to people's lives. OC's concept development and message testing for this initiative included the following activities.

Three values of medical research were selected for concept development:

1. Progress (e.g., we are achieving breakthroughs)
2. Benefits (e.g., prevention, detection, and treatment research are benefiting all of us)
3. Hope (e.g., we are hopeful that today's research will yield tomorrow's breakthroughs)

Based on these values, the following message concepts were developed and explored in focus groups with intended audience members:

- Research has led to real progress in the detection, diagnosis, treatment, and prevention of cancer.
- Everyone benefits from cancer research in some fashion.
- Cancer research is conducted in universities and medical schools across the country.
- Cancer research gives hope.
- At the broadest level, research priorities are determined by societal problems and concerns; at the project level, research priorities are driven primarily by past research successes and current opportunities.

The following messages were crafted after listening to intended audience members' reactions and their language and ideas about the importance of medical research:

A. Cancer Research: Discovering Answers for All of Us
B. Cancer Research: Because Cancer Touches Us All
C. Cancer Research: Discovering More Answers Every Day
D. Cancer Research: Because Lives Depend on It
E. Cancer Research: Only Research Cures Cancer

Mall intercept interviews were conducted to pretest them. Based on responses from the intended audience in these interviews, message D was selected as the program theme.

Source: U.S. National Cancer Institute and National Institute of Health. *Making Health Communication Programs Work.* National Institute of Health, Publication No. 02–5145, 2002, p. 56.

MESSAGE DEVELOPMENT

Once the type of message appeal has been selected, messages should be developed and pretested with intended audiences or their representatives (National Cancer Institute and National Institutes of Health, 2002). Several factors can influence message efficacy and need to be considered in message development. Effective messages are:

- *Concise and to the point.* There should be no more than two or three messages per audience; too many messages may be confusing.
- *Credible.* They are evidence based and delivered using reputable tools and spokespeople.
- *Relevant to the intended audience.* They need to address the, "So what?" and "What is in there for me?" questions.
- *Consistent* throughout the communication activities and materials as well as over reasonable periods of time.
- *Simple.* They should not use jargon or technical terms.
- *Easy to remember.* Whenever possible, they should include catchy language or evoke images that resonate with intended audiences.

If a health communication program has more than one message per audience, the most important message should be mentioned at the beginning and the end of each communication and activity. Communication trainers normally use a simple ten- to twelve-word exercise to prove this point. If a group hears a list of ten to twelve related words and then they are asked to recall the list in order, chances are that most people remember the first and the last word and fewer people remember the words in between.

Message retention is also another important topic in communication. Message frequency, vocal variety (in the case of interpersonal communications or live events), and a multichannel approach to message delivery, which creates the so-called resonance effect, can all have a positive influence on message retention by key audiences. A common model for information retention is Ebbinghaus's curve of forgetfulness, based on the work of Hermann Ebbinghaus, a pioneer researcher of the psychology of human memory who studied message retention in the late 1800s (Perlotto, 2005). Ebbinghaus's curve demonstrates that "75% of information learned in week one, and not reinforced afterwards, is forgotten in week two. 90% of it is gone in week three, and so on" (Nuzum, 2004, p. 23). This supports the importance of message repetition and consistency, a common practice in effective health communication. Finally, a cross-cultural approach to message development that incorporates audience feedback can improve the chances that messages will be understood, retained, remembered, and implemented.

Selecting Communication Channels and Vehicles

Communication channels refer to the path that is used to reach intended audiences with relevant information and communication. *Communication vehicles* are materials, events, activities, or other ways used to deliver a message through communication channels. This category (materials, events, and activities) is also called *tactics*. A variety of communication channels and vehicles are audience specific and should be researched as part of the situation analysis and audience profile (see Chapter Ten).

Selecting appropriate and culturally competent channels and vehicles is extremely important in making sure that specific health communication messages or programs stand out in the audience's mind. Formative research should set the stage for and guide the selection of adequate and audience-specific communication channels and tactics. At this point in program planning, health communicators should have a clear understanding of audience preferences for channels and vehicles that are most likely to be effective in carrying the message. Moreover, program planners should stay informed on new options and trends in the use of communication channels and vehicles, as well as trends in their acceptance. Media coverage, peer-reviewed studies, online resources, and informal conversations with colleagues and representatives of relevant health organizations are all excellent ways to stay informed. (Appendix A includes a menu of communication channels and venues as well as examples of related vehicles. See "Communication Channels and Venues and Examples of Related Vehicles.")

Some of the criteria that guide the selection of audience-specific channels and vehicles are message content and complexity, audience reach, cultural and issue appropriateness, and cost-effectiveness (see Chapter Ten). The efficacy of specific communication vehicles also depends on their ability to grab an audience's attention (Health Communication Unit, 2003b), which is often related to the graphic and visual appeal of the vehicles (as it applies, for example, to the case of printed materials, videos, or broadcast segments) as well as the credibility and appeal of the program's spokespeople. For example, the use of celebrities, well-known physicians, peer leaders, or other role models may enhance the ability of communication vehicles to capture audience attention.

Effective vehicles should also be easy to reproduce and disseminate (Health Communication Unit, 2003b). Since message consistency and repetition are key factors in message development and dissemination, communication vehicles should reflect and accommodate these attributes of effective messages and be selected to ensure widespread message circulation.

Ultimately, the final word on clear and culturally appropriate messages, channels, and vehicles is determined by the intended audiences or their representatives, who should be involved in the development and pre-testing of these essential communication tools. Box 12.2 features a case study by the Program for Appropriate Technology in Health (PATH) that highlights how the selection of culturally appropriate and research-based messages, channels, and vehicles can influence changes in knowledge, attitudes, and behavior.

Box 12.2

Community Theater in Benin: Taking the Show on the Road

Spacing births or limiting the number of children reduces risks to mothers' and children's health. Yet, women in northern Benin have an average of six children, and 20 percent of them have children dangerously close together—fewer than two years apart. Five women for every thousand children who are born die of complications from pregnancy and childbirth. Contraception prevents unwanted and high-risk pregnancies and can save women's health. Still, only seven percent of families used it.

PATH, an international non-profit organization, has found that theater is a highly effective way to address health issues—and even to begin to change social norms. In villages with no access to television or cinema, and in which many people cannot read, it's relatively easy to gather a large crowd—often up to 300 people—for a performance. The lack of competing media makes the play even more efficient at spreading ideas and getting youth, parents, and elders thinking and talking about the health topic.

PATH designed the play *Spacing Our Children* to instigate discussion and raise villagers' awareness of modern family planning methods. In the first year, more than 65,000 people in 232 villages in northern Benin attended the play, which was in the local Bariba language.

Constructing the Set

In preparation for the play, PATH assessed knowledge and attitudes of villagers. Research showed that men, who control the purse strings, often oppose their wives' wishes to use contraception. As a result, the play emphasized the husband's responsibility in family planning and the economic benefits of well-spaced, healthy children. The two central characters were brothers with divergent views and life situations. One had carefully nurtured his small family. The other had a large family that had fallen into poverty, disarray, and ill health.

An existing African theater troupe, Troupe Bio Guerra, helped PATH create and tour the production. Project staff trained the actors to administer oral surveys before and after the play and to hold short discussion groups with the villagers after each performance. The discussion groups, which were segmented by age and sex, were the first chance for villagers to freely exchange stories with their peers, ask questions, and clarify what they learned. The play's messages were reinforced by radio shows, printed materials, and home visits by community health volunteers.

Results

Data from surveys of villagers before and after the play indicated dramatic increases in the number of villagers who:

- Were able to describe several contraceptive methods.
- Said they would discuss contraception with their spouses.
- Said they planned to have no more than four children.

Use of contraceptives by married women increased from 7 percent prevalence in 2000 to 11 percent in 2002. The project continued to work to increase this percentage in 2003–2005. However, national statistics were not available at the time this book went to press.

Source: Program for Appropriate Technology in Health (PATH), "Community Theater in Benin: Taking the Show on the Road," unpublished case study, 2005b. Funding for this project was provided by the US Agency for International Development through an award to University Research Co., LLC. Copyright © 2005b, Program for Appropriate Technology in Health (PATH), www.path.org. All rights reserved. The material in this case study may be freely used for educational or noncommercial purposes, provided that the material is accompanied by this acknowledgment line. Used by permission.

PROGRAM LAUNCH

The tactical plan should also include a section that highlights the timing and the kinds of activities and materials that would be used to kick off the overall health communication program and introduce its messages and activities to intended audiences. The program launch plan should be determined by formative research findings. Launch messages should be the same as for the overall health communication program. Messages should be consistent until the evaluation and feedback phase is completed or has gathered significant results that point to the need for message refinement.

Launch activities and materials aim to spread the word about the program's core messages and implement its activities, potential services, and resources. A few practical suggestions can be used to develop effective launch plans:

- Make sure that program launch activities are audience, channel, and venue specific.
- Select communication channels and venues for maximum audience outreach. For example, if the audience is the general public, the mass media are effective channels, especially in developed countries. If the audience includes health care professionals, medical meetings and conferences as well as trade and medical publications are adequate venues or channels for launch activities. In the United States, a large percentage of patient groups and other kinds of audiences can also be reached at meetings and conferences. In the developing world, traditional communication channels (for example, theater) and venues (for example, the local village square or market) may be suitable for a crowd of community members to gather (see the example in Box 12.2).
- Be creative. Program launch activities should be designed to attract the attention of key audiences, as well as key **gatekeepers**, such as journalists, professional organizations, and other individuals and groups that may provide access to intended audiences.
- Whenever possible, use celebrities, community leaders, role models, or other well-known opinion leaders who are recognizable and respected by intended audiences to deliver

program messages at program launch as well as during follow-up activities.

- In all launch activities and materials, include information about where and how to obtain additional information or help about the specific health issue. For example, provide telephone numbers, Web site addresses, and the names and addresses of a specific community or health centers or organizations. Ask people to become involved in the solution of the health issue or specific program activities.

- Research activities, news, and events that may interfere with program launch and deflect attention from its core messages. Avoid scheduling launch activities in conjunction with other presentations or events that may be of greater interest to intended audiences.

Special considerations apply to each communication channel, venue, and country. For example, in designing communication activities and tools for a health communication program that relies on the mass media for its launch activities, communicators must consider different options for their cost-effectiveness and efficacy in achieving media coverage. In the United States, press conferences are an adequate communication vehicle for program launch only in the case of breakthrough news or the participation of extremely well-known political figures and celebrities. Competition for media coverage is fierce. Journalists do not attend press conferences or in-person media briefings unless there is breakthrough news or a celebrity is participating. If these criteria cannot be met, traditional media relations such a press release and a media alert announcing speaker availability for one-on-one telephone or in-person interviews may be a cost-effective option to secure coverage on the program's content and key messages.

PRETESTING OF COMMUNICATION CONCEPTS, MESSAGES, AND MATERIALS

Pretesting should be used to assess whether communication concepts, messages, and materials meet the needs of intended audiences and are culturally appropriate. As defined in Chapter Ten, pretesting is considered an essential part of formative research. As in other phases of formative research, if key audiences are multi-cultural, they should all be represented in pretesting studies.

Outside academia, many health organizations in the commercial and nonprofit sectors consider pretesting a costly and avoidable step in communication planning. This common misperception (National Cancer Institute and National Institutes of Health, 2002) may result in messages and materials that do not support key objectives and strategies and fail to meet audience preferences and needs. In fact, "pre-testing answers questions about whether your materials [and messages] are understandable, relevant, attention getting, attractive, credible, and acceptable to the target audiences" (Washington State Department of Health, 2000; Doak, Doak, and Root, 1995). In other words, pretesting helps assess if all the criteria that inspired the development of draft concepts, messages, and materials have been met.

Pretesting starts within the immediate environment of the health communication team. Colleagues, program partners, and professional acquaintances can provide initial feedback on draft concepts and materials. Actual pretesting with members of key audiences relies on traditional marketing and communication research methods (see Chapter Ten), including focus groups, one-on-one interviews, expert or gatekeeper interviews, and surveys. Methods should be selected according to materials format, size of target audiences, cost-effectiveness, and cultural preferences, to name a few criteria. Focus groups and one-on-one interviews tend to be most commonly used in pretesting.

Pretesting needs to be cost-effective. Obviously the cost should never exceed the cost of materials and activity development. A number of solutions can accommodate limited budgets and time concerns and make pretesting more affordable; examples are conducting stakeholder, expert, or gatekeeper interviews to validate program elements and adapting pretesting questions from previous studies.

In pretesting, "one of the most significant questions is: 'What can the readers do after reading this that they could not do before?'" (Matiella, Middleton, and Thaker, 1991; Washington State Department of Health, 2000). Messages and materials are more likely to encourage behavioral change when they are simple and do not try to accomplish too many objectives at the same time.

Finally, pretesting is important in assessing the overall level of comprehension of messages and materials by intended audiences. Low health literacy is a widespread issue in both developed and developing countries (see Chapter Two). A good communication practice is to write in simple and clear terms for low-literacy audiences. Communication messages and materials should be designed for the reading level of intended audiences, but "most materials should be written for no higher than sixth grade reading skills" (Washington State Department of Health, 2000). (For resources on readability tests as well as examples of pretesting questions, see Appendix A: "Health Literacy: Methods to Assess and Refine Readability Levels of Communication Messages and Materials" and "Pretesting Messages, Materials, and Activities: Sample Questions.")

PARTNERSHIP PLAN

Even if there are sufficient funds or human resources for program implementation, it is important to consider partnering with other organizations and stakeholders (see Chapter Eight). Partners can increase the possibilities for audience reach and add organizational skills competency in a specific area of program implementation, credibility, technical and medical expertise, spokespeople, or other knowledge and skills that can contribute to a program's outcome. Other authors and publications support the importance of sound partnership plans as a key component of health communication planning (National Cancer Institute and National Institutes of Health, 2002; O'Sullivan, Yonkler, Morgan, and Merritt, 2003).

The list of potential partners to be considered or involved in a health communication program is issue and audience specific. Potential partners range from public health departments to voluntary organizations, from state or national professional organizations to patient groups, from corporations and local businesses to universities and other educational institutions, from student associations to many other kinds of organizations and stakeholders. Partnerships, coalitions, and other forms of collaborative efforts often arise from good relationships, as well as organized constituency relations efforts. The partnership plan is the last step of these efforts.

In general, there are two phases in developing partnership plans. Phase One is part of the situation analysis and audience profile and continues with the evaluation of potential partners, as well as organizational constraints, barriers, and issues that should be considered prior to engaging a specific health organization or stakeholder. Often Phase One relies on preliminary conversations and meetings that may help potential partners assess the feasibility of a joint effort.

Phase Two is the actual partnership plan, which should be as comprehensive as possible in highlighting the time line of all activities for which partners are joining efforts, the roles and responsibilities of each partner, and other elements (see Table 12.2). This phase should be completed prior to the development of communication strategies, objectives, and activities. It is fundamental to the success of all partnerships to involve potential partners early in the planning process. The actual partnership plan is a way to formalize and record discussions and negotiations that should take place throughout the overall health communication process.

An important component of Phase Two is to develop and describe a standard process for ongoing communications among

TABLE 12.2. KEY ELEMENTS OF A PARTNERSHIP PLAN

Phase I	*Phase II*
• Program title	• Time line
• Overall program goal	• Steps to secure partnership
• Program objectives	• Names of partners' representatives
• Target audiences	
• Benefits of potential partnership	• Assigned roles and responsibilities
• Expected roles and responsibilities	• Frequency and methods of progress update and other routine communications among partners
• List of potential partners	
• Organizational constraints and policies	• Standard protocol for decision making
• Administrative issues	• Expected program outcomes and intermediate milestones
• Potential drawbacks	• Measures for program success

partners (for example, a weekly phone call or scheduled meetings). All partners must understand the process, as well as how decisions will be made, and agree to it. Mutual understanding and agreement on expected outcomes of the joint effort as well as related measurement parameters will keep the partnership healthy by minimizing misunderstandings, as well as setting and managing realistic expectations among all partners. Finally, partnership management requires funds and human resources that should be considered part of the overall program budget and resource allocation.

PROGRAM TIME LINE AND BUDGET ESTIMATE

The tactical plan should include a program time line and budget estimate for each communication activity as well as the development of all communication materials. Budget estimates should be based on actual price quotes from printers, graphic designers, creative or communication agencies, marketing research firms, consultants, and other potential vendors and include funds for contingency plans and potential crises. It is also helpful to include an estimate for each activity of the time spent by members of the communication team in the program. (Sample time lines and budget estimates are included in Appendix A. See examples 1 and 2 of "Program Time Line: Sample Forms" and "Budget Sample Form.")

THE EVALUATION PLAN: AN OVERVIEW OF MODELS AND TRENDS

This section provides an overview of evaluation trends, opinions, and topics in regard to their application to the field of health communication. It also includes a brief discussion of selected frameworks and models used to measure the outcomes of health communication programs.

Evaluation plans should be developed at the same time as tactical plans and should refer to the outcome (behavioral, social, or organizational) and communication objectives as well as the overall program goals that have been established. In fact, in designing messages, activities, and materials, health communicators should always ask themselves how these elements support the program's goals and objectives. Do they serve the communication strategy?

What were the theoretical assumptions and models that informed program planning, and how do they influence evaluation?

This kind of questioning lays the groundwork for a detailed evaluation plan in which all elements are interconnected and considered. In this phase, planners should also be aware of the limitations and costs of the evaluation process in health communication, so that all decisions made will enhance the objectivity of evaluation parameters.

The Language of Evaluation

Measurement, and specifically mathematics, is the language of science. We use mathematics and related measurement parameters in everyday life to evaluate quantity, size, shapes, relationships, and personal and professional achievements. Health communication incorporates mathematical principles in many evaluation models and metrics. Although this book does not go into the details of specific mathematical models used in health communication, we define common terms in evaluation:

- *Evaluation:* The science and process of appraising the value or worth of a health communication program.
- *Program assessment:* A general term used to indicate program-specific evaluation.
- *Metrics:* Another term for *evaluation parameters.* Metrics should be quantifiable and define a system of parameters to assess periodically specific program elements or outcomes (for example, process-related results or changes in attitude and behavior).
- *Return on investment (ROI):* The economic benefits that may derive from having invested funds in a program or activity. This parameter is commonly used in the commercial sector to assess the impact of marketing and communication activities on product sales. In public health, it may be useful in assessing the benefit of specific communication activities. For example, the return could be calculated in terms of the percentage of people who changed knowledge, attitude, or behavior or benefited from a specific change in social policies and practices.
- *Outcomes:* Changes in knowledge, comprehension, attitudes, skills, behavior, policies, or social norms as established by the program's outcome and communication objectives (Coffman, 2002; Freimuth, Cole, and Kirby, 2000). Outcomes are measured

in relation to the estimated influence the health communication program had on each change.

- *Impact:* Sometimes refers to outcome in relation to a specific change (for example, behavioral impact) influenced by a health communication program or activity. In other models (Coffman, 2002), it is used to refer only to the long-term change influenced by a program in relation to the overall program goal, such as changes in disease incidence, which are almost never directly used as an evaluation parameter in actual communication practice. This term may also have other connotations in different models (Bertrand, 2005).
- *Behavioral impact:* The specific behavioral results of a health communication program. This is measured in relation to specific behavioral indicators that have been established at the onset of planning.
- *Social change indicators:* Measures of changes in social interactions, norms, policies, and practices, as well as changes in the issues of concern (for example, poverty reduction, HIV/AIDS rates) (Rockefeller Foundation Communication and Social Change Network, 2001). Social indicators for evaluation are issue and audience specific. They are also a consequence of behavioral change within different groups and communities. For example, if the social indicator is the establishment of a new policy, this is the result of several changes in the beliefs and behavior of policymakers that led them to support and pass a new policy.

As these terms demonstrate, there are a variety of definitions as well as potential significances attributed to them. Using consistent theoretical assumptions and models throughout planning and evaluation helps ensure the accuracy of measurement and limits the possibility of misunderstandings on evaluation parameters and terminology.

WHY WE MEASURE

Measurement in health communication is needed for more than satisfying the requirements of donors, clients, partners, or other key stakeholders in a specific health issue or program. In fact, it is instrumental for a number of other reasons:

- Focusing health communication staff, partners, and key audiences on shared goals
- Clarifying the overall program goal and objectives
- Identifying and comparing effective health communication practices
- Improving service delivery (for example, in the case of health communication programs that also offer specific public or community services or communication consultants and agencies)
- Adjusting the program in progress by refining strategies and messages
- Assessing the overall cost-effectiveness of the program
- Determining program reproducibility and sustainability
- Communicating results to key program stakeholders and audiences
- Competing for economic and human resources

In short, measurement is a valuable tool not only in assessing results but also in achieving those results. Through different phases, research and evaluation methods help inform, focus, and refine health communication programs.

EVALUATION PHASES

Most authors (Bertrand, 2005; Freimuth, Cole, and Kirby, 2000) identify three phases in the evaluation of health communication interventions: formative, process, and summative. They correspond to the research phases described in Chapter Ten and are usually incorporated into effective health communication practices.

Formative Evaluation

Formative evaluation occurs prior to the program's development and implementation and includes the analysis of all research data gathered in the situation analysis, audience profile, and pretesting. Formative evaluation informs, guides, and helps validate all elements of a health communication program.

Process Evaluation

Process evaluation is used to compare key steps of the program's implementation with the original program plan. Frequently process evaluation is also used to measure expected results for specific

326 HEALTH COMMUNICATION: FROM THEORY TO PRACTICE

activities, materials, and messages. It refers to parameters such as audience reach, attendance, quality and tone of media coverage, message retention, ability to create alliances, community or stake-holder endorsement of the program's key concepts, circulation of materials, as well as short-term changes in knowledge and attitudes that may occur as a result of specific communication messages, ac-tivities, or materials. For example, some parameters for process evaluation of a communication workshop targeted to health care providers may include the number of attendees, message reten-tion, audience feedback on and level of interest in the workshop's content, and the provider's intention to translate new information into actual clinical practice. These parameters can be assessed with various tools, for example, a questionnaire or evaluation form dis-tributed to workshop attendees.

Process evaluation helps health communicators keep track of progress as well as the overall quality of the program's implemen-tation. This is directly connected to the need for spotless execution, which is one of the key characteristics of effective implementation and monitoring of the health communication process.

Finally, process evaluation should not be used to assess the di-rect impact of specific activities or materials on long-term changes in knowledge, attitudes, skills, or behavior. This direct cause-and-effect relationship is somewhat difficult to establish in health com-munication because "change does not often occur as a result of just one specific activity" (National Cancer Institute and National Institutes of Health, 2002, p. 45).

Summative Evaluation

Summative evaluation measures program efficacy in relation to the outcome and communication objectives initially established by the program. In other words, it "measures the extent to which change occurs. In health communication programs, the primary objective is usually a health-related behavior" (Bertrand, 2005). Behavioral im-pact is also the key evaluation parameter of WHO COMBI programs. (World Health Organization, 2003; see also Chapter Two).

In other cases, the primary objective may be a specific social or organizational outcome. However, since social or organizational outcomes are the result of gradual changes in behaviors by key stakeholders and members of different levels of society, behavioral impact is still a key measurement. Changes in behaviors that may lead to social or organizational change, as well as changes in other indicators (for example, knowledge, attitudes, or skills) that have been previously established by outcome or communication objectives, should also be measured as part of summative evaluation. In some mass media health communication campaigns, audience reach is part of summative evaluation. In this book, audience reach is considered one of the measurement parameters of process evaluation.

KEY FACTS AND TRENDS ON EVALUATING HEALTH COMMUNICATION OUTCOMES

Evaluation is considered an essential step by health communication theorists and practitioners. However, too many health organizations do not conduct evaluation of health communication programs. For example, "a study of 50 published nutrition and/or physical activity campaigns" showed that "fewer than 1/3 of the campaigns expressed goals in measurable terms" (Health Communication Unit, 2003c, pp. 28–29). Moreover, "goals were rarely formulated on the basis of data descriptive of target audiences" (p. 29). Similar findings also applied to audience segmentation, consumer research, and theory-based communication approaches. In fact, although the campaigns often mentioned social marketing as a planning framework, social marketing or behavioral theories concepts were rarely integrated into planning (Health Communication Unit, 2003b; Alcalay and Bell, 2000).

In practice, most health organizations are pressed for results and would like to conduct some kind of measurement and support the overall concept. Still, only rarely do annual budgets include funds for evaluating health communication programs or training human resources that in the long term may influence the cost-effectiveness of the evaluation process. When evaluation is part of program planning, this tends to be formative evaluation. Process and summative evaluation are often perceived as too costly or inconclusive. In addition, lack of adequate training and understanding of evaluation tools and methods may result in a series of barriers to evaluation that may be perceived as insurmountable.

Evaluation has several drawbacks (Table 12.3), some of which are more difficult to overcome than others. Recognizing evaluation

TABLE 12.3. DRAWBACKS OF EVALUATION

- Cost
- Time
- Chance of measuring the wrong variables and indicators
- Questionable accuracy for programs with limited scope, reach, and duration
- Potential bias in evaluation method or tool
- Hard to do if not planned ahead
- Results that may be affected by independent influences on key audiences and program's outcomes

---

barriers and drawbacks helps set realistic expectations among team members, partners, donors, clients, and key stakeholders about the program's results and the overall evaluation process.

A major limitation in the evaluation of health communication programs is related to the complexity of human behavior. Health communication efforts attempt to achieve behavioral or social change. However, since all people are influenced by multiple sources of information as well as personal and professional events, it may be difficult to make a direct connection between the actual health communication program (or, even more difficult, specific communication activities) and the behavioral or social outcome. It is important to remember that "communication programs generally occur in a real-world setting, where there are many other influences on the intended audiences. [In many cases], it can be impossible to isolate the effect of a particular communication activity, or even the effect of a communication program on a specific intended audience" (National Cancer Institute and National Institutes of Health, 2002, p. 45).

Say that a woman who is forty-five years old suddenly decides to change her previous behavior and see her physician for annual breast cancer screenings. It may be challenging to define with certainty to which degree her behavior has been influenced by an ongoing health communication program on this topic or that her best friend was just diagnosed with advanced breast cancer at age forty-three. Similarly, when a new law is passed to ban workplace discrimination of people who suffer from a specific medical condition, it may be difficult to ascertain which factors have weighed more in the legislators' decision: ongoing mass media and advocacy efforts, direct experiences of loved ones, professional observations, personal ambition, or something else. In both examples, chances are that all of these factors influenced the outcome. Being aware of the challenges of evaluation is fundamental to the design of adequate evaluation plans, which should include a combination of quantifiable parameters and qualitative analyses and sometimes rely on intermediate steps and other quantifiable measures to assess progress- and program-related results.

In spite of potential limitations, ignoring this fundamental step of health communication planning may harm the overall perception of the field's efficacy and contribution to health care issues, as well as the ability to secure funds and resources for subsequent health communication programs. Most important, it will leave health communicators without adequate instruments to evaluate the significance of their efforts.

Health organizations should find the optimal balance of evaluation, cost, and other factors that are related to measurement. This balance may vary from organization to organization. "Small nongovernmental organizations (NGOs) with limited resources may opt to perform only one of these types of evaluation [formative, process, or summative], whereas a major communication program with national scope would be remiss to exclude any of them" (Bertrand, 2005).

Still, in defining evaluation parameters, it is important to set realistic expectations. For example, impact measurement (if impact is defined as the effect of the program on the overall program goal, such as changes in disease incidence or mortality) may be difficult and take a long time to assess. Outcome evaluation such as behavioral impact or changes in knowledge, attitudes, and skills may include more realistic parameters. Therefore, it is important to select indicators that are strongly linked to the achievement of the overall program goal. This is already a common practice in many fields. For example, "increased immunization levels predict decreased child mortality. Increasing numbers of girls in school is often cited as a predictor of economic progress" (Rockefeller Foundation Communication and Social Change Network, 2001).

Since health communication never stops being a cycle, this brings us back to several of the initial questions of communication planning. What does the program want people to do? Do you want them to immunize their children? Send their girls to school and be proud of them? What are the intermediate steps to encourage these behaviors, and were they met by the program? Was the program well executed in relation to activities that supported intermediate objectives? Did the program reach the number of people originally estimated? Can you quantify the actual behavioral impact of the program?

In health communication, behavioral change at different levels of society is the ideal standard measurement. However, evaluation needs to set realistic parameters that vary from program to program and case to case. In doing so, it is important to take into account that the complexity of evaluation increases with the complexity of the parameter being measured (Freimuth, Cole, and Kirby, 2000). Key evaluation parameters need to be mutually agreed on with all program partners, team members, donors, clients, or other key stakeholders.

Finally, participatory evaluation, which complements and includes the practice of participatory research (described in Chapter Six), has emerged as an alternative evaluation approach (Bertrand, 2005) versus more traditional evaluation methodologies that normally rely on expert evaluation. In participatory evaluation, key audiences or their representatives lead or are part of the evaluation team. They contribute to the design of the evaluation plan and the analysis of key results as well as overall feedback. This approach is part of the participatory model of communication planning (see Chapter Nine).

The appropriate level of participation by key audiences, as well as the degree of expert input and involvement, should be influenced by several factors, including cultural preferences and the specific characteristics of the health issue, audience, or country. In general, even with more traditional approaches, it should be common practice of effective health communication to establish and analyze measurement parameters with representatives of intended audiences and program partners. This is frequently accomplished by involving or soliciting the opinion of professional organizations, patient groups, and other constituency groups that attend or represent intended audiences. Finally, it is important to be aware that "participatory evaluation may not meet the methodical rigor of the scientific community to measure effectiveness" (Bertrand, 2005). Therefore, the participation of health communication practitioners and other experts may be critical to preserve such rigor.

Quantitative and Qualitative Measurements

Measurement for each of the three types of evaluation uses traditional marketing and communication research methodologies. Some of them are described in Chapter Ten as part of the formative research phase that is needed to complete the situation analysis and audience profile.

For complex analyses, it is likely that health organizations and their audiences may require the help of evaluation experts. For example, assessing changes in attitudes and behaviors requires intensive efforts in a specific geographical area and period of time. Pre- and postintervention studies are needed to assess the baseline (in terms of frequent health behaviors or attitudes) as well as the impact of the communication program on such parameters. Since these studies require a significant financial commitment and specific skills, health organizations often turn to evaluation experts or health communication agencies. One word of caution is needed in this regard: behavioral change occurs only over time. Only long-term efforts can generate sustainable behavioral results. Therefore, measuring too soon after the program launch may show some modest changes but will not guarantee that these changes can be sustained over time. Ideally, measurement should take place at different intervals using tracking surveys or other methodologies described in Chapter Ten. If this is not possible, summative evaluation efforts should take place later in program implementation.

In general, measurement of health communication programs relies on qualitative and quantitative methods.

Qualitative Methods

- In-depth interviews of members of intended audiences, program participants, or other key stakeholders before and after the program
- Focus groups
- Completion of evaluation forms after specific activities (for process evaluation only)

- Evidence of endorsement, such as letters of support or actual program participation from key influentials (for formative and process evaluation only)
- Panel studies, that is, pre- and postintervention studies, which involve the same panel of key stakeholders or representatives of intended audiences

Quantitative Methods

- Pre- and postsurveys—most commonly telephone surveys (see Chapter Ten)
- Tracking surveys, which collect evaluation data at different time intervals
- Control and intervention groups in which groups are either randomized or selected in a way that one group will be exposed to the health communication intervention and the other will not

Most of these methods carry several limitations, such as in the case of control and intervention groups in which other differences may exist and have an impact on evaluation data (National Cancer Institute and National Institutes of Health, 2002).

The selection of specific measurement methods depends on several factors, including budget, purpose of the evaluation, audience characteristics, type of health organization, health issue–related factors, donor or client requirements as well as the theoretical assumptions or planning framework of the health communication program. For example, the theory of reasoned action (see Chapter Two) "is one of the most frequently used in campaign evaluation" (Coffman, 2002, p. 18). Logic models (see Chapter Two) are also increasingly used in the evaluation of health communication programs to organize and connect different program components with the program's outcomes (Coffman, 2002; University of Wisconsin, 2005).

ESTABLISHING EVALUATION PARAMETERS

Effective health communication programs include mutually agreed-on evaluation terms (Cole and others, 1995) and parameters. This is a common procedure in participatory evaluation and is important to focus everyone's efforts on common goals as well as to minimize the possibility for misunderstanding and unrealistic expectations about the potential program's outcomes. As Sarriot (2002) describes, "There can be benefits, particularly improved collective learning in agreeing on shared and critical dimensions of evaluation." This includes "the contextual definition and selection of indicators of progress" (p. 91). This general principle applies to all forms of evaluation, and more specifically to process and summative evaluation.

For process evaluation, the commercial sector as well as many health communication agencies have been using models that rely on mutually agreed-on parameters. Although this method may take different empirical formats, the overall premise is to set specific qualitative and quantitative parameters for each activity or material of a health communication program. Data collection methods are also included for each parameter. These criteria are discussed and agreed on by the program's sponsor, clients, health communication agencies, and all other key stakeholders involved in program planning. A written report is normally provided on the basis of the parameters previously agreed. (See Appendix A for a sample chart: "Process Evaluation: Establishing Mutually Agreed Parameters.")

Although this method is currently being used primarily for process evaluation, but also including intermediate steps to change, the overall principle of establishing mutually agreed parameters is important to all forms and phases of evaluation, even when conducted with different methods. Health communication is an integrated approach that frequently involves different stakeholders and uses multiple approaches. Potential evaluation parameters should reflect the diversity of approaches and stakeholders who may contribute to specific health programs and issues. Unifying these parameters under a mutually agreed-on principle helps meet the expectations that have been set with donors, partners, team members, clients, and intended audiences.

KEY CONCEPTS

Tactical Plan
- The tactical plan encompasses the communication messages, channels, and vehicles (materials and activities) that are designed to serve core communication strategies.

- All elements of the tactical plan are informed and guided by research findings of the situation analysis and audience profile. Messages, channels, and activities are audience specific and should be developed and tested with the input and participation of intended audiences. When multiple tactics can serve the same communication strategies and objectives, it is important to rank and prioritize them on the basis of several parameters that are discussed in this chapter (for example, message complexity, audience reach, cost-effectiveness).

Evaluation Plan

- The evaluation of health communication programs is a much debated and evolving topic.
- Evaluation starts with program planning and is an integral part of the overall health communication cycle. Outcomes objectives should be set at the onset of program planning. The evaluation plan should be developed at the same time as the tactical plan and include evaluation parameters and methods.
- In health communication, key evaluation parameters are behavioral and social outcomes. Behavioral impact is considered a primary parameter in the assessment of health communication programs.
- Evaluation of health communication programs presents several limitations and challenges, but should not prevent program planners from considering it as an essential step of effective health communication programs.
- Although evaluation should always be part of health communication, health organizations and programs may opt for different evaluation plans that represent diverse combinations of evaluation needs, costs, and other audience- or issue-specific factors.
- Given the variety of evaluation parameters and models, establishing mutually agreed measurement parameters with key program stakeholders, team members, partners, and donors is the latest wisdom in the evaluation of health communication programs. This helps focus everyone's efforts on common goals and limits the possibility for misunderstandings and unrealistic expectations about potential program outcomes.

- Other key trends in the evaluation of health communication programs are participatory evaluation and the use of consistent models. Maintaining the same theoretical assumptions and planning framework throughout the health communication cycle may be helpful in preserving the accuracy of program evaluation.

FOR DISCUSSION AND PRACTICE

1. Discuss the significance, pros and cons, and implications of current trends and core principles in the evaluation of health communication programs as described in this chapter (for example, participatory evaluation, mutually agreed-on parameters). Whenever possible, use practical examples or observations to support your discussion points.
2. Describe the key steps you would take to evaluate the cost-effectiveness of two different tactics you are proposing to influence the behavior of young adults and therefore to reduce the use of drugs and alcohol consumption in this age group (for example, a mass media campaign targeted to consumer media and college newspapers and publications versus a peer-to-peer series of interactive workshops at local colleges and universities). Focus on only cost-effectiveness parameters (for example, financial cost, human resources, time), and assume that both tactics have been validated by members of intended audiences in terms of audience suitability and cultural competence.
3. If you completed questions 2 and 3 of the "For Discussion and Practice" section of Chapter Eleven, think of examples of core communication concepts, messages, channels, and tactics to address the issue of skin cancer prevention among Luciana and her peers.
4. Think of recent health communication materials (print or online) you may have seen. Describe their content, key messages, graphic appearance, and intended audiences. Identify core questions of a potential focus group to pretest these materials with representatives of intended audiences.

CHAPTER THIRTEEN

IMPLEMENTING, MONITORING, AND EVALUATING A HEALTH COMMUNICATION PROGRAM

IN THIS CHAPTER

- Planning a Successful Program Implementation
- Monitoring: An Essential Element of Program Implementation and Evaluation
- Evaluation Report
- Key Concepts
- For Discussion and Practice

Finally, the communication program has been funded and is ready to be launched. All the building blocks in the health communication plan appear to be cohesive and have a strong evidence-based foundation. There are many great expectations about the program's implementation and potential outcomes. The plan seems to be stable and strong. Yet even sturdy and balanced plans may falter or even fail in the absence of adequate maintenance or in the case of unforeseen difficulties. Clearly it is important to maintain the health communication plan through management and monitoring of activities that ensure a spotless execution of all the plan elements.

Implementing a health communication plan is similar to implementing any other type of plan. It is a combination of managing economic and human resources with monitoring program activities and audience feedback (National Cancer Institute and National Institutes of Health, 2002) as well as measurement parameters and all the external factors and trends that can influence the program's potential outcomes. It requires hard work, perseverance, problem-solving skills, and a team-oriented mind-set. The implementation of the evaluation plan is part of this process.

This chapter focuses on the implementation and evaluation phases of the health communication cycle. It provides practical guidance on some of the considerations that go into executing a health communication program. It also highlights some resources on monitoring and guides readers on how to share and use evaluation data for program assessment and refinement.

PLANNING A SUCCESSFUL PROGRAM IMPLEMENTATION

Planning for a spotless program execution entails several steps that are related to establishing and maintaining standard practices for the management of funds, human resources, specific activities (for example, monitoring and data collection), and internal communications among all members of the extended health communication team. It is also related to anticipating and preparing for potential issues that may arise during program implementation and affect expected outcomes. A team-oriented mind-set, as well as attention to detail, is critical to the implementation of all practices and steps described in this section.

HUMAN RESOURCE ALLOCATION AND BUDGET MONITORING

The tactical plan should include a detailed budget estimate as well as a description of the roles and responsibilities of specific team members and partners. This should ideally incorporate an approximate evaluation of the time each team member is committing to the program. Tactical plans should also identify the program's management team. However, sometimes programs get funded long after they were planned and call for a reassessment of these elements.

The first step in program implementation is to make sure that no changes in the original program's team are necessary in the light of recent career moves, loss of interest in the project, or conflicting and unexpected priorities. Program staff substitutions should be strategic and look at the specific skills and contribution the original team member or partner was bringing to the program. Perhaps a patient group that is well known for its research and advocacy work in the field of mental illness decides to withdraw from a specific health communication program for a variety of reasons. In this case, program planners should identify another organization with similar reputation, skills, interests, expertise, and constituencies in the same disease area. In other words, human resources are allocated to a program on the basis of their skills and experience. The same principle should apply to potential substitutions or integration of partners and staff.

Finally, the program's team should include specific individuals who are responsible for budget monitoring, that is, making sure that all program tactics are implemented within the budget that has been estimated and allocated for each of them. This is normally the responsibility of the management team with the help of one or two additional team members. Budget reports, which includes itemized expenditures and remaining amounts, may be a useful tool to record and share budget status.

ESTABLISHING MONITORING TEAMS

Monitoring is an essential function in program implementation and is related primarily to four areas: (1) program activities and the related process; (2) audience and stakeholders' ongoing feedback on the program's elements, overall content, and messages; (3) news and trends about the specific disease areas, key policies, audiences, and other relevant facts and events; and (4) the collection and analysis of evaluation data. Different skills and collection methods are required for each of these areas. For example, monitoring program activities, which is part of process evaluation and serves to assess whether program implementation occurs within the parameters envisioned by the program plan, is frequently a management function. However, it also involves the participation of all team members dedicated to a specific activity. If a team member has strong relationships with, for example, the HIV patient and advocacy community, he or she is the best candidate to secure ongoing reactions to and feedback on the program's key elements and contents from this audience. Finally, evaluation data should be monitored and collected on the basis of the indicators and methods described in the evaluation plan. Early in program implementation, specific team members should be assigned to each of these areas of monitoring.

TECHNICAL SUPPORT AND ADVISORY GROUPS

If the program has the funds and the need to hire a specialized health communication, marketing research, or creative agency, chances are that these agencies have also been involved in program planning. In fact, involving agencies and consultants early in the process, and in any case not later than during the strategy development phase, is good practice in health communication and helps maximize the strategic contribution and dedication of all consultants.

Early in program implementation, all agencies that have participated in program planning should be invited to a team meeting to define the implementation process, confirm the program's time line, and develop a checklist of all logistics related to the execution of program activities. Finally, it is possible that additional consultants (for example, printers or mailing services) may need to be interviewed and hired in this phase of the program. Obviously, funds for hiring other consultants that are not part of the strategic communication process should have been included in the original budget estimate.

If specific needs arise or preliminary conversations with key stakeholders have confirmed the importance of a specific advisory group that could lend technical support to the program, these groups should be established and involved as early as possible. Advisory groups can serve multiple functions. For example, the Macy Initiative, a collaborative effort to enhance physician communication skills between the University of Massachusetts Medical School and the schools of medicine of New York University and Case Western Reserve University, have established an advisory group of faculty involved with the teaching and curriculum planning for the initiative

(UMass Medical School, 2006). In Zambia, a youth advisory group "consisting of 35–40 young people from 11 youth organizations" advised the program's design team and developed communication objectives and abstinence messages for the HEART (Helping Each Other Act Responsibly Together) program, an HIV/AIDS initiative targeted to young adults (Health Communication Partnership, 2004).

Advisory groups and consultants should also be involved in program implementation. In fact, they can be a valuable source of expertise and, in some cases, can function as a link with an intended audience to continue securing audience feedback on all program elements.

PROCESS DEFINITION

The process needed for program implementation should be defined in the first few team meetings of this phase. This should include a plan of all logistics—for example, who will be responsible for contacts with key stakeholders, the review process of key communication materials and related time lines, travel arrangements for workshops or other in-person communication activities, and lists of potential vendors and consultants that will be used for data collection for the evaluation report. Roles and responsibilities should be clear to each team member, who should also be aware of activity and logistic-specific deadlines. A specific time line should be developed for each activity and materials and be updated with new information and progress at periodic time intervals established by the team.

The implementation process should identify exact dates for team meetings and other kinds of in-person, telephone, or online communications that will be used for progress reporting, problem solving, or brainstorming with partners and team members.

ISSUES MANAGEMENT

Several chapters in this book have discussed issue management in the context of specific health communication areas (for example, public relations and constituency relations). However, issues management and the concept of preparedness that inspire this practice apply to the entire health communication cycle and have particular relevance in program implementation.

The issues that may arise in program implementation range from logistical issues (for example, the flight of a key speaker for a workshop is cancelled and the speaker is not able to attend the event; the materials intended for distribution at a local conference do not arrive on time) to more substantial and critical issues (for example, an article in a major newspaper attacks some of the fundamental premises of the program's approach; one of the key program partners withdraws a few days before the program's launch). It is important that the communication team is prepared to handle potential issues, is clear about the decision-making process that would be used in facing them (in other words, who should be involved or would have the final say on how the issue is addressed), and knows who is ultimately responsible to handle them.

As part of the process of considering potential issues and ways to address them, key program spokespeople should be identified to address issues that involve the mass media or other public forums, as well as for communications with key partners and stakeholders in case of potential crises.

MONITORING: AN ESSENTIAL ELEMENT OF PROGRAM IMPLEMENTATION AND EVALUATION

Monitoring primarily addresses four areas:

- News and trends on the disease area or health issue, intended audiences, and policies
- Ongoing feedback by key audience and stakeholders on program content or vehicles
- Process indicators for all program activities and materials
- Collection of summative evaluation data

Information from these four areas contributes to the program's implementation, potential success, and refinement in different ways. For example, monitoring of news and trends on the disease area or health issue, as well as related policies and audiences, may provide the health communication team with an opportunity to react promptly to emerging audience needs, new scientific data, health products, or services that need to be considered by or incorporated in the program. Monitoring news and trends can also help address and manage criticisms from other constituency groups or develop new alliances by being informed on current thinking and key players in a specific health care field.

Evaluation data should be monitored and collected in relation to the process indicators and the outcome parameters established by the evaluation plan. Since monitoring has different purposes, some of the methods to collect, share, and use data may be different, and others may overlap. For example, monitoring news and trends relies primarily on the review of relevant media coverage and online and peer-reviewed publications. Ongoing contacts and conversations with key opinion leaders and stakeholders in a specific health care field can point to emerging trends and information, which are used to secure ongoing audience and stakeholder feedback and reactions to program implementation, content, core messages, and materials.

In collecting data that will be used for process or summative evaluation, the health communication team should refer to the indicators and methods described in the original evaluation plan. Process evaluation data can be collected at different times in program implementation and for each specific activity (see Chapter Twelve). They can also be used to adjust the content or the process of specific communication vehicles and channels. For example, if the public relations component of a health communication program does not secure the expected media coverage (which should be quantified in terms of number of impressions or relevant articles on major publications; see Chapter Six), the team may need to consider different story angles or timing for the release of additional news about the program. Similarly, if a physician workshop does not attract the estimated number of attendees, several factors (including the workshop's venue, the appeal of key speakers, the event's timing, or the extent of publicity efforts to announce the workshop) should be evaluated and reconsidered in preparation for the next event. Specific process indicators (for example, audience reach, level of audience satisfaction with the logistics and appeal of a specific activity, message retention) should be included as part of the evaluation plan (see Chapter Twelve).

In-depth interviews, postevent questionnaires, surveys, focus groups, observation, and other methods described in Chapters Ten and Twelve are used to monitor and track summative evaluation data and process indicators. Sometimes specific services can be used to track process indicators such as audience reach. For example, in the United States, the reach of mass media campaigns that aim at securing television coverage can be assessed using the Nielsen Station Index, a TV audience service that generates data on the number of people or households who are watching a specific program in a given television market (geographical area). Also, several commercial companies provide press clipping services, which include the retrieval of all media articles on specific search terms as well as transcripts or broadcast clips of radio and television programs. Press clips can be helpful in analyzing the frequency and the tone with which the health communication program messages are covered by the media as well as new trends and facts on the specific health issue.

All monitoring data should be collected and discussed with key team members, partners, and stakeholders in the health communication program. This is usually accomplished through periodic reports and presentations that also provide a strategic analysis of the data being collected and their implications for the health communication program. The input and feedback of all recipients of these reports will contribute to the analysis of the data in relation to potential adjustments the program needs to make. The current tendency in health communication is to maximize participation of key stakeholders, team members, and audience representatives in the monitoring and analysis of all data collected during program implementation (Health Communication Partnership, 2003; Exchange, 2001). Table 13.1 gives examples of methods for the collection and reporting of different kinds of monitoring data.

EVALUATION REPORT

The evaluation report should include a detailed analysis of all data collected for process and summative evaluation in relation to the original evaluation plan, methods, and indicators. The evaluation framework as well as its theoretical basis should be consistent throughout the entire program. Program progress and summative evaluation reports should be addressed in different sections of the final evaluation report.

TABLE 13.1. EXAMPLES OF AREAS OF MONITORING WITH
RELATED DATA COLLECTION AND REPORTING METHODS

Monitoring	Data-Collection Methods	Reporting
News and Trends	Literature review (including peer-reviewed and trade publications, organizational newsletters, annual reports, and so on)	Periodic media-analysis reports (at least monthly)
	Review and analysis of mass media coverage	Presentation and discussion at team meetings
	Internet searches	E-mail summaries to all key program stakeholders and team members
	Informal conversations and meetings with key stakeholders, health organizations, colleagues, audience representatives, and others	
Ongoing Audience and Stakeholder Feedback	Informal conversations and meetings (see above)	Presentation and discussion at team meetings
	Activity-specific methods that are already part of process monitoring	E-mail summaries
		Can be incorporated in monthly media analysis reports
Process Indicators	Activity- or material-specific methods	
	Events	
	• Post-event questionnaires for audience feedback	Event evaluation summary for distribution to team members and program stakeholders*

TABLE 13.1. EXAMPLES OF AREAS OF MONITORING WITH
RELATED DATA COLLECTION AND REPORTING METHODS, CONT'D.

Monitoring	Data-Collection Methods	Reporting
	Mass-media campaigns	
	• Collection of media clips generated by the program to analyze message tone and frequency, audience reach, and so on	Monthly media coverage reports*
	• Use of specific services (Nielson Index Rating) for audience reach of television coverage	
	Online activities and materials	
	• Number of hits on home page or specific content pages of a program-related Web site (to assess Internet traffic)	Monthly reports*
	All	
	• Pre- and postactivity in-depth interviews with audience representatives, key stakeholders, and others	Can be incorporated as part of reports listed above*

---

*These reports can be summarized in a preliminary process report and should be included as part of the final evaluation report.

TABLE 13.1. EXAMPLES OF AREAS OF MONITORING WITH
RELATED DATA COLLECTION AND REPORTING METHODS, CONT'D.

Monitoring	Data-Collection Methods	Reporting
Summative Evaluation Data (in relation to the original evaluation plan and indicators)	Collection methods, including focus groups, in-depth interviews, panel studies, and surveys, vary and should reflect the evaluation plan.	Final evaluation report to be developed, shared, and discussed with all team members, key program stakeholders, and representatives of key audiences. Should include process and summative evaluation as well as data collected for other areas and phases of monitoring. Can be presented at professional conferences as well as distributed and publicized using different communication channels.

Evaluating can be a "moving target" (Kennedy and Abbatangelo, 2005, p. 13), at least in reference to process evaluation. Although potential revisions of the original evaluation plan should be always minimized, it is possible that some program corrections will be needed in response to specific process evaluation data (Kennedy and Abbatangelo, 2005). Such revisions are justified primarily by emerging audience needs or specific observations and data collected during program implementation.

Take the example of a town hall meeting, which included the participation of breast cancer prevention organizations and patient groups as well as breast cancer survivors. At the end of the town hall meeting, all participants were asked to complete an evaluation questionnaire about the quality, duration, content, venue, and format of the event. If participants' responses suggest that additional topics should be included or that the duration or venue of the town hall meeting may limit attendance, these points should be addressed in preparation for the next event. If adequately designed, evaluation models can accommodate changes in process indicators or in the program's materials and procedures (Kennedy and Abbatangelo, 2005).

Outcome indicators (for example, behavioral change) for summative evaluation should be consistent throughout the program. Changes in outcome indicators may complicate the overall evaluation process and compromise the accuracy of all analyses of the potential impact of the program on expected outcomes.

Evaluation reports should be customized to meet the program and audience needs. Special considerations should be given to the potential limitations of evaluation data (for example, sample size, limits of self-reported frequency of performing a recommended behavior, length of time dedicated to the evaluation process, organizational constraints), which should be described and considered as part of the report. In general, an evaluation report should (National Cancer Institute and National Institutes of Health, 2002; Office of Adolescent Pregnancy Programs, 2006):

- Refer to the key theoretical assumptions and models that have influenced the design of the health communication program as well as the evaluation plan
- Provide an overview of the health communication program
- Restate expected program outcomes
- Highlight formal research objectives in relation to expected outcomes
- Describe methods for data collection and analysis, as well as the composition of the evaluation and monitoring teams
- Provide a progress report in relation to process indicators and each program activity or material
- Report key evaluation findings and their implications for current or future programs in relation to expected outcomes and other evaluation indicators
- Highlight key lessons learned and future directions

- Discuss barriers to the achievement of expected outcomes and highlight how they can be minimized or eliminated in the future

Program evaluation serves multiple purposes. In fact, not only do evaluation data provide information on the efficacy and impact of a program on expected outcomes, but also define program refinement as well as future programs in the same health field (National Cancer Institute and National Institutes of Health, 2002). An example of a multifaceted health communication program was developed and implemented by the Hamilton-Wentworth Drug and Alcohol Awareness Committee in collaboration with the Health Communication Unit (2004) of the University of Toronto. The program aimed at "reducing the number of children born with Fetal Alcohol Spectrum Disorder" in Hamilton, Ontario, Canada. Summative evaluation showed that there was "still uncertainty among women of reproductive age regarding a safe level of alcohol consumption during pregnancy." These data and other postevaluation analyses contributed to the definition of many of the elements of the second phase of the campaign.

Because of their relevance to program reassessment and refinement, evaluation reports should be shared with as many key stakeholders as possible. These include members of key audiences, opinion leaders, partners, and professional organizations. Ideally, all of these stakeholders should participate in the evaluation design, data collection and analysis, and compilation of the final report. While most of the time evaluation reports rely on the expertise of communication consultants, agencies, or centers, securing the involvement of key stakeholders and members of the program's audiences may add to the accuracy and relevance of the evaluation analysis. As for other components of program planning, this is in line with the participatory model of communication planning (see Chapter Nine). Incentives for participation should be identified for all key stakeholders (Exchange, 2001) and audiences and may include organizational visibility, the ability of being part of a major health change at the community level, personal experiences about a specific disease or health issue, peer pressure, and access to special services. These incentives also apply to other areas of program planning and implementation.

Finally, evaluation reports should be used to showcase program results whenever possible, as well as the overall contribution of health communication to the solution of health issues. Evaluation reports should be presented at professional conferences and meetings, posted on relevant Web sites, distributed through direct mail and online summaries, and publicized through the mass media and all appropriate channels.

KEY CONCEPTS

Program Implementation

- The implementation of a health communication program is a combination of human resources and funds management with monitoring program activities and impact. It requires hard work, perseverance, and problem-solving skills.
- A spotless execution is a key attribute of the implementation and monitoring phase of the health communication cycle. Even well-designed programs can fail to achieve expected results if they are not adequately implemented.
- Several actions contribute to effective program implementation as well as process definition for all program's components.

Monitoring

- Monitoring, an essential component of program implementation, refers to the collection and analysis of data and information relevant to the implementation, evaluation, and potential success of the health communication program.
- Monitoring applies primarily to four areas:
  - News and trends on the disease area or health issue, intended audiences, and relevant policies
  - Ongoing feedback by key audiences and stakeholders on program content or vehicles
  - Process indicators for all program activities and materials
  - Collection of summative evaluation data
- Methods for data collection may vary and sometimes overlap for the different areas of monitoring.

Evaluation Report

- The evaluation report summarizes process and summative evaluation findings in relation to the original evaluation plan, methods, and indicators.
- An evaluation report includes a summary description of these elements:
  - Key theoretical assumptions and models used in program and evaluation design
  - Expected program outcomes
  - Formal research objectives in relation to expected outcomes
  - Methods for data collection and analysis as well as the composition of the evaluation team
  - Progress report in relation to process indicators and specific activities and materials
  - Key evaluation findings and their implications for current or future programs
  - Key lessons learned and future directions
  - Existing barriers to expected outcomes and potential approaches to overcome them
- Evaluation reports (as well as the overall evaluation process) are used not only to assess program results but also to inform program refinement and future programs. For this reason, participation of all key program stakeholders should be maximized in developing the evaluation report.
- Evaluation reports should be shared with all team members, partners, key audiences, and other key stakeholders. Publicity of the report's key findings should be used to showcase program results as well as the overall contribution of health communication to the health care field.

FOR DISCUSSION AND PRACTICE

1. Your communication team is establishing process indicators for a new Web site that focuses on increasing awareness of a vaccine-preventable childhood disease among parents and health care providers. The Web site includes sections for health care providers and parents (in both English and Spanish); a time line on the history of the disease; a section that highlights

testimonials of parents whose children suffered or died from the disease; a contact e-mail to submit case studies, testimonials, questions, or suggestions for professionals and parents; a media section with recent press releases, facts, and statistics on the disease; a list of available speakers or experts to address media questions; and a resources section with links to other organizations that work in this disease area and relevant publications. Identify examples of process indicators that could be established to evaluate the potential success of this Web site, and discuss which methods you would use to monitor them.

2. After reviewing the evaluation report section of this chapter, think of the outline of a potential evaluation report that is related to a health communication case study or program of which you are aware. List the categories your report should include.

3. What are some of the similarities or differences of program implementation in health communication when compared to program implementation in other health care or public health fields of which you are aware? How do some of the suggestions and practical examples in this chapter relate to your professional experience (if at all)?

Appendix A: Examples of Worksheets and Resources on Health Communication Planning

Topics in this resource are organized within two main categories: (1) examples of planning worksheets and sample questions and (2) online resources. Many of these resources refer to multiple chapters in the text.

Examples of Planning Worksheets and Sample Questions

A1: Situation Analysis and Audience Profile Worksheet: Sample Questions and Topics

This list of questions and topics is not all inclusive and may not apply to all health issues. Therefore, it should be used only as an example.

Category	Key Topics and Questions
Condition or health issue	Description
	Prevalence/incidence
	Trends (for example, decreasing, staying the same, increasing)
	Degree of severity in different groups
	Risk factors (for example, socioeconomic conditions, age, specific ethnic groups, regions, marital status, lifestyle, other conditions)

Category	*Key Topics and Questions*
	Overview of treatment or prevention methods
	Most common causes and symptoms
	Comorbidities (if relevant)
	Other relevant issues
Key audiences	Identify key primary and secondary audiences of the health communication program
	State reasons for audience selection (for example, in the case of multiple secondary audiences that cannot all be addressed by the program because of economic or other limitations)
Social, political, and other external influences	Predominant health beliefs, attitudes, and behaviors
	Social norms
	Existing laws and regulations
	Trends and other factors that may influence the program's ability to address the health issue (for example, social, economic, demographic, political)
	Other relevant issues or topics
Audience profile and segmentation	Key characteristics of primary and secondary audiences, including health beliefs, attitudes and behaviors, lifestyle issues, demographics, socioeconomic conditions, geographical factors
	Audience segments (by behavioral stage and other common characteristics)
	Professional organizations, patient support groups, other kinds of groups or associations

Category	*Key Topics and Questions*
	that already work on this health issue or represent or attend key audiences
	Key opinion leaders (for example, prominent physicians, health care providers, patients, celebrities who may be frequently quoted on the health issue)
	Preferred communication channels
Existing programs, initiatives, and resources	Top programs that seek to address the same health issue (for example, most reputable or most publicized programs, the largest programs)
	Existing coalitions or partnerships
	Existing resources (for example, books, Web sites)
	For all of the above: lessons learned, trends, key success factors, program assumptions and theoretical foundations, target audiences, key messages, activities and channels, key spokespeople, other relevant information
	Potential opponents to the program's approach or key premises and existing initiatives and groups (for example, animal rights activists in the case of a program supporting animal research)
Unmet communication needs	An analytical description of potential messages, topics, or activities that have not been covered yet (or have been only partially or ineffectively covered) by existing programs and should be addressed by the health communication program
	This topic could be covered as a stand-alone section of the situation analysis or integrated in other sections

Category	*Key Topics and Questions*
Barriers to program implementation or the adoption of the recommended change	Existing barriers that may complicate program implementation and should be addressed to achieve expected outcomes; examples are cost, time, socioeconomic factors, cost-cutting interventions, current beliefs and attitudes toward recommended health behavior
Program goals and outcome objectives	To be included at the beginning of the analysis and restated at the end of it. If research findings do not reinforce preliminary program goals and outcome objectives, changes should be made to reflect research findings.
References or bibliography	Primary and secondary sources of key data and research findings

A2: RANKING AND SELECTING COMMUNICATION STRATEGIES

	Communication Strategy Option 1	*Communication Strategy Option 2*	*Communication Strategy Option 3*
Does the strategy support communication objectives? If yes, how?			
Key benefits			
Disadvantages			
Barriers to strategy implementation			
Does the strategy have the potential to secure community			

	Communication Strategy Option 1	Communication Strategy Option 2	Communication Strategy Option 3
and stakeholder endorsement? If yes, why?			
Are available resources (for example, funds, staff) sufficient for strategy implementation?			
Organizational capability in relation to strategy execution (include strengths and weaknesses)			
Strategy ranking (with final comments)			

A3: COMMUNICATION CHANNELS AND VENUES AND EXAMPLES OF RELATED VEHICLES (TACTICS)

	Channels	Vehicles (Tactics)
Mass media	Print and broadcast media, the Internet, and other new media	Editorials, feature articles, letter to the editor, online quiz, online seminar, television documentary, public service announcement, illustrations, journal supplement
Interpersonal	Counseling, one-on-one meetings, peer education, provider-patient encounters, stakeholder-led	Presentations, courses, speeches, workshops, symposia, lectures, home visits, training, coaching, open discussions,

Channels	*Vehicles (Tactics)*
communications, or other interactive channels	questioning, meet-the-expert sessions
Other community-specific channels and venues (traditional channels)	Local or traditional media, poetry, traditional folk media, theater, existing community meetings, churches, local markets, annual conferences	Theater workshops, comedy, drama, rallies, presentations, lectures, workshops, sermons, poetry contexts, poetry books, health information kiosks, comic books

A4: PRETESTING MESSAGES, MATERIALS, AND ACTIVITIES: SAMPLE QUESTIONS

What is the key point or message of these materials?

What do you think people should do after reading them?

Is any relevant information missing from them?

What are the elements that you most dislike about this message or these materials, and why?

What are some of the strengths and weaknesses of the illustrations and images in the materials?

Will you use or distribute these materials? If yes, why, and in which kinds of situations or venues?

What do you think of the role models that have been used in this public service announcement? What do you like or dislike about them?

What do you think of the idea of appealing to people's hope for a cure? Will that work for you? If yes, why?

Is there anything you suggest to improve these materials or activities?

A5: Program Time Line: Sample Forms

Example 1

Activity	Estimated Time for Project Completion	Notes or Comments
Development of core communication materials for physician workshop	3 to 5 months	Time frame is contingent on a 4-week time line for approval of first draft by all program partners

Example 2

Use different colors for specific program phases—for example, yellow for project planning and development, red for project launch and implementation, and green for evaluation and reporting. Alternatively, use different patterns or shades of black and gray, as in the following example.

Activities for 200x	First Quarter	Second Quarter	Third Quarter	Fourth Quarter
Local media outreach	————	- - - - - - -	- - - - - - - — · — · —	— · — · —

Legend

———— Project planning and development

- - - - - - - Project launch and implementation

— · — · — Evaluation and reporting

A6: BUDGET SAMPLE FORM

Activity Description	Estimated Cost

Disease Awareness Kit for Local Hospitals

Assumes the following materials: cover sheet; fact sheet on disease symptoms, early signs, and diagnostic tools; camera-ready feature article for publication in hospital or organizational newsletters; list of online and peer-reviewed resources

Estimated costs include: research costs (database search; article fees); agency fee for materials development; printing and distribution costs (assumes 10,000 copies); binder, kit development, and design; assembly and shipment; cost of meetings with local hospitals or other relevant organizations (travel, refreshments, room rental)

A7: PROCESS EVALUATION: ESTABLISHING MUTUALLY AGREED PARAMETERS

Preimplementation Sample Chart

Activity	Anticipated Quantitative and Qualitative Results
Health care provider workshop series	Reach audience of 30 to 100 depending on venue
	80 percent positive response to evaluations
	70 to 80 percent speaker endorsement of key messages
	Message retention assessed using pre- and posttest survey with health care providers in target practices and hospitals
Radio public service announcement	20 to 25 million radio impressions over one-year period
	10,000 to 15,000 requests for additional information using the program's Web site or toll-free number

Activity	*Anticipated Quantitative and Qualitative Results*
School-based parental outreach	Program endorsement by five to seven schools per city
	Message retention assessed using pre- and posttest research with parents in target area
	Increase by 15 to 30 percent parental awareness and suspicion of disease (assessed using a pre- or postsurvey with health care providers attending families in target regions)
	5,000 to 10,000 requests for materials fulfilled in each city after initial distribution

ONLINE RESOURCES

HEALTH LITERACY: METHODS TO ASSESS AND REFINE READABILITY LEVELS OF COMMUNICATION MESSAGES AND MATERIALS

SMOG Readability Formula

- University of Utah Health Sciences Center, http://uuhsc.utah.edu/pated/authors/readability.html
- Minnesota Department of Health, http://www.health.state.mn.us/communityeng/groups/test.html

Other Formulas

- European Medicines Agency, http://www.emea.eu.int/pdfs/human/patientgroup/presentation7.pdf
- Agency for Healthcare Research and Quality, http://www.talkingquality.gov/docs/section5/5_1.htm

STRATEGIC PARTNERSHIPS AND COALITIONS

- National Council for Public-Private Partnerships, http://www.ncppp.org
- Communication Initiative, www.comminit.com (case studies on successful partnerships)

- American Marketing Association, www.marketingpower.com
- Centers for Disease Control and Prevention, http://www.cdc.gov/partners/

SUMMATIVE EVALUATION: LOGIC MODEL TEMPLATES

- Health Communication Unit, http://www.thcu.ca/infoandresources/publications/logic_model.pdf
- Harvard Family Research Project, http://www.gse.harvard.edu/hfrp/eval/issue32/logicmodel.html

APPENDIX B: SELECTED ONLINE RESOURCES ON HEALTH COMMUNICATION

All listings are in alphabetical order. For listings in the "Communication Centers" and "Graduate Program" sections, the alphabetical order is based on the organization's name.

WEB SITES

Ask Me 3, http://www.askme3.org/. A Web site of the Partnership for Clear Health Communication. It offers health literacy information for patients, providers, media, and health organizations.

CHANGE Project, http://www.changeproject.org/. Provides resources, publications, case studies on communication, and capacity-building interventions in several disease areas.

Coalition for Health Communication, http://www.healthcommunication.net/. The Web site of the Coalition for Health Communication, formed by the American Public Health Association's Health Communication Working Group, the Health Communication Division of the International Communication Association, and the Health Communication Division of the National Communication Association. It provides information on resources, job openings, conferences, and journals in the field.

Communication Initiative, www.comminit.com. A multidisciplinary partnership between U.S. and international organizations. Includes health communication–related articles, resources, planning models, programs, events, job openings, and links to other sources of information.

Exchange, http://www.healthcomms.org/. A multiorganizational partnership to strengthen communication processes and share learning from practical experience. Information on health communication definitions, news, case studies, and links to articles in the field.

HealthComm KEY, http://cfusion.sph.emory.edu/PHCI/Users/ LogIn.cfm. A database of health communication literature focusing on communication research and practice in the context of public health. Developed by the Emory Center for Public Health Communication, under the sponsorship of the Association of Schools of Public Health and the National Center for Health Marketing, Centers for Disease Control and Prevention.

Health Communication Partnership, http://www.hcpartnership. org/. A multidisciplinary partnership of educational institutions, national organizations, and international organizations to strengthen public health in the developing world through strategic communication programs. The content includes health communication theory and practice, case studies, news, and other resources and links.

JOURNALS

Cases in Public Health Communication and Marketing, http://www. casesjournal.org/. Online annual journal featuring peer-reviewed case studies in public health communication and marketing. Case studies are submitted by a team of authors led by a graduate student of advanced standing.

Health Communication, https://www.leaonline.com/loi/hc. Peer-reviewed bimonthly journal on health communication. Articles focus on topics such as provider-patient or family interaction, communication and cooperation, health information, health promotion, interviewing, and health public relations.

Journal of Health Communication, http://www.gwu.edu/~cih/ journal/. Peer-reviewed bimonthly journal on health communication issues and news, including research studies in risk communication, health literacy, social marketing, interpersonal and mass media communication, psychology, government, policymaking, and health education around the world.

ORGANIZATIONS AND GROUPS

American Public Health Association, Health Communication Working Group, http://www.healthcommunication.net/APHA.html. Information on working group activities and volunteer opportunities, as well as health communication resources, events, and links.

Centers for Disease Control and Prevention (CDC), http://www.cdc.gov/. Resources and links to CDC communication models and activities such as training opportunities, fellowships in health communication, health communication programs in specific disease areas, entertainment, education, and health literacy.

Communication for Social Change Consortium, http://www.communi cationforsocialchange.org/. Includes news, publications, resources, and case studies on communication for social change.

International Communication Association, http://www.healthcom munication.net/ICA.html. Information on association conferences, activities, publications, special events, and other areas. The International Communication Association has a Health Communication Division.

National Communication Association, http://www.healthcommu nication.net/NCA.html. Information on association conferences, activities, publications, special events, and other areas. The National Communication Association has a Health Communication Division.

Pan American Health Organization, http://www.paho.org/Project. asp?SEL=TP&LNG=ENG&ID=152#. Organization activities, publications, multimedia resources on social communication and several disease areas, and health statistics.

Rockefeller Foundation, http://www.rockfound.org/. News, publications, and case studies related to communication for social change.

World Health Organization, http://www.who.int/. News and case studies on Communication for Behavioral Impact programs, publications, resources; disease-related information and statistics; activities in different fields and disciplines.

COMMUNICATION CENTERS

Harvard School of Public Health, Center for Health Communication, http://www.hsph.harvard.edu/chc/. Information about the center's health communication projects and key activities. The center focuses primarily on researching and analyzing the contribution of mass communications to behavior change and policy.

Center for Public Health Communication, Rollins School of Public Health, Emory University, http://www.sph.emory.edu/healthcomm/pubs.htm. Provides information on the center's projects, publications, and presentations on health communication. The primary areas the center addresses are health information technology, risk communication, media relations, and health literacy.

Johns Hopkins University, Center for Communications Programs, http://www.jhuccp.org/topics/hc.shtml. The center partners with other organizations to design and implement strategic communication programs. This site includes publications and resources on population, health communications, and development.

John M. Eisenberg Clinical Decisions and Communications Science Center, U.S. Agency for Healthcare Research and Quality, http://effectivehealthcare.ahrq.gov/dsc/index.cfm. The center is dedicated to translating complex scientific and health-related information into understandable language and formats that can appeal to different audiences (patients, policymakers, health care providers, and others).

Health Communication Research Laboratory, Saint Louis University, School of Public Health, http://hcrl.slu.edu. The research laboratory is dedicated to developing, testing, and implementing tailored health communication programs. The site includes information on key communication programs and research studies.

Center for Health Communication and Marketing at the Center for Health, Intervention and Prevention, University of Connecticut, http://www.chcm.uconn.edu. The mission of this center is to conduct research informing the design and dissemination of health communication and marketing interventions. Special emphasis is placed on the relationship between at-risk populations and their contexts, communication strategies, messages, and behavior change.

Southern Center for Communication, Health and Poverty, University of Georgia, http://www.uga.edu/news-bin/artman/exec/view.cgi? archive=8&num=3830. A health marketing and health communication center that focuses primarily on research and interventions aimed at reducing health disparities in the southern United States and underserved populations.

Public Health Informatics Research Laboratory, University of Maryland, College of Health and Human Performance, http//www.phi. umd.edu. The research laboratory develops multimedia-based training and instructional systems, which include interactive health communication tools such as games and simulations.

Health Communication Unit, Center for Health Promotion, University of Toronto, Canada, http://www.thcu.ca. The Health Communication Unit provides training and information on health communication. The site includes resources on health communication, policy development, planning, sustainability, evaluation, Health Communication Unit case studies and projects, and audience profiles.

GRADUATE PROGRAMS

Master's Degree Program in Health Communication, Emerson College and Tufts University School of Medicine, http://www.emerson. edu/marketing_communication/index.cfm?doc_id=487 http:// www.tufts.edu/med/gpph/MPH/hcom.html. A collaborative effort between Emerson College and Tufts University School of Medicine. Information can be found on the Web sites of both universities.

Master of Public Health and Graduate Certificate in Public Health Communication and Marketing, George Washington University, School of Public Health and Health Services, http://www.gwumc.edu/sphhs/academicprograms/programs/MPH_Graduate_Certificate/PHCM.pdf.

Health Communication Concentration, Harvard School of Public Health, Harvard University, http://www.hsph.harvard.edu/hcc/.

Master's Degree Program in Health Communication, Michigan State University, http://cas.msu.edu/programs/masters/hcomm/.

CONFERENCES AND MEETINGS

American College of Physicians Foundation, Health Communication Conferences, http://foundation.acponline.org/healthcom/hcc.htm. Sponsored by the American College of Physicians Foundation.

American Public Health Association, http://www.apha.org/meetings/. Annual meeting with several presentations and events on health communication.

Kentucky Conference on Health Communication, http://www.uky.edu/CommInfoStudies/COM/news/conferences/kchc/index.html. Biannual conference.

National Communication Association, http://www.natcom.org/nca/Template2.asp. Annual meeting with presentations and events on health communication.

Society for Public Health Education, http://www.sophe.org/mtg_list.asp. Annual meeting with several presentations on health communication.

World Health Assembly, http://www.who.int/fch/fch_wha_docu
ments/en/. Sponsored by the World Health Organization.

JOB LISTINGS

American Public Health Association Public Health Career Mart, http://
apha.jobcontrolcenter.com/search.cfm. Lists positions in public
health, including health communication.

Association of Teachers of Preventive Medicine, http://www.atpm.
org/training/Prev_Med_Fellowship/prev_med_fellowship.html.
Information on the ATPM-CDC Preventive Medicine and Public
Health Fellowship Program, including several fellowships in specific areas of health communication.

CDC Health Communication Intern/Fellow Program, http://www.
cdc.gov/communication/opportunities/opps_fellowship.htm. Information on the Health Communication Intern/Fellow Program
at the Centers for Disease Control and Prevention.

Coalition for Health Communication, http://www.healthcommunica
tion.net/Jobs.html.

Communication Initiative, http://www.comminit.com/vacancies.
html.

International Jobs Center, http://www.internationaljobs.org/. A comprehensive source of international jobs for professionals, including international health care positions and jobs in international
understanding, education, communication, and exchange.

National Cancer Institute Internship in Health Communication, http://
internship.cancer.gov/. Information on internships offered in the
area of health communication by the National Cancer Institute.

Nonprofit Career Network, http://www.nonprofitcareer.com/.

Public Relations Society of America Job Center, http://www.prsa.org/
jobcenter/candidates/jobs.asp. Most positions advertised here are

in the public relations area but sometimes include other communication areas.

Riley Guide, http://www.rileyguide.com/firms.htm. A link to U.S. and international executive search firms that specialize in different fields including health care, public health, health communication, and related areas.

GLOSSARY

Attitudes: Positive or negative emotions or feelings toward a behavior, a person, or a concept or an idea that may affect health or social behavior (Health Communication Partnership, 2005d).

Audience profile: One of the key sections of the situation analysis. A comprehensive, research-based, and strategic description of all key audiences' characteristics, demographics, needs, values, attitudes, and behavior. It includes both primary and secondary audiences. *See also* primary audiences; secondary audiences; situation analysis.

Audience segmentation: The subdivision of key audiences into groups (segments) with similar characteristics and behavioral stages; one of the key steps of the situation analysis and completes the audience profile.

Behavioral impact: The specific behavioral results of a health communication program; measured in relation to specific behavioral indicators that have been established at the onset of planning.

Behavioral objectives: Outcome objectives that explicitly highlight what key audiences are expected to do as the result of the health communication program; can be synonymous with *behavioral indicators*. *See also* outcome objectives.

Channels: *See* communication channels.

Communication channels: The path selected by program planners to reach the intended audience with health communication messages and materials. There are three broad categories of communication channels: mass media channels, interpersonal channels, and community-specific channels and venues (traditional channels).

Communication concepts: Concepts that describe "ways of presenting the information to intended audiences" (National Cancer Institute and National Institutes of Health, 2002, p. 55) as well as the overall kind of appeal (fear, hope, action, progress) that will be used in reaching them. Concepts are preliminary to message and materials development.

Communication objectives: The intermediate steps that need to be achieved in order to meet the overall program goals as complemented by specific behavioral, social, and organizational objectives. They usually highlight changes in knowledge, attitudes, skills, and other intermediate and necessary steps to behavioral or social change.

Communication strategy: A statement describing the overall approach used to accomplish communication objectives.

Communication vehicles: A category that includes materials, events, activities, or other tools for delivering a message using communication channels (Health Communication Unit, 2003b). For example, if the communication channel is a consumer magazine, potential vehicles are feature articles and advertorials.

Community: Indicates a variety of social, ethnic, cultural, or geographical associations, for example, a school, workplace, city, neighborhood, organized patient or professional group, or association of peer leaders. Communities tend to share similar values, beliefs, and overall objectives and priorities.

Community mobilization: One of the key areas of health communication. A bottom-up and participatory process. Using multiple communication channels, it seeks to involve community leaders and the community at large in addressing a health issue, becoming part of the key steps to behavioral or social change or practicing a desired behavior.

Community-specific channels and venues (traditional channels): Local or traditional media, poetry, traditional folk media, theater, churches, local markets, existing community meetings, and annual conferences, for example.

Constituency relations: The process of convening, exchanging information, and establishing and maintaining strategic relationships with key stakeholders and organizations with the intent of identifying common goals that can contribute to the outcomes of a specific communication program or health-related mission.

Constituents or constituency groups: Individuals, communities, and groups that are influenced by or can influence a specific issue. In health care, they include patients, physicians, and other health care providers, hospital employees, professional and advocacy groups, nonprofit organizations, pharmaceutical companies, public health departments, the general public, and policymakers, as well as groups that have a stake in a health issue and can influence its solutions. *See also* stakeholders.

Evaluation plan: A detailed description of the behavioral, social, or organizational indicators as well as other parameters for assessing program outcomes. It should describe methods for data collection, analysis, and reporting, as well as related costs.

External or environmental factors: Political, social, market, and other external influences that shape or contribute to a specific situation or health problem as well as influence key program audiences.

Focus group: One of the most common marketing and communication research methodologies consisting of small group discussion. Participants in focus groups are representatives of key program audiences.

Formative evaluation: An evaluation phase that informs, guides, and helps validate all elements of a health communication program. It occurs prior to program development and implementation and includes the analysis of all research data gathered as part of the situation analysis, audience profile, and pretesting studies.

Gatekeeper: All individuals, groups, or organizations that may provide access to intended audiences. Sometimes they control access to specific communication channels (for example, journalists who control access to the mass media).

Health communication: A multifaceted and multidisciplinary approach to reach different audiences and share health-related information with the goal of influencing, engaging, and supporting individuals, communities, health professionals, special groups, policymakers, and the public to champion, introduce, adopt, or sustain a behavior, practice, or policy that will ultimately improve health outcomes.

Impact: An outcome in relation to a specific change or, alternatively, the long-term change influenced by a program in relation to the overall program goal.

In-depth interviews: A research method that consists of one-on-one interviews (for example, telephone or in-person interviews) with internal and external stakeholders, members of key audiences, or representatives of relevant health organizations.

Intended audiences: All audiences the health communication program is seeking to influence and engage in the communication process.

Interpersonal channels: Counseling, one-on-one meetings, peer education, provider-patient encounters, stakeholder-led meetings, or other interactive channels and venues that are used for interpersonal communications.

Interpersonal communications: A key health communication area that uses interpersonal channels. Includes personal selling and counseling, provider-patient communications, and other kinds of group or one-on-one interactions and communications.

Key program audiences: *See* intended audiences.

Low health literacy: "The inability to read, understand and act on health information" (Zagaria, 2004, p. 41).

Mass media channels: Print and broadcast media, the Internet, and other new media.

Media advocacy: *See* public advocacy.

Organizational objectives: Refers to the change that should occur within an organization in terms of its focus, priorities, or structure in relation to the specific health issue addressed by a health communication intervention.

Outcome objectives: The desired outcomes the health communication program is seeking to achieve: behavioral, social, and organizational objectives. These objectives are used as key indicators of change in the evaluation of health communication programs and should be set at the onset of program planning.

Outcomes: Changes in knowledge, comprehension, attitudes, skills, behavior, policies, and social norms as established by the program's outcome and communication objectives. These are measured in relation to the estimated influence the health communication program had on each change.

Overall program goal: Describes the overall "health improvement" (National Cancer Institute and National Institutes of Health, 2002, p. 22) or "overall change in a health or social problem" (Weinrich, 1999, p. 67) that the program is seeking to achieve.

Pretesting: An essential phase of formative research that uses several research methods to assess whether communication concepts, messages, and materials meet the needs of intended audiences; are culturally appropriate; and are easily understood.

Primary audiences: The people whom the program seeks to influence most directly—for example, people at risk for a certain medical condition or already suffering from it; parents or other caregivers responsible for pediatric care decisions for their children; or other audiences in the case of programs of limited scope that seek to influence only one audience.

Process evaluation: Used to compare key steps of the program's implementation with the original program plan and to measure expected results for specific activities, materials, and messages.

Professional medical communications: A key health communication area that describes a peer-to-peer approach intended for health care professionals. Professional medical communications aim to (1) promote the adoption of best medical and health practices; (2) establish new concepts and standards of care; (3) publicize recent medical discoveries, beliefs, parameters, and policies; (4) change or establish new medical priorities; and (5) advance health policy changes.

Program outcomes: Changes in knowledge, attitudes, skills, behavior, and other parameters measured against those anticipated in the program planning phase.

Public advocacy: "The act of influencing decision makers and promoting changes to laws and other government policies to advance the mission of a particular organization or group of people" (American Heart Association, 2006a). It relies on multiple tools and activities, including community or town hall meetings and one-on-one encounters with policymakers and decision makers. A fundamental component of public advocacy efforts is the use of the mass media. Also called *media advocacy,* reflecting public advocacy that heavily relies on the strategic use of the mass media.

Public relations (PR): One of the key health communication areas, defined as "the art and science of establishing and promoting a favorable relationship with the public" (*American Heritage Dictionary of the English Language,* 2004). Functions of PR include public affairs, community relations, issues or crisis management, media relations, and marketing PR. PR relies on the skillful use of culturally competent and audience-appropriate mass media, as well as other communication channels to place a health issue on the public agenda, advocate for its solutions, and highlight the importance that the government and other key stakeholders take action. *See also* public advocacy.

Qualitative research: Research methods and approaches that are used to collect data in relatively small groups. Qualitative data are not statistically significant and focus on opinions, trends, and insights.

Quantitative research: Research methods and data that are statistically significant and are usually collected from large samples. Its aim is to provide the health communication team with exact numbers about different kinds of external factors or audience-specific characteristics and behaviors.

Secondary audiences: All individuals, groups, communities, and organizations that can exert an influence on the decisions and behaviors of the primary audiences. *See also* primary audiences.

Situation analysis: The analysis of all individual, community, social, political, and behavior-related factors that can affect attitudes, behaviors, social norms, and policies about a health issue and its potential solutions.

Social change indicators: Indicators that measure changes in social interactions, norms, policies, and practices, as well as changes in the issues of concerns.

Social objective: An outcome objective that highlights the policy, practice, or social change that the program is seeking to achieve or implement.

Stakeholders: All individuals and groups that have an interest or share responsibilities in a given issue. They may represent the primary audience or influence them. *See also* constituency groups and constituents.

Summative evaluation: A phase of evaluation that measures the program's efficacy in relation to the outcome and communication objectives initially established by the program.

Tactical plan: A detailed description of all communication messages, materials, activities, and channels, as well as the methods that will be used to pretest them with key audiences. The plan is audience specific and relates to the different areas of health communication. It includes a detailed time line for the program implementation, an itemized budget for each communication activity or material, and a partnership plan with roles and responsibilities that have been agreed to by all team members.

Tactics: All communication activities, materials, and events that are strategically connected with other key communication elements and are described in the tactical plan. *See also* communication vehicles.

Target audiences: *See* intended audiences.

Vehicles: *See* communication vehicles.

REFERENCES

ABC News. "Poll: What Americans Eat for Breakfast." http://www.
abcnews.com/GMA/PollVault/story?id=762685. Retrieved Nov.
2005.

Adams, J. "Successful Strategic Planning: Creating Clarity." *Journal of
Healthcare Information Management,* 2005, *19*(3), 24–31.

Ad Council. "About Asthma." http://www.noattacks.org/about.html.
Retrieved Feb. 2006a.

Ad Council. "Preventing Attacks." http://www.noattacks.org/preventing.
html. Retrieved Feb. 2006b.

Ader, M., and others. "Quality Indicators for Health Promotion Programmes." *Health Promotion International,* 2001, *16*(2), 187–195.

Advertising Law Resource Center. "Children and Tobacco, Executive
Summary, Final Rule: U.S. Food and Drug Administration."
http://www.lawpublish.com/fdarule.html. Retrieved Mar. 2006.

Agunga, R. A. *Developing the Third World: A Communication Approach.* Com-
mack, N.Y.: Nova Science, 1997.

Ahorlu, C., and others. "Malaria-Related Beliefs and Behaviour in Southern Ghana: Implications for Treatment, Prevention and Control."
Tropical Medicine and International Health, 1997, *2*(5), 488–499.

Ajzen, I., and Fishbein, M. *Understanding Attitudes and Predicting Social
Behavior.* Upper Saddle River, N.J.: Prentice Hall, 1980.

Alcalay, R., and Bell, R. *Promoting Nutrition and Physical Activity Through Social Marketing: Current Practices and Recommendations.* For the Cancer
Prevention and Nutrition Section of California Department of
Health Services. Davis: Center for Advanced Studies in Nutrition
and Social Marketing, University of California, Davis, June 2000.
http://socialmarketing-nutrition.ucdavis.edu/Downloads/Alcalay-
Bell.pdf. Retrieved Sept. 2005.

Al-Khayat, M. H. *Health: An Islamic Perspective.* Alexandria: World Health
Organization, Regional Office for the Eastern Mediterranean, 1997.
http://www.emro.who.int/Publications/HealthEdReligion/
IslamicPerspective/Chapter1.htm. Retrieved Oct. 2006.

American Academy of Family Physicians. "Good Communication Is Sign of Good Medicine for FP of the Year." FP Report, Oct. 1999. http://www.aafp.org/fpr/991000fr/10.html. Retrieved June 2005.

American Academy of Pediatrics. "Periodic Survey of Fellows, Periodic Survey #43—Part 1, Characteristics of Pediatricians and Their Practices: The Socioeconomic Survey." http://www.aap.org/research/periodicsurvey/ps43aexs.htm. Retrieved Nov. 2005a.

American Academy of Pediatrics. "Periodic Survey of Fellows, Periodic Survey #54—Part 1, Characteristics of Pediatricians and Their Practices: The Socioeconomic Survey." http://www.aap.org/research/periodicsurvey/ps54aexs.htm. Retrieved Nov. 2005b.

American Association for the Advancement of Science. "Malaria and Development in Africa: A Cross-Sectoral Approach." http://www.aaas.org/international/africa/malaria91/rec6.html. Retrieved Feb. 2006.

American Association of Medical Colleges. "AAMC Report Aims to Enhance Communications Skills Training at U.S. Medical Schools, AAMC Issues Doctor-Patient Communications Fact Sheet, Launches 'Doctoring 101.'" 1999. http://www.aamc.org/newsroom/pressrel/1999/991026.htm. Retrieved Nov. 2005.

American Diabetes Association, "Diabetes and Your Weight." http://www.diabetes.org/weightloss-and-exercise/weightloss/diabetes.jsp. Retrieved Oct. 2005.

American Folklife Preservation Act. Public Law 94–201, 94th Congress, H.R. 6673, Jan. 2, 1976.

American Heart Association, "Public Advocacy: What Is Public Advocacy?" http://www.americanheart.org/presenter.jhtml?identifier=4758. Retrieved Mar. 2006a.

American Heart Association. Office of Tobacco Control. "The American Heart Association Youth Fitness and Tobacco Prevention/Education Project." http://www.fsu.edu/~ctl/Tobacco2.htm. Retrieved Mar. 2006b.

American Medical Association. "Partnership for Clear Health Communication—What Can Providers Do?" http:/www.askme3.org/PFCHC/what_can_provid.asp. Retrieved June 2005a.

American Medical Association. "Partnership for Clear Health Communication—What is Ask Me 3?" http:/www.askme3.org/PFCHC/what_is_ask.asp. Retrieved June 2005b.

American Medical Association. "Partnership for Clear Health Communication." http://www.ama-assn.org/ama/pub/category/11128.html. Retrieved June 2005c.

American Medical Association. "AMA to New York Times: Good Physician-Patient Communication Helps All Doctors." Dec. 2005d.

http://www.ama-assn.org/ama/pub/category/15788.html. Retrieved Mar. 2006.

American Medical Association. Young Physicians Section. "Guidelines for Physician-Patient Electronic Communications." http://www.ama-assn.org/ama/pub/category/2386.html. Retrieved Mar. 2006.

American Medical Student Association. "Cultural Competency in Medicine: A Project-in-a-Box." http://www.amsa.org/programs/gpit/cultural.cfm. Retrieved Oct. 2005.

American Public Health Association. "Media Advocacy Session." 133rd Annual Meeting and Exposition, Philadelphia, Dec. 2005.

American Public Health Association. Health Communication Working Group. "What Is Health Communication?" http://www.hehd.clemson.edu/Publichealth/PHEHP/HealthComm/define.htm. Retrieved Feb. 2006.

Amoah, S. O., "Mobilizing Community Support for a Radio Serial on HIV." Paper presented at the American Public Health Association's 129th Annual Meeting, Atlanta, Ga., Oct. 2001.

Andersen, M. R., and Lobel, M. "Predictors of Health Self-Appraisal: What's Involved in Feeling Healthy." *Basic and Applied Social Psychology Bulletin,* 1995, *16*(1–2), 121–136.

Andreasen, A. R. *Marketing Social Change: Changing Behavior to Promote Health, Social Development and the Environment.* San Francisco: Jossey-Bass, 1995.

Arias, J. R., Monteiro, P. S., and Zicker, F. "The Reemergence of Visceral Leishmaniasis in Brazil." *Emergency Infectious Diseases,* 1996, *2*(2), 145–146.

Atkin, C., and Schiller, L. "The Impact of Public Service Advertising." In Henry Kaiser Family Foundation, *Background Papers. Shouting to Be Heard: Public Service Advertising in a New Media Age.* Menlo Park, Calif.: Kaiser Family Foundation, Feb. 2002.

Babalola, S., and others. "The Impact of a Community Mobilization Project Knowledge and Practices in Cameroon." *Journal of Community Health,* 2001, *26*(6), 459.

Babrow, A. "Tensions Between Health Beliefs and Desires: Implications for a Health Communication Campaign to Promote a Smoking-Cessation Program." *Health Communication,* 1991, *3*(2), 93.

Balog, J. E. "An Historical Review and Philosophical Analysis of Alternative Concepts of Health and Their Relationship to Human Education." Unpublished doctoral dissertation, University of Maryland, 1978.

Bandura, A. "Self-Efficacy: Toward a Unifying Theory of Behavioral Change." *Psychological Review,* 1977, *84*, 191–215.

Bandura, A. *Social Foundations of Thought and Action: A Social Cognitive Theory.* Upper Saddle River, N.J.: Prentice Hall, 1986.

Bandura, A. *Self-Efficacy: The Exercise of Control.* New York: Freeman, 1997.

Baranick, E., and Ricca, J. "Community Mobilization Within a Multi-Channel Behavior Change C-IMCI Framework Has Rapid Impact in Diverse Settings." Paper presented at the American Public Health Association 133rd Annual Meeting, Philadelphia, Dec. 2005. http://apha.confex.com/apha/133am/techprogram/paper_110778.htm. Retrieved Oct. 2006.

Barbato, C. A., and Perse, E. M. "Interpersonal Communication Motives and the Life Position of Elders." *Communication Research,* 1992, *19*(4), 516–531.

Barbieri, C. "Your Mother Would Know." *New York Times,* Nov. 29, 2005.

Barney, L. J., Griffiths, K. M., Jorm, A. F., and Christensen, H. "Stigma About Depression and Its Impact on Help-Seeking Intentions." *Australian and New Zealand Journal of Psychiatry,* 2006, *40*(1), 51–54.

Beal, G. M., and Rogers, E. M. *The Adoption of Two Farm Practices in a Central Iowa Community.* Special report no. 26. Ames: Iowa State University, 1960.

Becker, M. H., Haefner, D. P., and Maiman, L. A. "The Health Belief Model in the Prediction of Dietary Compliance: A Field Experiment." *Journal of Health and Social Behaviour,* 1977, *18*, 348–366.

Belzer, E. J. "Improving Patient Communication in No Time." *Family Practice Management,* 1999, *6*(5), 3–28.

Bernhardt, J. M., and others. "Perceived Barriers to Internet-Based Health Communication on Human Genetics." *Journal of Health Communication,* 2002, *7*(4), 325–340.

Bernhardt, J. M. "Communication at the Core of Effective Public Health." *American Journal of Public Health,* 2004, *94*(12), 2051–2053.

Bertrand, J. T. "Evaluating Health Communication Programmes." *The Drum Beat,* no. 302, Communication Initiative, 2005. http://www.comminit.com/drum_beat_302.html. Retrieved Mar. 2006.

Blanchard, J., and others. "In Their Own Words: Lessons Learned from Those Exposed to Anthrax." *American Journal of Public Health,* 2005, *95*(3), 489–495.

Blot, W. J., and others. "Smoking and Drinking in Relation to Oral and Pharyngeal Cancer." *Cancer Research,* 1988, *48*(11), 3282–3287.

Bogen, K. "The Effect of Questionnaire Length on Response Rates—A Review of the Literature." Washington, D.C.: U.S. Bureau of the Census. http://www.census.gov/srd/papers/pdf/kb9601.pdf. Retrieved Mar. 2006.

Bongaarts, J., and Watkins, S. C. "Social Interactions and Contemporary Fertility Transitions." *Population and Development Review,* 1996, *22*(4), 639–682.

Borg, E. "Smoking Ban Near Dorms Not Enforced: University Police Not Ticketing Smokers by Residency Halls." 2004. http://www.spectatornews.com/media/paper218/news/2004/11/18/CampusNews/Smoking.Ban.Near.Dorms.Not.Enforced-809676.shtml?norewrite200603271326andsourcedomain=www.spectatornews.com. Retrieved Mar. 2006.

Boruchovitch, E., and Mednick, B. R. "Cross-Cultural Differences in Children's Concepts of Health and Illness." *Revista de Saude Publica,* 1997, *31*(5), 448–456.

Boruchovitch, E., and Mednick, B. R. "The Meaning of Health and Illness: Some Considerations for Health Psychology." *Psico-USF,* 2002, *7*(2), 175–183.

Bray, G. "Medical Consequences of Obesity." *Journal of Clinical Endocrinology and Metabolism,* 2004, *89*(6), 2583–2589.

Brennan, S. E. "Seeking and Providing Evidence for Mutual Understanding." Unpublished doctoral dissertation, Stanford University, 1990.

Brennan, S. E. "How Conversation Is Shaped by Visual and Spoken Evidence." In J. Trueswell and M. Tanenhaus (eds.), *World Situated Language Use: Psycholinguistic, Linguistic, and Computational Perspectives on Bridging the Product and Action Traditions.* Cambridge, Mass.: MIT Press, 2004.

Brennan, S. E., and Lockridge, C. B. "Computer-Mediated Communication: A Cognitive Science Approach." In K. Brown (ed.), *ELL2, Encyclopedia of Language and Linguistics.* (2nd ed.) New York: Elsevier, 2006. http://www.psychology.stonybrook.edu/sbrennan-/papers/BL_ELL2.pdf. Retrieved Nov. 2005.

Brown, R. *Social Psychology.* New York: Free Press, 1965.

Burson-Marsteller. "Constituency Relations." http://www.bm.com/pages/functional/relations. Retrieved Feb. 2006.

Burstall, M. L. "European Policies Influencing Pharmaceutical Innovations." In A. C. Gelijins and E. A. Halm (eds.), *The Changing Economics of Medical Technology.* Washington, D.C.: National Academies Press, 1991.

Calmy, A. "MSF and HIV/AIDS: Expanding Treatment, Facing New Challenges." 2004. http://www.doctorswithoutborders.org/publications/ar/i2004/hivaids.cfm. Retrieved Jan. 2006.

Campaign for Tobacco-Free Kids. "About the Campaign: Who We Are." http://www.tobaccofreekids.org/organization/. Retrieved Mar. 2006.

Campbell, J. D. "Illness Is a Point of View: The Development of Children's Concept of Illness." *Children's Development,* 1975, *46,* 92–100.

Canadian Public Health Association. "ParticipACTION: The Mouse That Roared a Marketing and Health Communications Success Story." http://www.cpha.ca/English/inside/mediarm/newsrel/mouse_e.htm. Retrieved Dec. 2005.

CancerBACKUP, "Why Improve Access to Cancer Information?" http://www.cancerbacup.org.uk/Healthprofessionals/Reaching-morecommunities/BeyondtheBarriers/Whyimproveaccess#6623. Retrieved Jan. 2006.

Caribbean Epidemiology Center. "Report of Communication Advisory Committee Meeting, Sub-Committee of the Technical Advisory Group." 2003. http://www.carec.org/documents/cccpcp/communication_advisory_report.doc. Retrieved Feb. 2006.

Carter, K. E. "Building a Constituency Through Outreach." 1994. http://www.stc.org/confproceed/1994/PDFs/PG5152.PDF. Retrieved Mar. 2006.

Castrucci, B. C., Gerlach, K. K., Kaufman, N. J., and Orleans, C. T. "Tobacco Use and Cessation Behavior Among Adolescents Participating in Organized Sports." *American Journal of Health Behavior,* 2004, *28*(1), 63–71.

Cave, L. "NIMH Establishes Outreach, Education Program." Bethesda, Md.: National Institutes of Health, n.d. http://www.namiohio.org/html/nimh_outreach.htm. Retrieved Feb. 2006.

Cendron, M. "Primary Nocturnal Enuresis: Current Concepts." *American Family Physician,* 1999, *59*(5), 1205–1213.

Center for Consumer Freedom. "Humane Society of the United States." http://www.activistcash.com/organization_overview.cfm/oid/136. Retrieved Mar. 2006.

Center, A. H., and Jackson, P. *Public Relations Practices: Management Case Studies and Problems.* (5th ed.) Upper Saddle River, N.J.: Prentice Hall, 1995.

Centers for Disease Control and Prevention. *Addressing Emerging Infectious Disease Threats: A Prevention Strategy for the United States.* Atlanta, Ga.: Public Health Service, 1994a.

Centers for Disease Control and Prevention. "Preventing Tobacco Use Among Young People: A Report of the Surgeon General AT-A-GLANCE." 1994b. http://www.cdc.gov/tobacco/sgr/sgr_1994/94oshaag.htm. Retrieved Jan. 2006.

Centers for Disease Control and Prevention. Office on Smoking and Health. National Center for Chronic Disease Prevention and Health Promotion. "State Laws on Tobacco Control—United States, 1998." *MMWR,* June 25, 1999, *48* (SS-03), pp. 21–62. http://www.cdc.gov/mmwr/preview/mmwrhtml/ss4803a2.htm. Retrieved Mar. 2006.

Centers for Disease Control and Prevention. "HealthComm Key: Unlocking the Power of Health Communication Research." http://www.cdc.gov/od/oc/hcomm. Retrieved May 2001.

Centers for Disease Control and Prevention. "From Data to Action: Infant Sleep Position." Centers for Disease Control and Prevention. 2002. http://www.cdc.gov/PRAMS/dataAct2002/infant_sleep.htm. Retrieved Feb. 2006.

Centers for Disease Control and Prevention. "Colorectal Cancer: About the CDC Program." 2004/2005. http://www.cdc.gov/colorectal-cancer/pdf/about2004.pdf. Retrieved Mar. 2006.

Centers for Disease Control and Prevention. "Pertussis—United States, 2001—2003." 2005. http://www.cdc.gov/mmwr/preview/mmwrhtml/mm5450a3.htm. Retrieved Feb. 2006.

Centers for Disease Control and Prevention. Foodborne and Diarrheal Diseases Branch. "Safe Water System Manual." http://hetv.org/India/mh/plan/safewater/manual/ch_7.htm. Retrieved Jan. 2006a.

Centers for Disease Control and Prevention. "Syphilis Elimination Effort (SEE) Toolkit." http://www.cdc.gov/std/see/description.htm. Retrieved Jan. 2006b.

Centers for Disease Control and Prevention. "Colorectal Cancer." http://www.cdc.gov/colorectalcancer/. Retrieved Mar. 2006c.

Centers for Disease Control and Prevention. "Malaria Control in Endemic Countries." http://www.cdc.gov/malaria/control_prevention/control.htm. Retrieved Feb. 2006d.

Centers for Disease Control and Prevention. "Heads Up: Brain Injury in Your Practice Tool Kit." http://www.cdc.gov/doc.do/id/0900f3ec80017619/. Retrieved Jan. 2006e.

Centers for Disease Control and Prevention. "CDC-Funded Asthma Activities by State and Type of Funding." http://www.cdc.gov/asthma/aag05.htm#control. Retrieved Feb. 2006f.

Centers for Disease Control and Prevention. "Physical Activity for Everyone: The Importance of Physical Activity." http://www.cdc.gov/nccdphp/dnpa/physical/importance/index.htm. Retrieved Mar. 2006g.

Centers for Disease Control and Prevention. "Got a Minute? Give It to Your Kid: Audience Profile." http://www.cdc.gov/tobacco/parenting/audience.htm. Retrieved Feb. 2006h.

Centers for Disease Control and Prevention. "Preventing Tetanus, Diphtheria, and Pertussis Among Adolescents: Use of Tetanus Toxoid, Reduced Diphtheria Toxoid and Acellular Pertussis Vaccines." MMWR, Feb. 23, 2006i, 55, 1–34. http://www.cdc.gov/mmwr/preview/mmwrhtml/rr55e223a1.htm. Retrieved Feb. 2006.

Centers for Disease Control and Prevention. "Fact Sheet: Leishmania

Infection (Leishmaniasis)." http://www.cdc.gov/ncidod/dpd/parasites/leishmania/factsht_leishmania.htm. Retrieved Mar. 2006j.

Center for Health Equity Research and Promotion. "Intro to Health Disparities." http://www.cherp.research.med.va.gov/introhd.php. Retrieved Oct. 2005.

Chan, S. "Parents of Exceptional Asian Children." In M. K. Kitano and P. C. Chinn (eds.), *Exceptional Asian Children and Youth*. Reston, Va.: Council for Exceptional Children, 1986.

Cherry, J. D., and others. "Defining Pertussis Epidemiology: Clinical, Microbiologic and Serologic Perspectives." *Pediatric Infectious Disease Journal*, 2005, *24*(5 Suppl.), S25-S34.

Chiu, C., Krauss, R. M., and Lau, I. Y. "Some Cognitive Consequences of Communication." In S. R. Fussell and R. J. Kreuz (eds.), *Social and Cognitive Approaches to Interpersonal Communication*. Mahwah, N.J.: Erlbaum, 1998.

Clark, H. H., and Brennan, S. E. "Grounding in Communication." In L. B. Resnick, J. Levine, and S. D. Teasley (eds.), *Perspectives on Socially Shared Cognition*. Washington, D.C.: APA Press, 1991.

Clark, H. H., and Schaefer, E. F. "Contributing to Discourse." *Cognitive Science*, 1989, *13*, 259–294.

Clark, H. H., and Wilkes-Gibbs, D. "Referring as a Collaborative Process." *Cognition*, 1986, *22*, 1–39.

Cleland, J., and Wilson, C. "Demand Theories of the Fertility Transition: An Iconoclastic View." *Population Studies*, 1987, *41*(1), 5–30.

Clift, E., and Freimuth, V. "Health Communication: What Is It and What Can It Do for You?" *Journal of Health Education*, 1995, *26*(2), 68–74.

Cline, R.J.W., and Haynes, K. M. "Consumer Health Information Seeking on the Internet: The State of the Art." *Health Education Research*, 2001, *16*(6), 671–692.

Coalition for Health Communication. "Coalition for Health Communication." www.healthcommunication.net. Retrieved Mar. 2006.

Coffman, J. "Public Communication Campaign Evaluation: An Environmental Scan of Challenges, Criticisms, Practice, and Opportunities." 2002. http://www.gse.harvard.edu/hfrp/pubs/onlinepubs/pcce/index.html. Retrieved Jan. 2006.

Cole, G. E., and others. "Addressing Problems in Evaluating Health Relevant Programs Through Systematic Planning and Evaluation." *Risk: Health, Safety and Environment*, 1995, *37*(1), 37–57.

Colle, R. D., and Roman, R. "A Handbook for Telecenter Staffs." 2003. http://ip.cals.cornell.edu/commdev/handbook.cfm. Retrieved Mar. 2006.

Colwill, J. M., and Cultice, J. M. "The Future Supply of Family Physicians: Implications for Rural America." *Health Affairs*, 2003, *22*, 190–198.

Communication Initiative. "Change Theories: Cultivation Theory of Mass Media." July 2003a. http://www.comminit.com/changetheories/ctheories/changetheories-24.html. Retrieved Sept. 2005.

Communication Initiative. "Change Theories Precede-Proceed." Nov. 2003b. http://www.comminit.com/changetheories/ctheories/changetheories-42.html. Retrieved Dec. 2005.

Constance, H. "Animal Wars." *Science,* 2005, *309*(5740), 1485.

Corrigan, P. "How Stigma Interferes with Mental Health Care." *American Psychologist,* 2004, *59*(7), 614–625.

Costas-Bradstreet, C. "Spreading the Message Through Community Mobilization, Education and Leadership: A Magnanimous Task." *Canadian Journal of Public Health,* 2004, *95*, S25-S29.

Coward, H., and Sidhu, T. "Bioethics for Clinicians: 19. Hinduism and Sikhism." *Canadian Medical Association Journal,* 2000, *163*(9), 1167–1170.

Crystalinks. "Hippocrates." http://www.crystalinks.com/hippocrates.html. Retrieved Jan. 2006.

Cutlip, S. M., Center, A. H., and Broom, G. M. *Effective Public Relations.* Upper Saddle River, N.J.: Prentice Hall, 1994.

Das, A. K., Olfson, M., McCurtis, H. L., and Weissman, M. M. "Depression in African Americans: Breaking Barriers to Detection and Treatment." *Journal of Family Practice,* 2006, *55*(1), 30–39.

Debus, M. *Methodological Review: A Handbook for Excellence in Focus Group Research.* Washington, D.C.: Academy for Educational Development, 1988.

DES Action Canada and Working Group on Women and Health Protection. "Protecting Our Health: New Debates." http://www.whp-apsf.ca/pdf/dtca.pdf. Retrieved Jan. 2006.

Deutsch, M. *The Resolution of Conflict: Constructive and Destructive Processes.* New Haven, Conn.: Yale University Press, 1973.

Deutsch, M. "Cooperation and Conflict." In M. Deutsch and P. Coleman (eds.), *The Handbook of Conflict Resolution.* San Francisco: Jossey-Bass, 2000.

Dillman, D., Sinclair, M. D., and Clark, J. R. "Effects of Questionnaire Length, Respondent-Friendly Design, and a Difficult Question on Response Rates for Occupant-Addressed Census Mail Surveys." *Public Opinion Quarterly,* 1993, *57*(3), 289–304.

DiMatteo, M. R., and others. "Physicians' Characteristics Influence Patients' Adherence to Medical Treatment: Results from the Medical Outcomes Study." *Health Psychology,* 1993, *12*(2), 93–102.

Doak, C. C., Doak, L. G., and Root, J. H. *Teaching Patients with Low Literacy skills.* Philadelphia: Lippincott, 1995.

Donovan, R. J. "Steps in Planning and Developing Health Communication Campaigns: A Comment on CDC's Framework for Health Communication." *Public Health Reports,* 1995, *110*(2), 215–217.

Drum Beat Chat Forum. "Health Communication vs. Related Disciplines." The Communication Initiative, 2005. http://forums.comminit.com/viewtopic.php?t=63257&style=2. Retrieved Dec. 2005.

Druss, B. G., and others. "Mental Disorders and Use of Cardiovascular Procedures After Myocardial Infarction." *Journal of American Medical Association*, 2000, *283*(4), 506–511.

Dumke, N. M. "Preventing Asthma Hospitalizations Among Children and Teens." *Journal of the National Medical Association*, 2006, *98*(2), 304.

Du Pré, A. *Communicating About Health: Current Issues and Perspectives.* Mountain View, Calif.: Mayfield Publishing Company, 2000.

Economic and Social Research Council. "Why Media Relations Is Important?" http://www.esrc.ac.uk/ESRCInfoCentre/Support/Communications_Toolkit/media_relations/Why_Media_Relations_is_Important/index.aspx?ComponentId=1540&SourcePageId=1615. Retrieved Dec. 2005a.

Economic and Social Research Council. "Top Ten Tips." http://www.esrcsocietytoday.ac.uk/ESRCInfoCentre/Support/Communications_Toolkit/media_relations/top_ten_tips/index.aspx?ComponentId=1539andSourcePageId=1609. Retrieved Dec. 2005b.

Eisenberg, J. M., Kitz, D. S., and Webber, R. A. "Development of Attitudes About Sharing Decision Making: A Comparison of Medical and Surgical Residents." *Journal of Health and Social Behavior*, 1983, *24*, 85–90.

Eiser, J. R., and Pancer, S. M. "Attitudinal Effects of the Use of Evaluatively Biased Language." *European Journal of Social Psychology*, 1979, *9*, 39–47.

Emanoil, P. "The Key to Public Health Is Community." *Human Ecology*, 2002, *28*(2), 16.

Emblen, J. D. "Religion and Spirituality Defined According to Current Use in Nursing Literature." *Journal of Professional Nursing*, 1992, *8*(1), 41–47.

Emerson College. "Integrated Marketing Communication." http://www.emerson.edu/marketing_communication/index.cfm?doc_id=488. Retrieved Mar. 2006.

Encarta Dictionary: English, North America. "Search Term: Communication." http://encarta.msn.com/dictionary_/communication.html.

Engel, G. E. "The Need for a New Medical Model: A Challenge for Biomedicine." *Science*, 1977, *196*, 129–136.

Ericson, R. V., Baranek, P. M., and Chan, J. B. *Visualizing Deviance.* Toronto: University of Toronto Press, 1987.

Erickson, J. G., Devlieger, P. J., and Sung, J. M. "Korean-American Female Perspectives on Disability." *American Speech-Language-Hearing Association*, 1999, *8*, 99–108.

European Network for Smoking Prevention. "Implementation of the EU Directive on Advertising Ban—Status on 1 July 2005 Implementation Deadline: 31 July 2005." 2005. http://www.ensp.org/files/ad_ban_implementation_01.07.05.doc. Retrieved Mar. 2006.

Exchange. "Health Communication." http://www.healthcomms.org/comms/. Retrieved July 2005.

Exchange. "Issues in Evaluation for Health and Disability Communication." Aug. 2001. http://www.healthcomms.org/comms/eval/le05.html. Retrieved Mar. 2006.

Exchange. "Integrated Communication." http://www.healthcomms.org/comms/integ/ict-integ.html. Retrieved Mar. 2006.

Eysenbach, G. "Consumer Health Informatics." *British Medical Journal,* 2000, *320,* 1713–1716.

Eysenbach, G. "What Is E-Health?" *Journal of Medical Internet Research,* 2001, *3*(2), e20.

Fadiman, A. *The Spirit Catches You and You Fall Down: A Hmong Child, Her American Doctors, and the Collision of Two Cultures.* New York: Farrar, Straus and Giroux, 1997.

Favin, M. "Strategic Thinking Lessons Learned from Five Country Studies of Communication Support for Polio Eradication and Routine." http://www.comminit.com/strategicthinking/stcommforpolio/thinking-1008.html. Retrieved Jan. 2004.

Figueroa, M. E., Kincaid, D. L., Rani, M., and Lewis, G. *Communication for Social Change: An Integrated Model for Measuring the Process and Its Outcomes.* New York: Rockefeller Foundation and Johns Hopkins University Center for Communication Programs, 2002.

Finerman, R. "The Burden of Responsibility: Duty, Depression, and Nervios in Andean Ecuador." *Health Care for Women International,* 1989, *10*(2–3), 141–157.

Fischer, J. E. "Current Status of Medicine in the USA: A Personal Perspective." *Journal of the Royal College of Surgeons of Edinburgh,* 2001, *46,* 71–75.

Fishbein, M., Goldberg, M., and Middlestadt, S. *Social Marketing: Theoretical and Practical Perspectives.* Mahwah, N.J.: Erlbaum, 1997.

Fisher, S. "Case Study—Viim Kuunga Radio Project—Burkina Faso." Communication Initiative, 2003. http://www.comminit.com/experiences/pdskdv32003/experiences-1261.html. Retrieved Feb. 2006.

Fog, A. *Cultural Selection.* Norwell, Mass.: Kluwer, 1999.

FoodNavigatorUSA.com. "Innova taps Trans Fat-Free Vegetable Oil Demand." http://www.foodnavigator-usa.com/news-by-product/news.asp?id=62898andk=innova-taps-trans. Retrieved Jan. 2006a.

FoodNavigatorUSA.com. "Seafood Producer Goes Trans Fat Free."

http://www.foodnavigator-usa.com/news-by-product/news.asp?id=
57372andk=seafood-producer-goes. Retrieved Jan. 2006b.

Frable, P. J., Wallace, D. C., and Ellison, K. J. "Using Clinical Guidelines
in Home Care: For Patients with Diabetes." *Home Healthcare Nurse,*
2004, *22*(7), 462–468.

Freeman, R. E. *Strategic Management: A Stakeholder Approach.* Boston: Pit-
man, 1984.

Freimuth, V., Cole, G., and Kirby, S. *Issues in Evaluating Mass Mediated
Health Communication Campaigns.* Copenhagen: WHO Regional Office for Europe, 2000.

Freimuth, V., Linnan, H. W., and Potter, P. "Communicating the Threat
of Emerging Infections to the Public." *Emerging Infectious Diseases,*
2000, *6*(4), 337–347.

Freimuth, V. S., and Quinn, S. C. "The Contributions of Health Communication to Eliminating Health Disparities." *American Journal of
Public Health,* 2004, *94*(12), 2053–2055.

Friedman, H. S., and DiMatteo, M. R. "Health Care as an Interpersonal
Process." *Journal of Social Issues,* 1979, *35,* 1–11.

Gaebel, W., Baumann, A. E., and Phil, M. A. "Interventions to Reduce the
Stigma Associated with Severe Mental Illness: Experiences from the
Open the Doors Program in Germany." *Canadian Journal of Psychi-
atry,* 2003, *48*(10), 657–662.

Gallus, S., and others. "Effects of New Smoking Regulations in Italy." *An-
nals of Oncology,* 2006, *17,* 346–347.

Gans, H. *Deciding What's News: A Study of CBS Evening News, NBC Nightly
News, Newsweek and Time.* New York: Random House, 1980.

Gantenbein, R. E. "E-Health: Using Information and Communication
Technology to Improve Health Care." Presentation at the IRI Conference, Las Vegas, Nev., Nov. 2001. http://hive.cs.uwyo.edu/
~rex/eHealth.ppt. Retrieved June 2006.

Gardenswartz, L., and Rowe, A. *Managing Diversity: A Complete Desk Reference and Planning Guide.* New York: McGraw-Hill, 1993.

Garrity, T. F., Haynes, R. B., Mattson, M. E., and Engebretson, J. T. (ed.).
Medical Compliance and the Clinical-Patient Relationship: A Review.
Washington, D.C.: Government Printing Office, 1998.

Gay Men's Health Crisis. "The Gay Men's Health Crisis HIV/AIDS Timeline." New York: Gay Men's Health Crisis, 2006.

Gerbner, G. "Toward Cultural Indicators—Analysis of Mass Mediated Public Message Systems." *AV Communication Review, 1969, 17*(2), 137–148.

Gerbner, G., Gross, L., Morgan, M., and Signorielle, N. "The Main-
streaming of America: Violence Profile No. 11." *Journal of Communication,* 1980, *30,* 10–29.

Gillis, D. "Beyond Words: The Health-Literacy Connection." 2005. http://www.canadianhealthnetwork.ca/servlet/ContentServer?cid= 1059684393879&pagename=CHN-RCS/CHNResource/CHN ResourcePageTemplate&c=CHNResource&lang=En. Retrieved Oct. 2005.

Glucksberg, S., and Weisberg, R. W. "Verbal Behavior and Problem Solving: Some Effects of Labeling in a Functional Fixedness Problem." *Journal of Experimental Psychology,* 1963, *71,* 659–664.

Godfrey, F. "The Right Time for Europe to Stop Smoking." *Breathe,* 2005, *2*(1), 12–14.

Goodwin, J. S., Black, S. A., and Satish, S. "Aging Versus Disease: The Opinions of Older Black, Hispanic, and Non-Hispanic White Americans About the Causes and Treatment of Common Medical Conditions." *Journal of the American Geriatrics Society,* 1999, *47*(8), 973–979.

Gray-Felder, D., and Dean, J. *Communication for Social Change: A Position Paper and Conference Report.* New York: Rockefeller Foundation Report, 1999.

Green, L. W., and Kreuter, M. W. *Health Promotion Planning: An Educational and Environmental Approach.* (2nd ed.) Mountain View, Calif.: Mayfield, 1991.

Green, L. W., and Kreuter, M. W. *Health Promotion Planning: An Educational and Environmental Approach.* (3rd ed.) Mountain View, Calif.: Mayfield, 1999.

Green, L. W., and Ottoson, J. M. *Community and Population Health.* (8th ed.) New York: McGraw-Hill, 1999.

Greenberg, D. P., von Konig, C. H., and Heininger, U. "Health Burden of Pertussis in Infants and Children." *Pediatric Infectious Disease Journal,* 2005, *24*(5 Suppl.), S39-S43.

Greenes, R. A., and Shortliffe, E. H. "Medical Informatics: An Emerging Academic Discipline and Institutional Priority." *Journal of the American Medical Association,* 1990, *263*(8), 1114–1120.

Grimley, D., Gabrielle, R., Bellis, J., and Prochaska, J. "Assessing the Stages of Change and Decision-Making for Contraceptive Use for the Prevention of Pregnancy, Sexually Transmitted Diseases, and Acquired Immunodeficiency Syndrome." *Health Education Quarterly,* 1993, *20,* 455–470.

Grimshaw, J. M., Eccles, M. P., Walker, A. E., and Thomas, R. E. "Changing Physicians' Behavior: What Works and Thoughts on Getting More Things to Work." *Journal of Continuing Education in the Health Professions,* 2002, *22,* 237–243.

Grol, R. "Beliefs and Evidence in Changing Clinical Care." *British Medical Journal,* 1997, *315*(7105), 418–421.

Grol, R. "Changing Physicians' Competence and Performance: Finding the Balance Between the Individual and the Organization." *Journal of Continuing Education in the Health Professions,* 2002, *22,* 244–251.

Gross, A. "Overview of Asia, Healthcare Markets and Regulatory Issues in the Region." Aug. 2001. http://www.pacificbridgemedical.com/publications/html/AsiaAugust01.htm. Retrieved in Oct. 2005.

Haider, M. (ed.). *Global Public Health Communication: Challenges, Perspectives, and Strategies.* Sudbury, Mass.: Jones and Bartlett, 2005.

Harris, G. "Five Cases of Polio in Amish Group Raise New Fears." *New York Times,* Nov. 8, 2005.

Harvard Family Research Project. "Learning from Logic Models in Out-of-School Time." http://www.gse.harvard.edu/hfrp/projects/afterschool/resources/learning_logic_models.html. Retrieved Dec. 2005.

Hayes, R. B., and others. "Tobacco and Alcohol Use and Oral Cancer in Puerto Rico." *Cancer Causes Control,* 1999, *10*(1), 27–33.

Health Canada, "What Do Canadians Think About Nutrition?" 2002. http://www.hc-sc.gc.ca/fn-an/surveill/facts-faits/factsheet_canada_thinks-dossier_canada_pense_e.html. Retrieved Oct. 2005.

Health Canada and Schizophrenia Society of Canada. "Schizophrenia: A Handbook for Families." 1991. http://www.mentalhealth.com/book/p40-sc01.html#Head_5. Retrieved Jan. 2006.

Health Communication Partnership. "The New P-Process: Steps in Strategic Communication." Dec. 2003. http://www.hcpartnership.org/Publications/P-Process.pdf. Retrieved Mar. 2006.

Health Communication Partnership. "HEART Program Offers Zambian Youth Hope for an HIV/AIDS-Free Future." Dec. 2004. http://www.jhuccp.org/pubs/ci/17/17.pdf. Retrieved Mar. 2006.

Health Communication Partnership. "CCP Graduate Seminar Series Convergence and Bounded Normative Influence Theory." http://www.hcpartnership.org/Topics/Communication/theory/2004–04–16.ppt. Retrieved Sept. 2005a.

Health Communication Partnership. "Introduction to Theories of Communication Effects: Diffusion Theory." http://www.hcpartnership.org/Topics/Communication/theory/2004–04–02.ppt. Retrieved Sept. 2005b.

Health Communication Partnership. "Introduction to Theories of Communication Effects: Social Learning Theory." http://www.hcpartnership.org/Topics/Communication/theory/256,1,Slide 1. Retrieved Sept. 2005c.

Health Communication Partnership. "Introduction to Theories of Communication Effects: The Theory of Reasoned Action." http://www.

hcpartnership.org/Topics/Communication/theory/2004–03–19.ppt. Retrieved Sept. 2005d.

Health Communication Partnership. "About the Health Communication Partnership (HCP)." http://www.hcpartnership.org/About/about. php /. Retrieved Sept. 2005e.

Health Communication Partnership. "How to Mobilize Communities for Health and Social Change." http://www.hcpartnership.org/ Publications/comm_mob/htmlDocs/cac.htm. Retrieved Jan. 2006a.

Health Communication Partnership. "Africa, Namibia, Community Mobilization/Participation." http://www.hcpartnership.org/Programs/ Africa/Namibia/community_mobilization.php. Retrieved Jan. 2006b.

Health Communication Partnership. "About the Health Communication Partnership (HCP): Using Strategic Communication, Engaging Communities for Change." http://www.hcpartnership.org/ About/about.php. Retrieved Jan. 2006c.

Health Communication Unit. Center for Health Promotion. University of Toronto. "Overview of Health Communication Campaigns: Step 5 Set Communication Objectives." 1999. http://www.thcu.ca/ infoandresources/publications/OHC_Master_Workbook_v3.1. format.July.30.03_content.apr30.99.pdf. Retrieved Feb. 2006.

Health Communication Unit. Center for Health Promotion. University of Toronto. "Setting Communication Objectives Lecturette." Oct. 2003a. http://www.thcu.ca/infoandresources/publications/Step FiveSettingObjectivesForWebOct9–03.pdf. Retrieved Mar. 2006.

Health Communication Unit. Center for Health Promotion. University of Toronto. "Selecting Channels and Vehicles Lecturette." Oct. 2003b. http://www.thcu.ca/infoandresources/publications/StepSixSelect ChannelsVehiclesForWebOct9-03.pdf. Retrieved Mar. 2006.

Health Communication Unit. Center for Health Promotion. University of Toronto. "Lecturette on Health Communication Evaluation, Effectiveness and Why Campaigns Fail." Oct. 2003c. http://www. thcu.ca/infoandresources/publications/StepTwelveEvaluationEf- fectivenessWhyCampaignsFailForWebOct9–03.pdf. Retrieved Mar. 2006.

Health Communication Unit. Center for Health Promotion. University of Toronto. "Implementing THCU's Twelve Steps. PACE: A Campaign Preventing and Addressing FASD from the Hamilton-Wentworth Drug and Alcohol Awareness Committee." Nov. 2004. http:// www.thcu.ca/infoandresources/publications/CaseStudy2.pace.v1. 02.pdf. Retrieved Mar. 2006.

Health Communication Unit. Center for Health Promotion. University of Toronto. "Health Communication." http://www.thcu.ca/

infoandresources/health_communication.htm. Retrieved Mar. 2006.

Hester, E. L. *Successful Marketing Research.* Hoboken, N.J.: Wiley, 1996.

Heurtin-Roberts, S. "High-pertension: The Uses of a Chronic Folk Illness for Personal Adaptation." *Social Science Medicine,* 1993, *37,* 285–294.

Heurtin-Roberts, S., and Reisin, E. "The Relation of Culturally Influenced Lay Models of Hypertension to Compliance with Treatment." *American Journal of Hypertension,* 1992, *5,* 787–792.

Hodge-Gray, E., and Caldamone, A. A. "Primary Nocturnal Enuresis: A Review." *Journal of School Nursing,* 1998, *14*(3), 38–42.

Hofstede, G. *Culture's Consequences: International Differences in Work-Related Values.* Thousand Oaks, Calif.: Sage, 1984.

Hofstede, G. *Culture's Consequences: Comparing Values, Behaviors, and Organizations Across Nations.* (2nd ed.) Thousand Oaks, Calif.: Sage, 2001.

Holtzman, D., and Rubinson, R. "Parent and Peer Communication Effects on AIDS-Related Behavior Among U.S. High School Students." *Family Planning Perspectives,* 1995, *27*(6), 235–240, 268.

Hornik, R. "Speaking of Health: Assessing Health Communication Strategies for Diverse Populations." 2003. http://foundation.acponline. org/healthcom/hcc2/hornik.ppt. Retrieved Feb. 2006.

Houston, S. D. "The Archaeology of Communication Technologies." *Annual Review of Anthropology,* 2004, *33,* 223–250.

Hsu, V. P., and others. "Opening a *Bacillus anthracis*-Containing Envelope, Capitol Hill, Washington, D.C.: Public Health Response." *Emergency Infectious Diseases,* 2002, *8*(10), 1039–1043.

Hufford, M. "American Folklife: A Commonwealth of Cultures." http://www.loc.gov/folklife/cwc. Retrieved Oct. 2005.

Hustig, H. H., and Norrie, P. "Managing Schizophrenia in the Community." *Medical Journal of Australia.* 1998. http://www.mja.com.au. http://www.mja.com.au/public/mentalhealth/articles/hustig/ hustig.html. Retrieved Feb. 2006.

Hwa-Froelich, D. A., and Vigil, D. "Three Aspects of Cultural Influence on Communication: A Literature Review." *Communication Disorders Quarterly,* 2004, *25*(3), 107.

Institute of Medicine. *Crossing the Quality Chasm.* Washington, D.C.: National Academies Press, 2001.

Institute of Medicine. *Speaking of Health Assessing Health Communication Strategies for Diverse Populations.* Washington, D.C.: National Academies Press, 2002.

Institute of Medicine. *Who Will Keep the Public Healthy?* Washington, D.C.: The National Academies Press, 2003.

Institute of Medicine. "Report Brief. Apr. 2004. Health Literacy: A Prescription to End Confusion." Washington D.C.: National Academies Press. http://www.iom.edu/report.asp?id=19723. Retrieved Oct. 2004.

Institute for Public Relations. "Dictionary for Public Relations Measurement and Research." 2002.http://www.instituteforpr.com/pdf/Dictionary.pdf. Retrieved Dec. 2005.

Institute for Public Relations. "Guidelines for Measuring the Effectiveness of PR Programs and Activities." http://www.instituteforpr.com/pdf/2002_Guidelines_Standards_Book.pdf. 1997, 2003. Retrieved Dec. 2005.

International Center for Research on Women. "Disentangling HIV and AIDS Stigma in Ethiopia, Tanzania and Zambia." 2003. http://www.icrw.org/docs/stigmareport093003.pdf. Retrieved Feb. 2006.

Issue Management Council. "What Is Issue Management?" http://www.issuemanagement.org/documents/im_details.html#clarification%20of%20terms. Retrieved Dec. 2005.

Janz, N. K., and Becker, M. H. "The Health Belief Model: A Decade Later." *Health Education Quarterly*, 1984, *11*(1), 1–47.

Javidi, M., Long, L. W. , Long, P. N., and Javidi, A. "An Examination of Interpersonal Communication Motives Across Age Groups." Paper presented at the meeting of the Speech Communication Association, Chicago, Nov. 1990.

Jernigan, D. B., and others. "Investigation of Bioterrorism-Related Anthrax, United States, 2001: Epidemiologic Findings." *Emergency Infectious Diseases*, 2002, *8*(10), 1019–1028.

Jitaru, E., Moisil, I., and Jitaru, M. C. "Criteria for Evaluating the Quality of Health Related Sites on Internet." Paper presented at the Twenty-Second Romanian Conference on Medical Informatics Towards the Millennium, Nov. 1999. http://atlas.ici.ro/ehto/medinf99/papers/criteria_for_evaluating_the_qual.htm. Retrieved Feb. 2006.

Johnson and Johnson. "Campaign for Nursing's Future Initiative." Unpublished case study, 2005.

Joppe, M. "The Research Process." http://www.ryerson.ca/~mjoppe/ResearchProcess/. Retrieved Feb. 2006.

Joyner, A. M. "Eradication of a Disease: Keys to Success." July-Sept. 2001. http://www.prb.org/PrintTemplate.cfm?Section=July-September_2001andTemplate=/ContentManagement/HTMLDisplay.cfmand-ContentID=6233. Retrieved Mar. 2006.

Kapoor, S. C. "DOTS, NTP AND HIV." *Indian Journal of Pediatrics*, 1996, *43*(4), 177–222.

Kaur, H., Hyder, M. L., and Poston, W. S. "Childhood Overweight: An Expanding Problem." *Treatments in Endocrinology*, 2003, *2*(6), 375–388.

Kellermann, K., and Reynolds, R. "When Ignorance Is Bliss: The Role of Motivation to Reduce Uncertainty in Uncertainty Reduction Theory." *Human Communication Research*, 1990, *17*, 5–75.

Kennedy, M. G., and Abbatangelo, J. "Guidance for Evaluating Mass Communication Health Initiatives: Summary of an Expert Panel Discussion." 2005. http://www.cdc.gov/communication/practice/epreport.pdf. Retrieved Mar. 2006.

Kim, P., Eng, T., Deering, M. J., and Maxfield, A. "Published Criteria for Evaluating Health Related Web Sites: Review." *British Medical Journal*, 1999, *318*(7184), 647–649.

Kimbrell, J. D. "Coalition, Partnership, and Constituency Building by a State Public Health Agency: A Retrospective." *Journal of Public Health Management and Practice*, 2000, *6*(2), 55–61.

Kincaid, D. L. *The Convergence Model of Communication.* Honolulu: East-West Communication Institute, 1979.

Kincaid, D. L., and Figueroa, M. E. "Ideation and Communication for Social Change." Health Communication Partnership Seminar. Apr. 23, 2004. http://www.hcpartnership.org/Topics/Communication/theory/2004-04-23.ppt. Retrieved Oct. 2006.

Kincaid, D. L., Figueroa, M. E., Storey, D., and Underwood, C. *Communication and Behavior Change: The Role of Ideation.* Baltimore, Md.: Johns Hopkins University, Bloomberg School of Public Health, Center for Communication Programs, 2001.

Kotler, P., and Roberto, E. L. *Social Marketing: Strategies for Changing Public Behavior.* New York: Free Press, 1989.

Krauss, R. M., and Fussell, S. R. "Social Psychological Models of Interpersonal Communication." In E. T. Higgins and A. W. Kruglanski (eds.), *Social Psychology: Handbook of Basic Principles.* New York: Guilford Press, 1996.

Kraut, R. E. "Social and Emotional Messages of Smiling: An Ethological Approach." *Journal of Personality and Social Psychology,* 1979, *37*, 1539–1553.

Kreps, G. L., and Thornton, B. C. *Health Communication: Theory and Practice.* (2nd ed.) Prospect Heights, Ill.: Waveland Press, 1992.

Kreuter, M. W., and McClure, M. S. "The Role of Culture in Health Communication." *Annual Review of Public Health,* 2004, *25*, 439–455.

Kreuter, M. W., and Skinner, C. "Tailoring: What's in a Name?" *Health Education Research,* 2000, *15*, 1–4.

Krisberg, K. "Millions of Americans Suffer from Low Health Literacy." *Nation's Health,* June–July 2004. http://www.apha.org/journal/nation/literacycover0604.htm. Retrieved Aug. 2006.

Krugman, D. M., Fox, R. J., and Fischer, P. M. "Do Cigarette Warnings

Warn? Understanding What It Will Take to Develop More Effective Warnings." *Journal of Health Communication,* 1999, *4,* 95–104.

Laine, C., and Davidoff, F. "Patient Centered Medicine: A Professional Evaluation." *JAMA,* 1996, *275*(2), 152–156.

Lara, M., Allen, F., and Lange, L. "Physician Perceptions of Barriers to Care for Inner-City Latino Children with Asthma." *Journal of Healthcare for the Poor and Underserved,* 1999, *10*(1), 27–44.

Lavery, S. H., and others. "The Community Action Model: A Community-Driven Model Designed to Address Disparities in Health." *American Journal of Public Health,* 2005, *95*(4), 611–616.

Ledingham, J. A. "Explicating Relationship Management as a General Theory of Public Relations." *Journal of Public Relations Research,* 2003, *15*(2), 181–198.

Lewis, A. "Health as a Social Concept." *British Journal Society,* 1953, *4,* 110–115.

LexisNexis. "Search Terms: Baby and Sleep." http://www.lexisnexis.com/. Retrieved Mar. 27, 2006.

Li, K. UNICEF. "African Immunization Campaign Strikes Back Against Global Polio Epidemic." http://www.unicefusa.org/site/apps/nl/content2.asp?c=duLRI8O0Handb=39284andct=879135. Retrieved May 2005.

Lind, P., and Finley, D. "County Commissioners as a Key Constituency for Public Health." *Journal of Public Health Management and Practice,* 2000, *6*(2), 30–38.

Lipkin, M. J. "Patient Education and Counseling in the Context of Modern Patient-Physician-Family Communication." *Patient Education and Counseling,* 1996, *27*(1), 5–11.

Lukoschek, P., Fazzari, M., and Marantz, P. "Patient and Physician Factors Predict Patients' Comprehension of Health Information." *Patient Education and Counseling,* 2003, *50,* 201–210.

Maibach, E. "Pan-Canadian Healthy Living Strategy: The Roles of Communication and Social Marketing." Presentation at the Pan-Canadian Healthy Living Strategy, Public Information Strategic Direction: Social Marketing Roundtable, Sept. 23–24, 2003. http://www.phac-aspc.gc.ca/hl-vs-strat/ppt/ed_maibach/index.htm. Retrieved Oct. 2006.

Maibach, E., and Holtgrave, D. R. "Advances in Public Health Communication." *Annual Review of Public Health,* 1995, *16,* 219–238.

Marcus J. *Mesoamerican Writing Systems: Propaganda, Myth, and History in Four Ancient Civilizations.* Princeton, N.J.: Princeton University Press, 1992.

Mashberg, A., and Samit, A. "Early Diagnosis of Asymptomatic Oral and

Pharyngeal Squamous Cancers." *CA: A Cancer Journal for Clinicians,* 1995, *45*(6), 328–351.

Matiella, A. C., Middleton, K., and Thaker, N. *Guidebook to Effective Materials Development for Health Education.* Scotts Valley, Calif.: Tobacco Education Clearinghouse of California, California Department of Health Services, Tobacco Control Section, 1991.

Matsunaga, D. S., Yamada, S., and Macabeo, A. "Cross-Cultural Tuberculosis Manual." Kalihi-Palama Health Center, Association of Asian and Pacific Community Health Organizations, U.S. Centers for Disease Control, Oct. 1998. http://ethnomed.org/clin_topics/tb/tbmanual.pdf. Retrieved Nov. 2005.

McDivitt, J. A., Zimicki, S., and Hornik, R. C. "Explaining the Impact of a Communication Campaign to Change Vaccination Knowledge and Coverage in the Philippines." *Health Communication,* 1997, *9,* 95–118.

McEwen, E., and Anton-Culver, H. "The Medical Communication of Deaf Patients." *Journal of Family Practice,* 1988, *13,* 51–57.

McGuire, W. J. "Public Communication as a Strategy for Inducing Health-Promoting Behavioral Change." *Preventive Medicine,* 1984, *13*(3), 299–313.

McQuail, D. *Mass Communication Theory.* (3rd ed.) Thousand Oaks, Calif.: Sage, 1994.

Medscape. "How Stigma Interferes with Mental Healthcare: An Expert Interview with Patrick W. Corrigan, PsyD." *Medscape Psychiatry and Mental Health,* 2004, *9*(2). http://www.medscape.com/viewarticle/494548. Retrieved Jan. 2006.

Mercer, S. L., Potter, M. A., and Green, L. W. "Participatory Research: Guidelines and Lessons from the CDC's Extramural Prevention Research Program." Paper presented at the American Public Health Association 130th Annual Meeting, Philadelphia, Nov. 2002.

Mintzes, B., and Baraldi, R. "Direct-to-Consumer Prescription Drug Advertising: When Public Health Is No Longer a Priority." http://www.whp-apsf.ca/en/documents/dtca_priority.html. Retrieved Jan. 2006.

Mintzes, B., and others. "Influence of Direct to Consumer Pharmaceutical Advertising and Patients' Requests on Prescribing Decisions: Two Site Cross Sectional Survey." *British Medical Journal,* 2002, *324,* 278–279.

Mokhtar, N., and others. "Diet, Culture and Obesity in Northern Africa." *Journal of Nutrition,* 2001, *131,* 887S-892S.

Moment, D., and Zaleznik, A. *The Dynamics of Interpersonal Behavior.* Hoboken, N.J.: Wiley, 1964.

Monfrecola, G., Fabbrocini, G., Posteraro, G., and Pini, D. "What Do Young People Think About the Dangers of Sunbathing, Skin Cancer, and Sunbeds? A Questionnaire Survey Among Italians." *Photo-dermatology, Photoimmunology and Photomedicine*, 2000, *16*, 15–18.

Montecino, V. "Criteria to Evaluate the Credibility of WWW Resources." Aug. 1998. http://mason.gmu.edu/~montecin/web-eval-sites.htm. Retrieved Feb. 2006.

Morris, J. N. (ed.). *The Socio-Ecological Model: Uses of Epidemiology*. New York: Churchill Livingstone, 1975.

Morzinski, J. A., and Montagnini, M. L. "Logic Modeling: A Tool for Improving Educational Programs." *Journal of Palliative Medicine*, 2002, *5*(4), 566–570.

MSNBC. "Trans Fat Free—The Next Food Fad? Companies Rush to Get Rid of Artery-Clogging Ingredient." http://www.msnbc.msn.com/id/6840122/. Retrieved Jan. 2006.

Mueller, P. S., Plevak, D. J., and Rummans, T. A. "Religious Involvement, Spirituality and Medicine: Implications for Clinical Practice." *Mayo Clinic Proceedings*, 2001, *76*, 1225–1235.

Murray, D. M., Prokhorov, A. V., and Harty, K. C. "Effects of a Statewide Antismoking Campaign on Mass Media Messages and Smoking Beliefs." *Preventive Medicine*, 1994, *23*(1), 54–60.

Museum of Public Relations, "1992: The Case for PR Licensing." http://www.prmuseum.com/bernays/bernays_1990.html. Retrieved Nov. 2005.

Muturi, N. "Communication for HIV/AIDS Prevention in Kenya: Socio-Cultural Considerations." *Journal of Health Communication*, 2005, *10*, 77–98.

National Association of Pediatric Nurse Practitioners. "HIB Disease." http://www.hibdisease.com. Retrieved Nov. 2005.

National Cancer Institute. "Theory at a Glance: A Guide for Health Promotion Practice." http://www.cancer.gov/aboutnci/oc/theory-at-a-glance/page7. Retrieved Oct. 2005a.

National Cancer Institute. "What You Need to Know About Skin Cancer: Cause and Prevention." http://www.cancer.gov/cancertopics/wyntk/skin/page5. Retrieved Oct. 2005b.

National Cancer Institute and National Institutes of Health. *Making Health Communication Programs Work*. Bethesda, Md.: National Institutes of Health, 2002.

National Council for Public-Private Partnerships. "How Partnerships Work." http://ncppp.org/howpart/index.html. Retrieved Mar. 2006.

National Foundation for Infectious Diseases. "NFID Urges Use of New Childhood Vaccine Schedule." *Double Helix*, 1997, *22*(2).http://www.nfid.org/%5Fold/publications/helix/jun97/helix3.html. Retrieved Oct. 2005.

National Foundation for Infectious Diseases. "Flu Fight for Kids." Unpublished case study, 2005.

National Institute of Child Health and Human Development. "Safe Sleep for Your Baby: Reduce the Risk of Sudden Infant Death Syndrome (SIDS) (African American Outreach)." Oct. 2005. http://www.nichd.nih.gov/sids/sleep_risk.htm. Retrieved Feb. 2006.

National Institutes of Health. "Improving Health Literacy." http://www.nih.gov/icd/od/ocpl/resources/improvinghealthliteracy.htm. Retrieved Oct. 2005.

National Institutes of Health. "NIH News Release, February 28, 2003." 2003. http://www.nichd.nih.gov/new/releases/infant_sids_risk.cfm. Retrieved Feb. 2006.

National Institutes of Health. "Human Subjects Research and IRBs." http://www.nih.gov/sigs/bioethics/IRB.html. Retrieved Mar. 2006.

National Planning Council, Colombia. "Traditional vs. Participatory Planning." Communication Initiative, 2003. http://www.comminit.com/planningmodels/pmodels/planningmodels-93.html. Retrieved Sept. 2005.

National Public Radio. "Profile: How Sigmund Freud's Ideas Helped to Create the New Field of Public Relations." *Morning Edition*, Apr. 22, 2005.

National SIDS/Infant Death Resource Center. "SIDS Deaths by Race and Ethnicity 1995–2001." http://www.sidscenter.org/Downloads/S148.htm. Retrieved Feb. 2006.

New South Wales Department of Health, Australia. "Health Promotion Glossary." http://www.health.nsw.gov.au/public-health/health-promotion/abouthp/glossary.html. Retrieved Feb. 2006.

New York Times Company. "Circulation Data." http://www.nytco.com/investors-nyt-circulation.html. Retrieved Dec. 2005.

New York University. "Integrated Marketing Communication for Behavioral Impact in Health and Social Development 2006." http://education.nyu.edu/summer/imc/. Retrieved Mar. 2006.

Ngo-Metzger, Q., and others. "Surveying Minorities with Limited-English Proficiency: Does Data Collection Method Affect Data Quality Among Asian Americans?" *Medical Care,* 2004, *42*(9), 893–900.

Nowak, G., and others. "The Application of 'Integrated Marketing Communications' to Social Marketing and Health Communication: Organizational Challenges and Implications." *Social Marketing Quarterly,* 1998, *4*(4), 12–16.

Nuzum, E. "On-Air Program Promotions Insight Study—Final Report." May 2004. http://www.aranet.com/library/pdf/doc-0111.pdf. Retrieved Mar. 2006.

Office of Adolescent Pregnancy Programs. "Instructions for Completing the Adolescent Family Life Prevention Demonstration Project End of Year Report Template." http://www.hhs.gov/ocio/infocollect/ pending/EOYInstructionsPrev.doc. Retrieved Mar. 2006.

Office for Human Research Protections. "Office for Human Research Protections." http://www.hhs.gov/ohrp/about/ohrpfactsheet.pdf. Retrieved Mar. 2006.

101PublicRelations.com. "Public Relations: How to Make Your Story Pitch Stand Out in the Email Jungle." http://101publicrelations. com/blog/cat_marketing_and_sales.html. Retrieved Dec. 2005.

O'Sullivan, G. A., Yonkler, J. A., Morgan, W., and Merritt, A. P. *A Field Guide to Designing a Health Communication Strategy.* Baltimore, Md.: Johns Hopkins Bloomberg School of Public Health, Center for Communication Programs, 2003.

Painter, A. F., and Lemkau, J. P. "Turning Roadblocks into Stepping Stones: Teaching Psychology to Physicians." *Teaching of Psychology,* 1992, *19*(3), 183–184.

Paletz, D. L. *The Media in American Politics: Contents and Consequences.* New York: Longman, 1999.

Pang, C. "The Koreans." In N. Palafox and A. Warren (eds.), *Cross Cultural Caring: A Handbook for Health Care Professions in Hawaii.* Honolulu: Transcultural Healthcare Forum, 1980.

Parkin, D. M., and others (eds.). *Cancer Incidence in Five Continents.* Lyon: IARC, 1997.

Partnering for Patient Empowerment Through Community Awareness (PPECA). "PPECA Home Page." http://www.galter.northwestern. edu/ppeca/. Retrieved June 2005.

Patel, D. "Social Mobilization as a Tool for Outreach Programs in the HIV/AIDS Crisis." In M. Haider (ed.), *Global Public Health Communication: Challenges, Perspectives, and Strategies.* Sudbury, Mass.: Jones and Bartlett, 2005.

Paunio, M., and others. "Increase of Vaccination Coverage by Mass Media and Individual Approach: Intensified Measles, Mumps, and Rubella Prevention Program in Finland." *American Journal of Epidemiology,* 1991, *133*(11), 1152–1160.

Pearson, J. C., and Nelson, P. E. *Understanding and Sharing.* (5th ed.) Dubuque, Iowa: Wm. C. Brown, 1991.

Pechmann, C. "A Comparison of Health Communication Models: Risk Learning Versus Stereotype Priming." *Media Psychology,* 2001, *3*(2), 189–210.

Perlotto, M. "The Invisible Partner: How the Marketing Department Supports Your Sales Efforts." 2005. http://www.pharmrep.com/pharmrep/ article/articleDetail.jsp?id=160030. Retrieved Mar. 2006.

Pernice, D., and others. "Italian Validation of the Royal Free Interview for

Religious and Spiritual Beliefs." *Functional Neurology*, 2005, *20*(2), 77–84.

Physicians for Human Rights. "An Action Plan to Prevent Brain Drain: Building Equitable Health Systems in Africa." Health Action AIDS, June 2004. http://www.phrusa.org/campaigns/aids/pdf/brain drain.pdf. Retrieved Mar. 2006.

Pikoulis, E., Waasdorp, B. S., Leppaniemi, A., and Burris, D. "Hippocrates: The True Father of Medicine." *American Surgeon*, 1998, *64*(3), 274–275.

Pinto E. "KAP Study: Common Practices and Attitudes toward Malaria, 1998." Unpublished report. UNICEF, Angola.

Piotrow, P. T., Kincaid, D. L., Rimon, J. G., and Rinehart, W. *Health Communication: Lessons from Family Planning and Reproductive Health.* Westport, Conn.: Praeger, 1997.

Piotrow, P. T., Rimon, J. G. II, Payne Merritt, A., and Saffitz, G. *Advancing Health Communication: The PCS Experience in the Field.* Baltimore, Md.: Johns Hopkins Bloomberg School of Public Health, Center for Communication Programs, 2003.

Porter, R. W., and others. "Role of Health Communications in Russia's Diphtheria Immunization Program." *Journal of Infectious Diseases,* 2000, *181*(Supp. 1), S220-7.

Prochaska, J., and DiClemente, C. C. "Stages and Process of Self-Change of Smoking: Toward an Integrative Model of Change." *Journal of Consulting and Clinical Psychology*, 1983, *51*, 390–395.

Prochaska, J. O., and Vleicer, W. F. "The Transtheoretical Model of Health Behavior Change." *American Journal of Health Promotion*, 1997, *12*(1), 38–48.

Program for Appropriate Technology in Health. "How Bingwa Changed His Ways." Unpublished case study, 2005a.

Program for Appropriate Technology in Health. "Community Theater in Benin: Taking the Show on the Road." Unpublished case study, 2005b.

Prue, C. E., Lackey, C., Swenarski, L. and Gantt, J. M. "Communication Monitoring: Shaping CDC's Emergency Risk Communication Efforts." *Journal of Health Communication*, 2003, *8*(Suppl. 1), 35–49.

Public Relations Society of America. "The Public Relations Profession: About Public Relations." http://www.prsa.org/_Resources/Profession/index.asp?ident=profl. Retrieved Nov. 2005a.

Public Relations Society of America. "PRSA Member Code of Ethics 2000." http://www.prssa.org/downloads/codeofethics.pdf. Retrieved Nov. 2005b.

QuickMBA. "Marketing Research." http://www.quickmba.com/marketing/research/. Retrieved Feb. 2006.

Ramirez, A. G., and others. "Advancing the Role of Participatory Communication in the Diffusion of Cancer Screening Among Hispanics." *Journal of Health Communication*, 1999, *4*(1), 31–36.

Randall, V. R. "Racial Discrimination in Health Care and CERD." Dayton, Ohio: Institute on Race, Health Care and the Law, University of Dayton School of Law. http://academic.udayton.edu/health/07Human Rights/racial01.htm. Retrieved Mar. 2006.

Ratzan, C., and others. "Education for the Health Communication Professional." *American Behavioral Scientist*, 1994, *38*(2), 361–380.

Rednova. "Explanatory Models of Diabetes Among Asian and Caucasian Participants." http://rn-c.rednova.com/news/health/131170/explanatory_models_ of_diabetes_among_asian_and caucasian participants/index.html. Retrieved Oct. 2005.

Reeves, P. M. "Coping in Cyberspace: The Impact of Internet Use on the Ability of HIV-Positive Individuals to Deal with Their Illness." *Journal of Health Communication*, 2000, *5*(Suppl.), 47–59.

Renganathan, E., and others. "Communication-for–Behavioral-Impact (COMBI): A Review of WHO's Experiences with Strategic Social Mobilization and Communication in the Prevention and Control of Communicable Diseases." In M. Haider (ed.), *Global Public Health Communication: Challenges, Perspectives, and Strategies*. Sudbury, Mass.: Jones and Bartlett, 2005.

Rhode Island Department of Health. "Office of Minority Health African-American/Black Culture and Health." http://www.health.ri.gov/chic/minority/afr_cul.php. Oct. 2005a.

Rhode Island Department of Health. "Office of Minority Health Latino/Hispanic Culture and Health." http://www.health.ri.gov/chic/minority/lat_cul.php. Oct. 2005b.

Rhode Island Department of Health. "Office of Minority Health Native American Culture and Health." http://www.health.ri.gov/chic/minority/natcul.php. Oct. 2005c.

Rhode Island Department of Health. "Office of Minority Health Southeast Asian Culture and Health." http://www.health.ri.gov/chic/minority/asi_cul.php. Oct. 2005d.

Rienks, J., and others. "Evidence That Social Marketing Campaigns Can Effectively Increase Awareness of Infant Mortality Disparities." Paper presented at the Annual Meeting of the American Public Health Association, Philadelphia, Dec. 13, 2005.

Rimon, J. G. "Behaviour Change Communication in Public Health.

Beyond Dialogue: Moving Toward Convergence." The Communi-cation Initative, 2002. http://www.comminit.com/strategicthink ing/stnicroundtable/sld-1744.html. Retrieved Nov. 2005.

Robert Graham Center. Policy Studies in Family Practice and Primary Care. "Patterns of Visits to Physicians' Offices, 1980 to 2003." Sept. 2005, n. 35. American Academy of Family Physicians. http://www. graham-center.org/x587.xml. Retrieved Feb. 2006.

Robinson, T. N., Patrick, K., Eng, T. R., and Gustafson, D. "An Evidence-Based Approach to Interactive Health Communication: A Challenge to Medicine in the Information Age." *Journal of the American Medical Association,* 1998, *280,* 1264–1269.

Rockefeller Foundation Communication and Social Change Network. "Measuring and Evaluating Communication for Social Change." Communication Initiative, June 2001.http://www.comminit.com/ socialchange/measure_eval/sld-2076.html. Retrieved Mar. 2006.

Rogers, E. M. *Diffusion of Innovations.* New York: Free Press, 1962.

Rogers, E. M. "Communication and Development: The Passing of the Dominant Paradigm." *Communication Research,* 1976, *3*(2), 213–240.

Rogers, E. M. *Diffusion of Innovations* (3rd ed.) New York: Free Press, 1983.

Rogers, E. M. *Diffusion of Innovations.* (4th ed.) New York: Free Press, 1995.

Rogers, E. M., and Kincaid, D. L. *Communication Networks: Towards a New Paradigm for Research.* New York: Free Press, 1981.

Rogers, R. W. "A Protection Motivation Theory of Fear Appeals and Atti-tude Change." *Journal of Psychology, 91,* 93–114, 1975.

Rogers, R. W. "Cognitive and Physiological Processes in Fear Appeals and Attitude Change: A Revised Theory of Protection Motivation." In J. Cacioppo and R. Petty (eds.), *Social Psychophysiology.* New York: Guilford Press, 1983.

Roloff, M. E. *Interpersonal Communication: The Social Exchange Approach.* Thousand Oaks, Calif.: Sage, 1987.

Rosenstock, I. M., and Kirscht, J. P. "The Health Belief Model and Per-sonal Health Behavior." *Health Education Monographs,* 1974, *2,* 470–473.

Rubin, R. B., Perse, E. M., and Barbato, C. A. "Conceptualization and Measurement of Interpersonal Communication Motives." *Human Communication Research,* 1988, *14,* 602–628.

Ruxin, J., and others. "Emerging Consensus in HIV/AIDS, Malaria, Tu-berculosis, and Access to Essential Medicines." *Lancet,* 2005, *356*(9459), 618–621.

Saba, W. "Why Invest in Health Communication?" Feb. 21, 2006. The Communication Initiative. http://forums.comminit.com/view

topic.php?t=60061andpostdays=0andpostorder=ascandandstart=45 andsid=e3887d65f69451e3949aae2a487b9601andstyle=1. Retrieved Mar. 2006.

Sarriot, E. "Sustaining Child Survival: Many Roads to Choose, But Do We Have a Map. Background Document for the Child Survival Sustainability Assessment (CSSA)." Sept. 2002. http://www.childsurvival. com/documents/CSTS/csts_new.pdf. Retrieved Mar. 2006.

Saunders, M.N.K., Lewis, P., and Thornhill, A. *Research Methods for Business Students*. (3rd ed.) Upper Saddle River, N.J.: Prentice Hall, 2003.

Schepens Eye Research Institute. "Media and Public Relations." 2003. http://www.theschepens.org/pr.htm. Retrieved Nov. 2005.

Schiavo, R. "UNICEF Marketing and Production Study Preliminary Analysis/Research Protocol: The Marketing and Distribution of Insecticide-Treated Mosquito Nets in Angola—A National Program." Unpublished report. Luanda, Angola: UNICEF, National Malaria Control Program, Dec. 18, 1998.

Schiavo, R. "Marketing and Production Study Final Report/Research Results: The Marketing and Distribution of Insecticide-Treated Mosquito Nets in Angola—A National Program." Unpublished report. Luanda, Angola: UNICEF, National Malaria Control Program, May 4, 2000.

Schiavo, R. "Why Invest in Health Communication?" The Communication Initiative. http://forums.comminit.com/viewtopic.php?t= 60061andpostdays=0andpostorder=ascandandstart=60andstyle=1. Retrieved Mar. 2006.

Schiavo, R., and Robson, P. *Workshop sobre Éstrategias de Proteção Contra a Malária em Angola* [Workshop on malaria protection strategies in Angola]. Unpublished report. Luanda, Angola: UNICEF, National Malaria Control Program, 1999.

Schober, M. F., and Clark, H. H. "Understanding by Addressees and Observers." *Cognitive Psychology,* 1989, *21,* 211–232.

Scholl, H. J. "Applying Stakeholder Theory to E-Government: Benefits and Limits." Paper presented at the First IFIP Conference on E-commerce, E-business, E-government, Zurich, Switzerland. Oct. 2001. http:// www.albany.edu/~hjscholl/Scholl_IFIP_2001.pdf. Retrieved July 2006.

Schultz, D., and Schultz, H. *IMC: The Next Generation.* New York: McGraw-Hill, 2003.

Schultz, D., Tannerbaum, S. I., and Lauterborn, R. F. *The New Marketing Paradigm: Integrated Marketing Communications.* Chicago: NTC Business Books, 1994.

Schuster, M., McGlynn, E., and Brook, R. "How Good Is the Quality of Care in the United States?" *Milbank Quarterly,* 1998, *76,* 517–563.

Schutz, W. C. *The Interpersonal Underworld.* Palo Alto, Calif.: Science and Behavioral Books, 1966.

Selden, C. R., and others (eds.). *Health Literacy, January 1990 Through 1999.* Bethesda, Md.: National Library of Medicine, Feb. 2000.

Sellors, J. W., and others. "Incidence, Clearance and Predictors of Human Papillomavirus Infection in Women." *Canadian Medical Association Journal,* 2003, *168*(4), 421–425.

Sheikh, A. "Book of the Month: Religion, Health and Suffering." *Journal of the Royal Society of Medicine,* 1999, *92,* 600–601.

Slater, M. D. "Theory and Method in Health Audience Segmentation." *Journal of Health Communication,* 1996, *1,* 267–283.

Slotnick, H. B., and Shershneva, M. B. "Use of Theory to Interpret Elements of Change." *Journal of Continuing Education in the Health Professions,* 2002, *22,* 197–204.

Smith, R. D. "Psychological Type and Public Relations: Theory, Research, and Applications." *Journal of Public Relations Research,* 1993, *5*(3), 177–199.

Smith, W. A., and Hornik, R. "Marketing, Communication, and Advocacy for Large-Scale STD/HIV Prevention and Control." In K. K. Holmes and others (eds.), *Sexually Transmitted Diseases.* New York: McGraw-Hill, 1999.

Society for Neuroscience. "Programs." http://web.sfn.org/Template.cfm?Section=Programs. Retrieved Mar. 2006.

Solomon, D. "Conducting Web-Based Surveys. ERIC Digest." *ERIC Digest,* 2001. http://www.ericdigests.org/2002–2/surveys.htm. Retrieved Mar. 2006.

Solomon, M. Z. "The Enormity of Task: Support and Changing Practice." *Hastings Center Report,* 1995, *25*(6), S28-S32.

Solomon, M. Z., and others. "Toward an Expanded Vision of Clinical Ethics Education: From the Individual to the Institution." *Kennedy Institute of Ethics Journal,* 1991, *1*(3), 225–245.

Soul Beat Africa. "Situation Analysis Report on STD/HIV/AIDS in Nigeria." Communication Initiative. http://www.comminit.com/healthecomm/research.php?showdetails=178. Retrieved Feb. 2006.

Southwest Center for the Application of Prevention Technologies. "Community Based Social Marketing." 2001. http://captus.samhsa.gov/southwest/resources/documents/307,12,Slide 12. Retrieved Feb. 2006.

Spickard, A., Jr., and others. "Changes Made by Physicians Who Misprescribed Controlled Substances." Nashville, Tenn.: Vanderbilt University Medical Center. 2001. http://www.mc.vanderbilt.edu/root/vumc.php?site=cph&doc=1094. Retrieved Feb. 2006.

Spiegel, A. "Freud's Nephew and the Origins of Public Relations." http://www.npr.org/templates/story/story.php?storyId=4612464. Retrieved Nov. 2005.

Springston, J. K., Keyton, J., Leichty, G., and Metzger, J. "Field Dynamics and Public Relations Theory: Toward the Management of Multiple Publics." *Journal of Public Relations Research,* 1992, *4*(2), 81–100.

Springston, J. K., and Lariscy, R. A. "Health as Profit: Public Relations in Health Communication." Paper presented at the American Public Health Association 129th Annual Meeting, Atlanta, Ga., Oct. 2001. http://apha.confex.com/apha/129am/techprogram/paper_26391. htm. Retrieved Jan. 2006.

Standing Committee of European Doctors. "On Information to Patients and Patient Empowerment." July 2004. http://cpme.dyndns. org:591/adopted/CPME_AD_Brd_110904_080_EN.pdf. Retrieved Nov. 2005.

Steenholdt, D. "Enhancing Patient Outcomes Through the Utilization of Evidenced Based Best Practices." http://www.sdfmc.org/ClassLibrary/ Page/Information/DataInstances/235/Files/1235/Enhancing_ Patient_Outcomes_through_Utilization_of_Evidenced_Based_Best_ Practices.pdf. Retrieved Jan. 2006.

Step, M. M., and Finucane, M. O. "Interpersonal Communication Motives in Everyday Interactions." *Communication Quarterly,* 2002, *50*(1), 93–109.

Stock-Iwamoto, C., and Korte, R. "Primary Health Workers in North East Brazil." *Social Science and Medicine,* 1993, *36*(6), 775–782.

Strecher, V. J., and Rosenstock, I. M. *The Health Belief Model.* San Francisco: Jossey-Bass, 1997.

Sullivan, D. "Nielsen NetRatings Search Engine Ratings." Search EngineWatch, http://searchenginewatch.com/reports/article. php/2156451. Retrieved Feb. 2006.

Tan, T. "Summary: Epidemiology of Pertussis." *Pediatric Infectious Disease Journal,* 2005, *24*(5 Suppl.), S35-S38.

Tannebaum, R. D. "Emergency Medicine in Brazil." *Emedicine.* http:// www.emedicine.com/emerg/topic930.htm. Retrieved Feb. 2006.

Tufts University Student Services. "Exploring the Health Professions Handbook." http://studentservices.tufts.edu/hpa/handbook.shtm. Retrieved Feb. 2006.

TV-Turnoff Network. "Facts and Figures About Our TV Habit." http:// www.tvturnoff.org/images/factsandfigs/factsheets/FactsFigs.pdf. Retrieved Nov. 2005.

Twaddle, A. G., and Hessler, R. M. *A Sociology of Health.* New York: Auburn House, 1987.

UCLA Department of Epidemiology. School of Public Health and CNN.

"Six Months Later: Anthrax Lessons Learned." http://www.ph. ucla.edu/epi/bioter/sixmoanthraxlessons.html. Retrieved Mar. 2002.

Ukrainian Catholic Church in Australia, New Zealand and Oceania. "What Is the Meaning of Illness?" http://catholicukes.org.au/ tiki/tiki-print_article.php?articleId=160. Retrieved Jan. 2006.

UMass Medical School. "Macy Initiative in Health Communication." http://www.umassmed.edu/macy/. Retrieved Mar. 2006.

UNAIDS. "Community Mobilization." http://www.unaids.org/en/ Issues/Prevention_treatment/community_mobilization.asp. Retrieved Sept. 2005.

UNICEF. Division of Communication, Health Communication Materials. "Communication Programme Planning Work Sheet." Communication Initiative, 2001. http://www.comminit.com/planningmodels/ pmodels/planningmodels-22.html. Retrieved Sept. 2005.

UNICEF. "Right to Know Initiative: Communication Strategy Development Handbook." http://www.actforyouth.net/documents/comstrat_ toolkit.pdf. Retrieved Mar. 2006.

Unilever. "Unilever to Make Country Crock Soft Spreads Trans-Fat-Free." http://www.unileverna.com/ourcompany/newsandmedia/ pressreleases/2005_PressReleases/Country_Crock_TFF.asp. Retrieved Jan. 2006.

United Nations Development Programme. "The Legislature and Constituency Relations." http://www.undp.org/governance/docs/ Parl-Pub-constrelat.htm. Retrieved Feb. 2006.

University of Michigan Health System. Program for Multicultural Health. http://www.med.umich.edu/multicultural/ccp/africanamerican. htm. Retrieved Oct. 2005.

University of Utah. "IMC: Integrated Marketing Communication Certificate Program. Communication Institute. University of Utah." http://www.communication.utah.edu/certificate/imc/imcinfo.pdf. Retrieved Mar. 2006.

University of Wisconsin-Extension. "Program Development and Evaluation." http://www.uwex.edu/ces/pdande/evaluation/evallogicmodel. html. Retrieved Dec. 2005.

U.S. Agency for International Development. "Behavior Change Interventions." 1999. http://www.comminit.com/planningmodels/ pmodels/planningmodels-95.html. Retrieved Feb. 2006.

U.S. Department of Health and Human Services. *The Health Consequences of Using Smokeless Tobacco. A Report of the Advisory Committee to the Surgeon General.* Washington, D.C.: U.S. Department of Health and Human Services, 1986.

U.S. Department of Health and Human Services. *Preventing Tobacco Use*

Among Young People: A Report of the Surgeon General. Washington, D.C.: U.S. Department of Health and Human Services, 1994.

U.S. Department of Health and Human Services, National Committee on Vital and Health Statistics. *Information for Health: A Strategy for Building the National Health Information Infrastructure.* Washington, D.C.: U.S. Department of Health and Human Services, 2001. http://aspe.hhs.gov/sp/nhii/Documents/NHIIReport2001/default.htm. Retrieved Oct. 2006.

U.S. Department of Health and Human Services. Office of Disease Prevention and Health Promotion. *Healthy People 2010.* Volumes 1 and 2. http://www.healthypeople.gov/document/HTML/Voume1/11 HealthCom.htm. 2005.

U.S. Department of Health and Human Services. Office of Disease Prevention and Health Promotion. "Making Better Health Communication a Reality: A Midcourse Check on Healthy People 2010 Objectives." *Prevention Report,* 2006a, *20*(3, 4). http://odphp.osophs.dhhs.gov/pubs/prevrpt/Volume20/Issue3pr.htm. Retrieved July 2006.

U.S. Department of Health and Human Services. Office of Minority Health. "What Is Cultural Competence?" 2006b. http://www.omhrc.gov/templates/browse.aspx?lvl=2&lvlID=11. Retrieved Oct. 2006.

U.S. Food and Drug Administration. "FDA Licenses New Vaccine for Prevention of Cervical Cancer and Other Diseases in Females Caused by Human Papillomavirus." *FDA News,* June 8, 2006. http://www.fda.gov/bbs/topics/NEWS/2006/NEW01385.html. Retrieved Oct. 2006.

Vanderford, M. L. "Communication Lessons Learned in the Emergency Operations Center During CDC's Anthrax Response: A Commentary." *Journal of Health Communication,* 2003, *8*(Suppl. 1), 11–12.

VanLeeuwen, J. A., Waltner-Toews, D., Abernathy, T., and Smit, B. "Evolving Models of Human Health Toward an Ecosystem Context." *Ecosystem Health,* 1999, *5*(3), 204–219.

Viswanathan, M., and others. *Community-Based Participatory Research: Assessing the Evidence.* Rockville, Md.: Agency for Healthcare Research and Quality, Aug. 2004.

Vlassoff, C., and Manderson, L. "Incorporating Gender in the Anthropology of Infectious Diseases." *Tropical Medicine and International Health,* 1998, *3*(12), 1011–1019.

Waisbord, S. "Family Tree of Theories, Methodologies and Strategies in Development Communication." May 2001. Prepared for the Rockefeller Foundation. The Communication Initiative. http://www.comminit.com/pdf/familytree.pdf. Retrieved Dec. 2005.

Waisbord, S. "Communication Lessons Learned in Polio Eradication."

Jan. 2004. The Communication Initiative. http://www.comminit. com/strategicthinking/stcommforpolio/thinking-1005.html. Retrieved Dec. 2005.

Waisbord, S., and Larson, H. *Why Invest in Communication for Immunization: Evidence and Lessons Learned.* Baltimore, Md.: Johns Hopkins Bloomberg School of Public Health, Center for Communication Programs, and New York: United Nations Children's Fund, June 2005.

Wang, S. S., Brownell, K. D., and Wadden, T. A. "The Influence of the Stigma of Obesity on Overweight Individuals." *International Journal of Obesity,* 2004, *28*(10), 1333–1337.

Washington State Department of Health. "Guidelines for Developing Easy-to-Read Health Education Materials." June 2000. http:// www3.doh.wa.gov/here/howto/images/easy2.html. Retrieved Mar. 2006.

Watson, S. "Using Results to Improve the Lives of Children and Families: A Guide for Public-Private Child Care Partnerships." Fairfax, Va.: National Child Care Information Center, 2000. http://nccic.org/ ccpartnerships/results.pdf. Retrieved Dec. 2005.

Weinrich, N. K. *Hands-on Social Marketing: A Step-by-Step Guide.* Thousand Oaks, Calif.: Sage, 1999.

Weinstock, H., Berman, S., and Cates, W., Jr. "Sexually Transmitted Diseases Among American Youth: Incidence and Prevalence Estimates, 2000." *Perspectives on Sexual and Reproductive Health,* 2004, *36*(1), 6–10.

White House. "Biodefense for the 21st Century." Apr. 2004. http://www. whitehouse.gov/homeland/20040430.html. Retrieved Mar. 2006.

Wiggins, B. B., and Deeb-Sossa, N. "Conducting Telephone Surveys." 2000. http://www.irss.unc.edu/irss/bwiggins/shortcourses/telephone-handout.pdf. Retrieved Mar. 2006.

Winau, R. "The Hippocratic Oath and Ethics in Medicine." *Forensic Science International,* 1994, *9*(3), 285–289.

Witte, K., and Allen, M. "A Meta-Analysis of Fear Appeals: Implications for Effective Public Health Campaigns." *Health Education and Behavior,* 2000, *27*(5), 591–615.

Woods, J. E., and Kiely, J. M. "Short-Term International Medical Services." *Mayo Clinics Proceedings,* 2000, *75,* 311–313.

World Health Organization. "Constitution of the World Health Organization." New York, July 22, 1946. http://w3.whosea.org/about-searo/pdf/const.pdf. Retrieved Oct. 2005.

World Health Organization. Mediterranean Centre for Vulnerability Reduction. "Mobilizing for Action, Communication-for-Behavioural-Impact (COMBI)." 2003. The Communication Initiative. http://

www.comminit.com/pdf/Combi4-pager_Nov_14.pdf. Retrieved Oct. 2005.

World Health Organization and Global Polio Eradication Initiative. "Polio Eradication in India." http://www.polioeradication.org/content/videoaudio/diary/index.asp. Nov. 2004a.

World Health Organization. Mediterranean Center for Vulnerability Reduction. "COMBI in Action: Country Highlights." 2004b. http://wmc.who.int/pdf/COMBI_in_Action_04.pdf. Retrieved Nov. 2005.

World Health Organization. "Social Mobilization to Fight Ebola in Yambio, Southern Sudan." Action Against Infection, 2004c. http://wmc.who.int/pdf/Action_Against_Infection.pdf. Retrieved Jan. 2006.

World Health Organization. Social Mobilization and Training Team. "Guidelines for Social Mobilization, Planning Communication-for-Behavioural-Impact (COMBI) in TB Control." http://www.stoptb.org/wg/advocacy_communication/assets/documents/TB-COMBI%20Guide%202.pdf. Retrieved Nov. 2005.

World Health Organization. "Malaria and Travelers." http://www.who.int/malaria/preventionmethods.html. Retrieved Feb. 2006.

World Health Organization and Joint United Nations Programme on HIV/AIDS. "Access to HIV Treatment Continues to Accelerate in Developing Countries, But Bottlenecks Persist, Says WHO/UNAIDS Report." 2005. http://www.who.int/3by5/progressreportJune2005/en/. Retrieved Jan. 2006.

Zagaria, M.A.E. "Low Health Literacy: Raising Awareness for Optimal Health Communication." *U.S. Pharmacist*, 2004, *10*, 41–48.

Zaman, F., and Underwood, C. *The Gender Guide for Health Communication Programs*. Baltimore, Md.: Johns Hopkins Bloomberg School of Public Health, Center for Communication Programs, Mar. 2003.

Zorn, M., Allen, M. P., and Horowitz, A. M. (comps.). "Understanding Health Literacy and Its Barriers: Bibliography on the Internet." Bethesda, Md.: National Library of Medicine, May 2004. http://www.nlm.nih.gov/pubs/cbm/healthliteracybarriers.html. Retrieved July 2006.

Zuger, A. "Doctors Learn How to Say What No One Wants to Hear." *New York Times*, Jan. 10, 2006.

Zunker, C., Rutt, C., and Meza, G. "Perceived Health Needs of Elderly Mexicans Living on the U.S.–Mexico Border." *Journal of Transcultural Nursing*, 2005, *16*(1), 50–56.

NAME INDEX

A

Abbatangelo, J., 346, 347
Abernathy, T., 23
Adams, J., 215
Ader, M., 219
Ahorlu, C., 83
Ajzen, I., 40
Al-Khayat, M. H., 80
Alcalay, R., 44, 327
Allen, F., 233
Allen, M., 308, 309
Allen, M. P., 63
Amoah, S. O., 161
Andersen, M. R., 73
Andreasen, A. R., 38, 46, 47, 48, 153, 265, 268
Anton-Culver, H., 20
Arias, J. R., 310
Atkin, C., 233

B

Babalola, S., 149, 150, 157
Babrow, A., 84, 85
Balog, J. E., 73
Bandura, A., 39
Baraldi, R., 134
Baranick, E., 166
Barbato, C. A., 96, 97
Barbieri, C., 143
Barney, L. J., 300
Baumann, A. E., 246
Beal, G. M., 33
Becker, M. H., 37
Belfiori, J., 50
Bell, R., 44, 327
Bellis, J., 43
Belzer, E. J., 105, 110, 115

Berman, S., 243
Bernhardt, J. M., 6, 7, 10, 13, 23, 24, 30, 258
Bertrand, J. T., 324, 325, 326, 329, 330, 331
Black, S. A., 76, 81
Blanchard, J., 20
Blot, W. J., 60
Bogen, K., 277
Bongaarts, J., 41
Borg, E., 289
Boruchovitch, E., 73, 80
Bray, G., 84
Brennan, S. E., 116, 117
Brook, R., 181
Broom, G. M., 125
Brown, R., 98
Brownell, K. D., 84
Burris, D., 177
Burstall, M. L., 181

C

Caldamone, A. A., 179, 180
Calmy, A., 143
Campbell, J. D., 73
Carter, K. E., 200
Castrucci, B. C., 294
Cates, W., Jr., 243
Cave, L., 201
Cendron, M., 180, 310
Center, A. H., 125, 126
Chan, S., 83
Cherry, J. D., 287
Chiu, C., 98, 100
Christensen, H., 300
Clark, H. H., 116, 117
Clark, J. R., 277

413

SUBJECT INDEX

H

Hamilton-Wentworth Drug and Alcohol Awareness Committee, 348

Harvard Family Research Project, 56–57

Health: balance concept of, 74; comparative analysis of concept of, 75–78, 79*t*–81*t*, 134; cultural differences in definitions of, 72–73; medical model definition of, 73; WHO model of, 73–75. *See also* Illness

Health behavior: communication for persuasion theory, 44–45; convergence theory, 41–43; diffusion of innovation theory on, 33–37; health belief model (HBM) on, 37–38; ideation theory, 41, 42*fig*; power of mass media influencing, 132–139; social cognitive theory (SCT) on, 39; stages of behavior change model, 43–44; theory of reasoned action (TRA) on, 40–41. *See also* Behavior; Motivation

Health belief model (HBM), 37–38

Health beliefs: cultural differences in, 74–75, 79*t*–81*t*; gender influences on, 78, 81–82; HBM on, 37–38; religious/spiritual influences on, 75–76, 80*t*; as situation analysis factor, 244–246; tensions between desires and, 82–85. *See also* Attitudes; Beliefs

Health care providers: obstacles to changing behavior of, 184*t*; professional medical communication by, 177–182, 184*t*–191; relationship between patient and, 105–118; theoretical basis for behavior of, 182–184

Health communication: areas of, 24–26; cycle of, 220–221*fig*; definitions of, 4–7, 8*t*–10*t*; effective and efficient, 84; four "eras" of, 14; global, 24–25, 157; health is-

sues/topics affecting, 57–69; increasing importance of, 3–4; interpersonal, 25, 91–120; key characteristics and defining features of, 7, 10–22; key concepts of, 28; marketing mix role of, 22–23*fig*; professional medical, 175–198; public health role of, 23–24; what it can and cannot do, 26–27*t*. *See also* Communication; Messages

Health communication cycle, 220–221*fig*

Health communication features: aimed at behavioral and social change, 21–22; audience centered, 12; audience and media specific, 19–20; cost-effective, 18; creative in support of strategy, 19; listed, 12*t*; multidisciplinary, 13–15; overview of, 7, 10–11; process oriented, 16–18; relationship building, 21; research based, 13; strategic, 15–16

Health Communication Partnership: on community action cycle model, 154; on community action model, 171–172; on community mobilization, 153; on diffusion of innovation theory, 33, 34; on global health communication, 24; on multidisciplinary health communication, 30–31; on primary and secondary audiences, 41; on social cognitive theory (SCT), 39

Health communication planning: approaches to, 218–220; communication objectives guiding the, 290–291; developing tactical and evaluation, 298–335; importance of, 217–218; phases of, 220–221*fig*; for program implementation, 327–341; steps of, 222–226; traditional versus participatory, 219–220

biopsychosocial, 55–56, 73; health defined under, 73
Medicus Mundi, 69
Medline, 269
MEDLINE quality of care studies, 181
Mental illness, 245–246
Mental retardation, 83*t*
Merck Frosst Canada, 148
Messages: audience reach factor, 258; communication concepts used in, 308–311; content and complexity of, 257–258; cost-effectiveness of, 258–259; cultural and issue appropriateness of, 258; development of, 312–313; health literacy required to understand, 63–64, 111*t*; launching, 317–318; NCI's Cancer Research Awareness Initiatives, 311*b*–312*b*; pretesting, 318–320; retention of, 313; selecting communication channels and vehicles for, 314–316*b*. *See also* Audience; Communication channels; Health communication
Methodologies. *See* Research methodologies
Metrics (evaluation parameters): definition of, 323; establishing, 332–333; health communication program, 227–228; public relation program, 141–142
Minority populations: African Americans, 48*b*–50*b*, 79*t*, 111, 214; Hispanics, 74–75, 79*t*–80*t*; Hmong, 77–78; Koreans, 79*t*; Native Americans, 80*t*; religious, 80*t*; Vietnamese, 79*t*. *See also* Racial/ethnic differences
Models. *See* Health communication theories
Monitoring: data-collection/reporting on areas for, 345*t*–346*t*; establishing teams for, 338–339; four primary areas addressed by, 341–343; summary on, 349

Morality rates, 242
Morbidity factors, 242–243
Morbidity rates, 242
Motivation: factors affecting interpersonal communication, 96–98; social cognitive theory (SCT) on, 39; stages of behavior change model on, 43–44. *See also* Behavior; Health behavior
MSNBC, 143
MTBI (mild traumatic brain injury), 187
Museum of Public Relations, 121, 122
Muslim health beliefs, 80*t*

N

National Association of Pediatric Nurse Practitioners, 66
National Cancer Institute: on behavior reciprocal factors, 39; Cancer Research Awareness Initiative of, 311*b*–312*b*; on communication concepts to present information, 300, 308–309; on communication outcome objectives, 233, 282; on communication for persuasion theory, 44; on diffusion of innovation theory, 33, 36; on ethical issues of focus group research, 276; on evaluations, 302, 328, 332, 347, 348; on health belief model (HBM), 37; on health communication importance, 24, 26; on health communication planning, 217, 222, 224; message development approach by, 311–312; on partnerships, 320; on planning frameworks, 15; on precede-proceed model, 53; on pretesting, 319; on process evaluation, 326; public-private partnerships with, 129, 208, 210*b*–211*b*; on social cognitive theory, 39; on social marketing, 47; on stages of behavior change model, 43–44; on survey research, 276

Organizational outcome objectives: health communication program, 222, 232–233; pediatric asthma, 234*e*; SMART approach to, 285; understanding connections to other program elements, 286*e*

Outcome objectives: health communication program, 228–229, 232–233, 282–290; pediatric asthma program, 234*e*; SMART approach to, 285; social, behavioral, organizational, 222, 232–233, 234*e*, 285, 286*e*. *See also* Communication objectives

Outcomes: cultural impact on, 85; definition of, 323–324; health communication program agreement on, 227–228; health communication programs impact on, 85; objectives of health communication program, 228–229, 232–233, 282–290; PR (public relations), 142; trends in evaluating, 327–331

Outreach Partnership Program (NIH), 201

P

Parents: childhood immunization campaigns aimed toward, 133, 188–189, 189*b*–191*b*, 257–258, 309*t*; childhood immunization complacency by, 66; comparing peer influence to that of, 259; "Got a Minute? Give It to Your Kids!" campaign (CDC) focus on, 252*b*–255*b*; snapshot of less-involved, 254. *See also* Children

Parents (magazine), 190*b*

ParticipACTION: community mobilization used by, 147–148, 149; public service announcements of, 147; "Walk a Block a Day" event of, 148

Participatory health communication planning, 219–220

Participatory needs assessment, 169

Participatory research: community action cycle (or model) approach to, 154, 171–173; community group meetings to share, 170; community mobilization through, 169

Partnering for Patient Empowerment Through Community Awareness, 59

Partnership for Clear Health Communication, 113, 114

Partnership meetings, 170–171

Partnerships. *See* Public-private partnerships

PATH (Program for Appropriate Technology in Health), 158*b*–159*b*, 160*b*, 315–316*b*

Patients: empowerment of, 58–59; professional medical communication with, 177–182, 184*t*–191; quality of care gaps for, 181; relationship between health care providers and, 105–118. *See also* Provider-patient relationships

Pediatric asthma outcome objectives, 233, 234*e*

Performance, 39

Personal selling: lymphatic filariasis (LF) elimination through, 102*b*–103*b*; public health applications of, 100–104

Pertussis incidence, 257–258, 287

Physicians: day-to-day demands and tasks faced by, 176; obstacles to changing behavior of, 184*t*; patient behavior impacted by attitudes of, 108*b*–109*b*; professional medical communication by, 177–182, 184*t*–191; relationship between patient and, 105–118; theoretical overview of influencing behavior of, 182–184. *See also* Nurses; Professional medical communications

Physicians for Human Rights (PHR), 68, 204, 206*b*–207*b*

Place (marketing), 47

Key Organisations 2012

The up-to-date guide to organisations

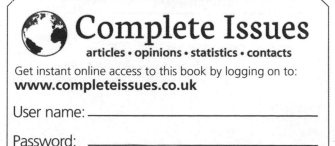

Complete Issues

articles • opinions • statistics • contacts

Get instant online access to this book by logging on to:

www.completeissues.co.uk

User name: _____

Password: _____

Introduction

Welcome to Key Organisations – the essential, annually updated, contact list.

Always updated

More than 3,000 addresses have been carefully checked and more than 1,000 important changes have been made.

More organisations have been added. In particular, we've included many new websites. 'Dead' sites have been removed. Where we know that an organisation is likely to change in the near future that too has been noted.

Organised with you in mind

We list organisations by the key word in their name eg Adoption and Fostering (British Association for), but we make an exception when reorganising the name would make the details less easy to find or would make a well-known name unfamiliar eg British Museum.

When an organisation changes its name, we include a cross-reference from the previous name eg ASBAH is now known as Shine. When the name of an organisation does not describe what it does, we include a brief description.

The Thematic Guide

When you are interested in a particular area or subject, but do not know any specific names, you can look under the appropriate theme. So the Children's Orchestra appears under both Music and Children/Young People. The themes are listed opposite.

New and improved

With Key Organisations you can access our fantastically helpful, new searchable database. Enter a key word here and generate a list of useful, current, relevant organisations – live and ready to go. See **www.completeissues.co.uk/ko**

You can make this available to everyone with an inexpensive site licence. See **www.carelpress.co.uk/keyorganisations**.

We have now integrated our major publications in the Complete Issues website. Key Organisations is combined with Essential Articles and Fact File to bring you a complete source of opinions, facts, figures and further research. Go to: **www.completeissues.co.uk**

13859072

Publication information
© 2012 Carel Press Ltd, 4 Hewson Street, Carlisle, CA2 5AU, UK
Tel 01228 538928 Fax: 591816
office@carelpress.co.uk
www.carelpress.co.uk
Editorial team: Anne Louise Kershaw, Debbie Maxwell, Christine A Shepherd, Chas White
Database: Debbie Maxwell
Subscription manager: Ann Batey

Cover design: Anne Louise Kershaw
Logos: Craig Mitchell
Printed by: Finemark, Poland
British Library Cataloguing in Publication Data
Is available for this publication
ISBN-13: 978-1-905600-28-1